WORKBOOK to accompany

EMT
Prehospital Care

WORKBOOK to accompany

EMT Prehospital Care

Third Edition

Mark C. Henry, MD

Professor and Chairman
Department of Emergency Medicine
School of Medicine
State University of New York, Stony Brook
Stony Brook, New York

Edward R. Stapleton, EMT-P

Assistant Professor of Clinical Emergency Medicine
Director of Prehospital Education
Department of Emergency Medicine
State University of New York, Stony Brook
Stony Book, New York

Eric Niegelberg, MS, NREMT-P

Assistant Professor of Clinical Emergency Medicine
Department of Emergency Medicine
Emergency Department Administrator/EMS Director
Stony Brook University Hospital
State University of New York, Stony Brook
Stony Brook, New York

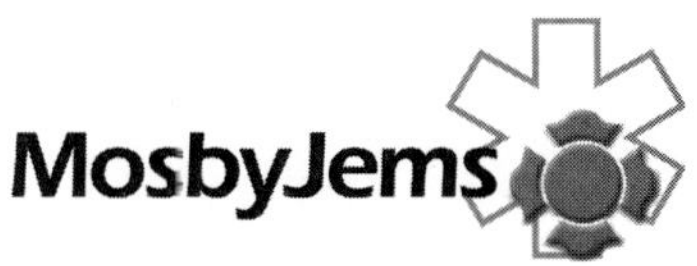

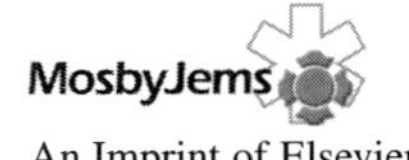

An Imprint of Elsevier

11830 Westline Industrial Drive
St. Louis, Missouri 63146

WORKBOOK TO ACCOMPANY EMT PREHOSPITAL CARE, THIRD EDITION 0-323-01649-9

NOTICE

EMS is an ever-changing field. Standard safety precautions must be followed, but as new research and clinical experience broaden our knowledge, changes in treatment and drug therapy may become necessary or appropriate. Readers are advised to check the most current product information provided by the manufacturer of each drug to be administered to verify the recommended dose, the method and duration of administration, and contraindications. It is the responsibility of the licensed prescriber, relying on experience and knowledge of the patient, to determine dosages and the best treatment for each individual patient. Neither the publisher nor the editor assumes any liability for any injury and/or damage to persons or property arising from this publication.

Previous editions copyrighted 1992, 1997

International Standard Book Number 0-323-01649-9

Publishing Director: Andrew Allen
Acquisitions Editor: Linda Honeycutt
Associate Developmental Editor: Kristin Armstrong
Publishing Services Manager: Linda McKinley
Project Manager: Judy Ahlers
Senior Designer: Julia Dummitt

KI/MVB
Printed in the United States of America
Last digit is the print number: 9 8 7 6 5 4 3 2 1

Preface

This student workbook was developed to be a learning and reinforcement tool for use by the EMT-Basic. The material in this workbook reinforces the concepts presented in *EMT Prehospital Care*, third edition.

Each chapter in the workbook corresponds to a chapter in the textbook. Before completing the workbook, read the corresponding chapter in the textbook and attend the classroom session in which the chapter material is presented to you by your instructor. When you complete the workbook, you should allow sufficient time to properly read each question and choose the most correct answer. After you have completed the chapter in the workbook, use the answer key to grade yourself and to identify any areas that require further study. The answers to all of the questions in the workbook can be found in the textbook.

As an EMT-Basic you will be working in an ever-changing environment that can be both challenging and rewarding. Each chapter in the workbook contains brief scenarios that allow you to "put it all together." These scenarios require that you identify the treatment order and priority for simulated patients. This allows you to think as a "street EMT" who is responsible for the complete care of the patient. An added feature in this workbook is a challenging crossword puzzle that contains key terms and ideas from the chapter.

This workbook contains questions that cover all of the EMT-Basic National Standard Curriculum cognitive objectives. These are the objectives that involve knowledge and analytical skills. Throughout your EMT class you will also be exposed to multitude psychomotor or hands-on practical skills. At the end of the workbook are the critical performance skill sheets that are used by the National Registry of Emergency Medical Technicians. Your instructor may use these identical forms or regionally approved skill sheets during your practical skill training.

Although this workbook contains multiple-choice, fill-in, matching, and true/false questions, the certification examination will contain only multiple-choice questions. When you sit for the certification examination, you should try and follow the following guidelines:

- Prepare well in the weeks leading up to the test. Do not cram the night before the test. This workbook is a critical preparation tool that will instill confidence; use it.
- Get a good night's sleep the night before the exam so that you are alert and in a state of readiness to focus on the exam items.
- Eat a good meal the day of the exam to optimize your concentration abilities.
- Read each item carefully and make your selection.
- Guess the right answer before looking at the choices. This will lead you to the correct choice and instill confidence in your final selection.
- Do not spend excessive time on a particular question. Skip it and make sure you return later to finish the questions. Often an answer will be found in a later question.
- As a rule, do not change an answer unless you are absolutely certain that the answer is incorrect. More times than not the original choice is correct.
- Don't become overwhelmed. If you feel stressed, take a few slow breaths and refocus.

Eric Niegelberg

Publisher's Acknowledgments

The editors wish to acknowledge and thank the following reviewers. Their comments were enlightening and invaluable in helping develop this workbook.

Steve Hazelton, EMT-P
EMS Educator
Rutland Regional Medical Center
Rutland, Vermont

Scot Phelps, JD, MPH, Paramedic
Assistant Clinical Professor of Cardiopulmonary Science
University of Medicine & Dentistry of New Jersey
New Brunswick, New Jersey

James M. Floyd, Jr., AS, EMT-B, PI, CTC
St. Vincent Hospitals and Health Services
Indianapolis, Indiana

Edward R. Stapleton III, NREMT-P
Paramedic
Stony Brook Volunteer Ambulance Corps
Stony Brook, New York

Table of Contents

Chapter 1 Introduction to Emergency Medical Care, 1

Chapter 2 Well-Being of the EMT-Basic, 10

Chapter 3 Medicolegal and Ethical Issues, 18

Chapter 4 The Human Body, 25

Chapter 5 Baseline Vital Signs and SAMPLE History, 42

Chapter 6 Lifting and Moving Patients, 50

Chapter 7 Airway, 57

Chapter 8 Scene Size-up, 66

Chapter 9 Initial Assessment, 71

Chapter 10 Focused History and Physical Examination of Trauma Patients, 77

Chapter 11 Focused History and Physical Examination of Medical Patients, 84

Chapter 12 Detailed Physical Examination, 92

Chapter 13 Ongoing Assessment, 97

Chapter 14 Communications, 103

Chapter 15 Documentation, 112

Chapter 16 General Pharmacology, 120

Chapter 17 Respiratory Emergencies, 127

Chapter 18 Cardiovascular Emergencies, 136

Chapter 19 Altered Mental Status, 148

Chapter 20 Allergies, 156

Chapter 21 Poisoning and Overdoses, 164

Chapter 22 Environmental Emergencies, 172

Chapter 23 Behavioral Emergencies, 184

Chapter 24 Obstetrics and Gynecology, 192

Chapter 25 Bleeding and Shock, 204

Chapter 26 Soft Tissue Injuries, 214

Chapter 27 Chest and Abdominal Trauma, 226

Chapter 28 Musculoskeletal Care, 234

Chapter 29 Injuries to the Head and Spine, 244

Chapter 30 Infants and Children, 256

Chapter 31 Ambulance Operations, 268

Chapter 32 Gaining Access, 276

Chapter 33 Disasters and Hazardous Materials, 283

Chapter 34 Advanced Airway Management, 292

Chapter 35 Weapons of Mass Destruction and the EMT, 302

Chapter 36 Geriatric Emergencies, 312

Appendix A Cardiopulmonary Resuscitation, 321

Appendix B National Registry Skill Sheets, 327

Chapter 1 Introduction to Emergency Medical Care

1. A system of resources and personnel necessary to provide immediate care to the ill and injured describes a(n):

   a. Emergency medical services (EMS) system
   b. Ambulance service
   c. Enhanced 911 dispatching system
   d. Hospital emergency service

2. Most of the growth and technical development of prehospital emergency care emerged from:

   a. Disaster drills
   b. Outpatient programs
   c. War
   d. Laboratory animal research

3. The Civil War is noted for the first use in the United States of:

   a. Military anti-shock trousers
   b. Mobile army surgical hospital units
   c. Ambulances
   d. A formal system of triage

4. The Korean War saw the first use of:

   a. Large-bore intravenous lines to stabilize the patient in the field
   b. Large hospital ships to provide definitive care to all patients
   c. Physicians assigned to every platoon
   d. Helicopters to provide rapid transport of casualties

5. Michael Reese Hospital in Chicago is credited with the first use of:

   a. Horse-drawn ambulances
   b. Motorized ambulances
   c. Military anti-shock trousers
   d. Emergency medical technicians (EMTs)

6. Trauma is the leading cause of death in which of the following age groups:

   a. 1 to 40 years
   b. 40 to 50 years
   c. 50 to 60 years
   d. Over 60 years

7. The National Academy of Sciences published a landmark paper entitled "Accidental Death & Disability: The Neglected Disease of Modern Society" in:

   a. 1966
   b. 1970
   c. 1945
   d. 1973

8. The leading cause of death in the United States is:

   a. Cancer
   b. Diabetes
   c. Heart disease
   d. Accidents

9. Ambulances, medical direction, human resources, evaluation, and hospitals are all components of a(n):

   a. EMS system
   b. Health care agency
   c. Emergency network
   d. Crisis intervention team

10. Primary responsibilities of an EMT at the scene of a trauma incident include all of the following *except:*

    a. Emergency care
    b. Patient assessment
    c. Disentanglement
    d. Patient advocacy

11. The hospital's emergency department, which is a component of an EMS system, is the "intersection of care" for the critical patient because it:

    a. Provides definitive care to a patient before discharge
    b. Trains the public in cardiopulmonary resuscitation (CPR) and first aid
    c. Provides stabilizing measures to prehospital patients before transfer to the operating room or critical care unit
    d. Coordinates multiple components of every EMS system

12. The lay rescuer is someone who:

    a. Is not a part of the EMS system
    b. Can never provide CPR and first aid for the patient
    c. Treats the patient in the emergency department
    d. Is often the first to help the patient

13. ___________ is a method of hospital designation and an essential part of an EMS system that uses capabilities in different areas of care such as trauma, burns, neonatology, and replantation.

    a. Specialty facilities
    b. Standardization
    c. Systemization
    d. Alteration

14. This aspect of an EMS system brings to the scene the first medical personnel that patients are likely to encounter. These individuals may use either basic or advanced skills to support and stabilize the critical patient:

    a. Lay rescuer
    b. Emergency departments
    c. EMS providers
    d. Intensive care units

15. This stage of an EMS system provides long-term care designed to restore the function of the body:

    a. Rehabilitation units
    b. Emergency departments
    c. Operating room
    d. Outpatient units

16. This stage of an EMS system provides definitive care and is cited as the end point of the "golden hour":

    a. Rehabilitation units
    b. Emergency departments
    c. Operating room
    d. Outpatient units

17. Physician involvement and participation in all phases of the EMS system to ensure quality care best define the concept of:

    a. Categorization
    b. Standardization
    c. Systemization
    d. Medical direction

18. Patient assessment, patient care, and transfer of the patient to hospital staff are:

    a. Beyond the scope of practice of the EMT
    b. Primary roles of the EMT in most systems
    c. Acts that must be completed and documented to prevent an act of negligence
    d. Taken together to form the basis for malfeasance

Indicate which of the roles of the EMT listed in column A are primary versus secondary (other) in most systems. Column B items can be used more than once.

Column A	Column B
19. ____ Patient assessment	a. Primary
20. ____ Extrication	b. Secondary (other)
21. ____ Personal safety and safety of others	
22. ____ Transfer of the patient to hospital staff	
23. ____ Lifting and moving of patients	

24. A serious effort to acquire the requisite skills taught in the initial EMT training program, as well as a continued effort to prevent deterioration of knowledge, is the best way to maintain:

    a. Respect
    b. Competence
    c. Certification
    d. Analytical skills

25. "Acting requisite to the body of knowledge which defines the service and abilities of the professional . . . according to the oath of the profession. Historically first applied to religious vows. . . ." This definition best describes the term:

    a. Competence
    b. Professionalism
    c. Ethics
    d. Honor

26. The person who usually is the first medical person to see the patient best describes the:

    a. Physician
    b. EMT-Basic
    c. Lay rescuer
    d. Nurse

27. The person who interprets the electrocardiogram, performs invasive airway skills, and has a more broadly based knowledge of pharmacology best describes the:

    a. EMT-Paramedic
    b. EMT-Basic
    c. EMT-Defibrillation
    d. First responder

28. Quality improvement programs are designed to:

    a. Provide a system of internal and external reviews
    b. Provide immunity from liability for the EMT
    c. Review ambulance runs and allow for continuing medical education
    d. Both a and c

29. The EMT:

    a. Practices medicine without medical direction
    b. Is not responsible to physician directors
    c. Is a designated agent of the physician
    d. Is not responsible for quality improvement issues

Match the appropriate personal protective equipment in column B with the potential hazard in column A.

Column A	Column B
30. ____ Bandaging a minor bleeding wound	a. Gloves
31. ____ Bandaging a spurting wound	b. Goggles
32. ____ Suctioning a patient's airway	c. Both a and b
33. ____ Emergency childbirth	d. Neither a nor b

34. Running reviews, audits, and gathering feedback from patients and hospital staff are all components of:

    a. The EMT recertification process
    b. Initial EMT training
    c. Medical direction
    d. The quality improvement process

35. Speaking directly with a physician for advice, by telephone or radio from the patient's side, is known as:

    a. Offline physician control
    b. Quality improvement
    c. Medical communications
    d. Online medical direction

36. Standing orders, written protocols, and quality improvement review are all components of:

    a. Offline medical direction
    b. Online medical control
    c. Physician control
    d. Hospital direction

37. The first link in the American Heart Association's "chain of survival" is:

    a. EMT training courses
    b. 911 access
    c. CPR
    d. Defibrillation

38. The ____ provides initial care such as CPR to the patient with minimal equipment before the arrival of the ambulance.

39. The ____ system is responsible for notification, prioritization of calls, and dispatch.

40. List six methods that the EMT may use as part of his or her role in quality improvement.

____

____

____

____

____

____

TRUE OR FALSE

41. ____ Documenting all aspects of prehospital care on a call report is an essential aspect of protection against lawsuits.

42. ____ Effective communication with a family member at the scene of an incident is not an important role for the EMT because the hospital staff are responsible for keeping the family informed about the status of the patient.

43. __F__ The National Registry of Emergency Medical Technicians was developed to standardize treatment protocols on a national level.

44. __T__ The American Heart Association establishes standards and guidelines for emergency cardiac care for both hospital and prehospital care providers.

Questions 45 to 47 refer to the following scenario.

You receive a call to respond to a motor vehicle crash at the intersection of Main Street and Washington Avenue. When you arrive you find a single car that went out of control and struck a utility pole. There is minor damage to the front end of the vehicle. You determine that there was only one person in the car and this driver is sitting on the curb. A bystander is applying direct pressure to a minor laceration on the patient's thigh. The patient tells you that he does not want to go to the hospital. After taking a complete set of vital signs you call your base physician who speaks directly to the patient in an attempt to convince him to go to the hospital.

45. The bystander that began treatment of the patient before your arrival can be classified as a:

    a. Lay rescuer
    b. Technician
    c. EMT
    d. Paramedic

46. The contact that you make with medical control is considered __Online__ medical control.

47. The appropriate personal protection devices to use when bandaging this patient's wound are:

    a. Disposable medical gloves, goggles, and a gown
    b. Disposable medical gloves and goggles
    c. Goggles and a face mask
    d. Disposable medical gloves

Across

1. Serves as team leader for in-hospital and prehospital personnel
5. Bystander who provides initial first aid to a victim
9. Sorting according to medical need
10. Helicopters were first used to evacuate the wounded during this war
11. Military hospitals are referred to as _____ units
12. Facility that provides on-line medical direction
13. Transmission of patient data by radio or telephone
15. _____ medical direction is medical guidance in the form of written protocols
17. _____ 911 allows the dispatcher to track the caller's exact location
18. Serves as the intersection of care in the EMS system
19. System through which emergency vehicles are summoned to respond

Down

2. Systematic collection and analysis of information obtained through examination
3. The physician's responsibility for the medical conduct of EMS personnel
4. Leading cause of trauma deaths
6. Process by which entrapped patients are rescued
7. System of reviews and audits of all aspects of an EMS system
8. Written policies or procedures that delineate patient care
14. Highest level of training for EMS workers
15. _____ medical direction involves real-time contact with a physician
16. Type of mask worn when treating a patient with suspected tuberculosis

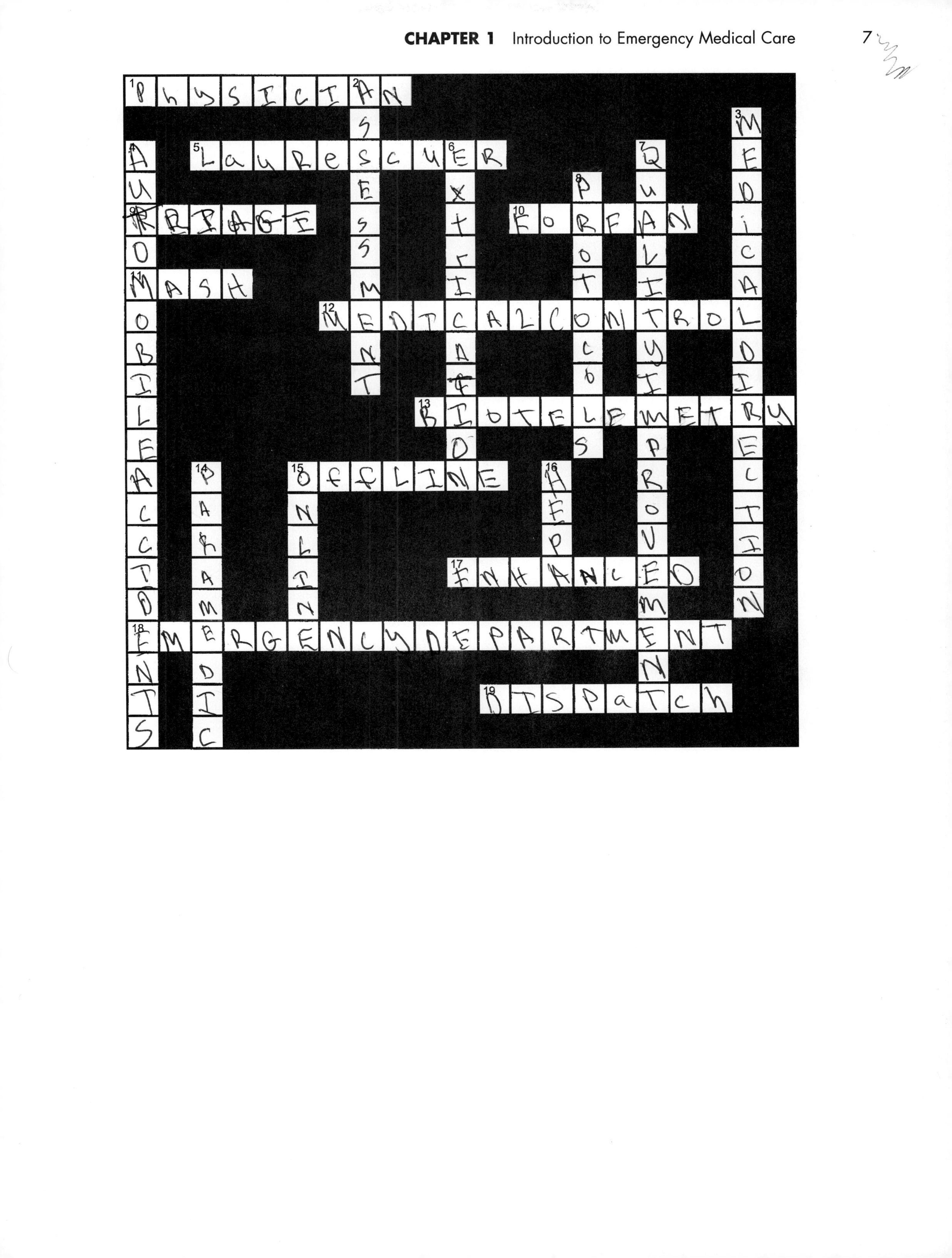

ANSWER KEY

1. a
2. c
3. c
4. d
5. b
6. a
7. a
8. c
9. a
10. c
11. c
12. d
13. a
14. c
15. a
16. c
17. d
18. b
19. a
20. b
21. a
22. a
23. a
24. b
25. b
26. b
27. a
28. d
29. c
30. a
31. c
32. c
33. c
34. d
35. d
36. a
37. b
38. Lay rescuer
39. Communications
40. 1. Reviewing prehospital documentation to ensure appropriate record keeping
    2. Reviewing ambulance runs to determine the type of care provided and the quality of care
    3. Gathering feedback from patients and hospital personnel on the quality of care
    4. Continuing education
    5. Performing preventive maintenance of the vehicle and equipment
    6. Maintaining personal skills
41. True
42. False
43. False
44. True
45. a
46. Online
47. d

1 P	H	Y	S	I	C	I	2 A	N												
							S												3 M	
4 A		5 L	A	Y	R	E	S	C	U	6 E	R					7 Q			E	
U							E			X				8 P		U			D	
9 T	R	I	A	G	E		S			T		10 K	O	R	E	A	N		I	
O							S			R				O		L			C	
11 M	A	S	H				M			I				T		I			A	
O						12 M	E	D	I	C	A	L	C	O	N	T	R	O	L	
B							N			A				C		Y			D	
I							T			T				O		I			I	
L									13 B	I	O	T	E	L	E	M	E	T	R	Y
E										O				S		P			E	
A		14 P			15 O	F	F	L	I	N	E		16 H			R			C	
C		A			N								E			O			T	
C		R			L								P			V			I	
I		A			I					17 E	N	H	A	N	C	E	D		O	
D		M			N											M			N	
18 E	M	E	R	G	E	N	C	Y	D	E	P	A	R	T	M	E	N	T		
N		D														N				
T		I									19 D	I	S	P	A	T	C	H		
S		C																		

Chapter 2 Well-Being of the EMT-Basic

1. Which of the following emotional reactions are common for the EMT to experience when dealing with death, dying, and illness?

   a. Loss of appetite
   b. Feelings of success
   c. Feeling appreciated
   d. Increased appetite

2. Emotions of guilt, grief, anger, loss of appetite, and increased alcohol or drug use experienced by the EMT are related to:

   a. Pain
   b. Organic illness
   c. Dealing with death and illness
   d. Phobias

3. When a family member wants to view the body of a deceased loved one, you should:

   a. Encourage them to avoid it to prevent hysterical reactions
   b. Tell them that they can view it at a later time
   c. Allow them to view the body
   d. Make them wait until the physician arrives

4. When dealing with the family of a patient who has just died, the EMT should:

   a. Attend strictly to the patient's needs
   b. Be supportive and nonjudgmental
   c. Point out to the family that they should have called EMS sooner
   d. Leave the scene because your services are not required

5. When arriving at the scene, the EMT should:

   a. Disregard the family member if he or she does not need medical attention
   b. Ask the family about the patient's condition
   c. Ignore the family member because he or she is not the patient
   d. Not acknowledge the family member's concern about his or her loved one

6. Which of the following represents an emotion that may be experienced by a family member of the EMT?

   a. A complete understanding of the EMT work
   b. No fear of being ignored or left out
   c. No feelings of competition with the job
   d. Resentment and feelings of being left out

7. To fulfill a commitment to his or her family, the EMT should:

   a. Overlook the needs of loved ones
   b. Organize a work schedule to include time for family needs
   c. Keep experiences inside because family members won't understand
   d. Separate work and family for the family's benefit

8. A simple approach that the EMT can exercise when faced with a particularly stressful incident, such as the death of a child, is to:

   a. Share the feelings with a colleague or a family member
   b. Take a strict clinical approach to avoid such feelings
   c. Ignore it through positive thinking
   d. Not think about it to avoid the stress

9. A sense of hopelessness, loss of appetite, and feelings of isolation are all signs of:

   a. Debriefing sickness
   b. Psychological emergencies
   c. Denial
   d. Stress induced by job-related activities

10. Major disasters such as the death of a child may require a more organized response by the EMT to resolve negative feelings. This process is called a(n):

    a. Critical incident stress debriefing
    b. Encounter group
    c. Catharsis
    d. Exchange session

11. The primary reason an EMT is responsible for scene safety is because:

    a. The patient may have sustained additional injury
    b. The patient has already sustained enough
    c. The family may take legal action against you
    d. The EMT is trained in safety procedures for himself or herself and others at the scene

12. The EMT is faced with hazards that include communicable disease, hazardous materials, and personal threats of violence. The first way the EMT can protect himself or herself after arriving at the scene is to:

    a. Perform an initial assessment
    b. Call for backup assistance
    c. Perform a scene safety size-up
    d. Use community resources

13. Gloves should be worn when:

    a. There is a cut on the EMT's finger
    b. Handling blood or other bodily fluids
    c. Equipment needs to be decontaminated
    d. All the above

14. Body substance isolation (universal precautions) considers:

    a. All body fluids from all patients as potentially infectious
    b. Blood from sick patients as potentially infectious
    c. Blood from high-risk patients as potentially infectious
    d. All body fluids from patients with HIV as potentially infectious

15. When confronted with an open wound oozing blood, the EMT should:

    a. Avoid the patient, only touching as necessary
    b. Wipe the blood with a sterile bandage
    c. Put on disposable medical gloves before treating the patient
    d. Place a surgical face mask on the patient

Match the personal protective equipment in column B to the hazard in column A.

Column A	**Column B**
16. ____ Bleeding laceration	a. HEPA respirator
17. ____ Psychiatric emergency	b. Disposable medical gloves
18. ____ Hazardous materials scene	c. Binoculars
19. ____ Patient with tuberculosis	d. Soft restraints

20. Diseases capable of being spread from one person to another are called:

    a. Communicable
    b. Endocrine
    c. Genetic
    d. Syndromes

21. Universal precautions are used with:

    a. Patients with AIDS
    b. All patients
    c. Patients with infections
    d. Patients with hepatitis

22. The routine practice of wearing protective clothing (e.g., gloves, protective eyewear) when performing certain procedures (e.g., bleeding control, airway control) is called:

    a. General infection prevention
    b. Barrier model
    c. Immunization
    d. Body substance isolation (universal precautions)

23. The simplest and most effective way to block the spread of infection is:

    a. Avoiding physical contact with patients
    b. Using alcohol wipes on infection sites
    c. Handwashing before and after every patient contact
    d. Wearing a gown with every patient contact

24. All the following are sources of information at a hazardous materials transportation trauma site *except*:

    a. The color of the vehicle
    b. The shipping papers
    c. The driver of the vehicle
    d. Placards on the vehicle

25. The primary responsibility of an EMT at the scene of a hazardous materials fire is:

    a. Containment
    b. Removal
    c. Decontamination
    d. Emergency medical care

26. The first priority with a potentially dangerous patient is:

    a. The patient's protection
    b. Self-protection
    c. The legal implications
    d. Restraining the patient

27. In general, the best way to deal with a violent patient is to be:

    a. Firm and authoritative
    b. Aggressive and self-assured
    c. Calm and reassuring
    d. Light-hearted and carefree

28. Securing items of potential importance at a crime scene is part of the Chain of evidency

29. The time period in which a person can transmit an infectious disease to others is called the communicable period

30. The stage of dying in which patients are profoundly sad and experience immense grief is called Depression

31. The patient's final words about his or her condition, or statements to others, are called his or her __________

32. The system in the body that protects against microorganisms is called the __________ system.

33. The time between contact with an infectious agent and the onset of symptoms is called the __________

34. __________ is the mode of disease transmission that occurs when the EMT touches a contaminated instrument.

35. Infections are caused by __________ that are toxic to the body, such as bacteria and viruses.

36. The receptacle used for the safe disposal of used needles is a __________

37. At the scene of a hazardous incident, a __________ should be established for the location of ambulances and personnel before on-scene patient care and decontamination.

38. __________ that incorporate universal precautions and body substance isolation should be used in all situations to avoid transmission from both recognized and unrecognized sources of infection.

39. __________ is spread by droplets and the airborne route and requires the EMT to wear a high-efficiency particulate air respirator mask to minimize the risk of disease transmission.

40. Transmission of disease by a tick or mosquito is called __________

Across

1. The body's protection against microorganisms
2. The most important measure for blocking the spread of infection
6. An early intervention that occurs shortly after a disaster to stop the negative stress process
8. German measles
11. Your first concern when responding to a call
15. Government agency that sets rules regarding exposure of emergency personnel to communicable diseases in the course of their work
17. The ability to resist the development of pathogenic microorganisms or their toxic effects
18. A person who is infected with an illness that may be spread
21. Stage of dying when patients may negotiate with God to extend their life
22. Illnesses that are capable of being spread from one person to another
23. Identification and assistance of distressed emergency workers
24. A susceptible person who if exposed to a source may become ill
27. Free from germs
28. Type of disease transmission that occurs when an infected person coughs or sneezes
29. ____ ____ education sessions designed to familiarize emergency responders with the nature of emergency service stress
31. Term used when a patient refuses to believe the seriousness of a situation
32. Government agency that creates guidelines to standardize infection control practices
33. Person who shows no signs of disease, but may be a source of infection to others
34. Lockjaw
35. The coming in contact with, but not necessarily being infected by, a disease-causing agent
36. Infection of the liver caused by viruses

Down

1. Transmission of infection through a contact of the susceptible host with a contaminated intermediate object
3. Acquired immunodeficiency syndrome
4. Stage of dying when patients project irate feelings onto others
5. High-efficiency particulate air respirator used in the prevention of transmission of tuberculosis
7. Transmission of disease by means of an organism, such as tick or mosquito
9. Time period during which a person can transmit an infectious disease to others
10. Final stage of dying when patients ultimately accept the situation
12. Stage of dying when patients are profoundly sad and experience immense grief
13. A national telephone resource that provides advice on how to handle chemical emergencies
14. Varicella
16. Method by which an infectious agent travels from the source to the host
19. Rigidity of the muscles that occurs at death
20. Physical transmission of infection between a susceptible host and an infected person
21. Precaution designed to reduce the risk of transmission of pathogens from moist body substances
25. Whooping cough
26. A sign that identifies hazardous materials
27. Transmission of microorganisms carried in the air and inhaled by a susceptible host
30. Specialized mask and regulator with portable air supply used by rescue personnel in environments that might contain hazardous materials

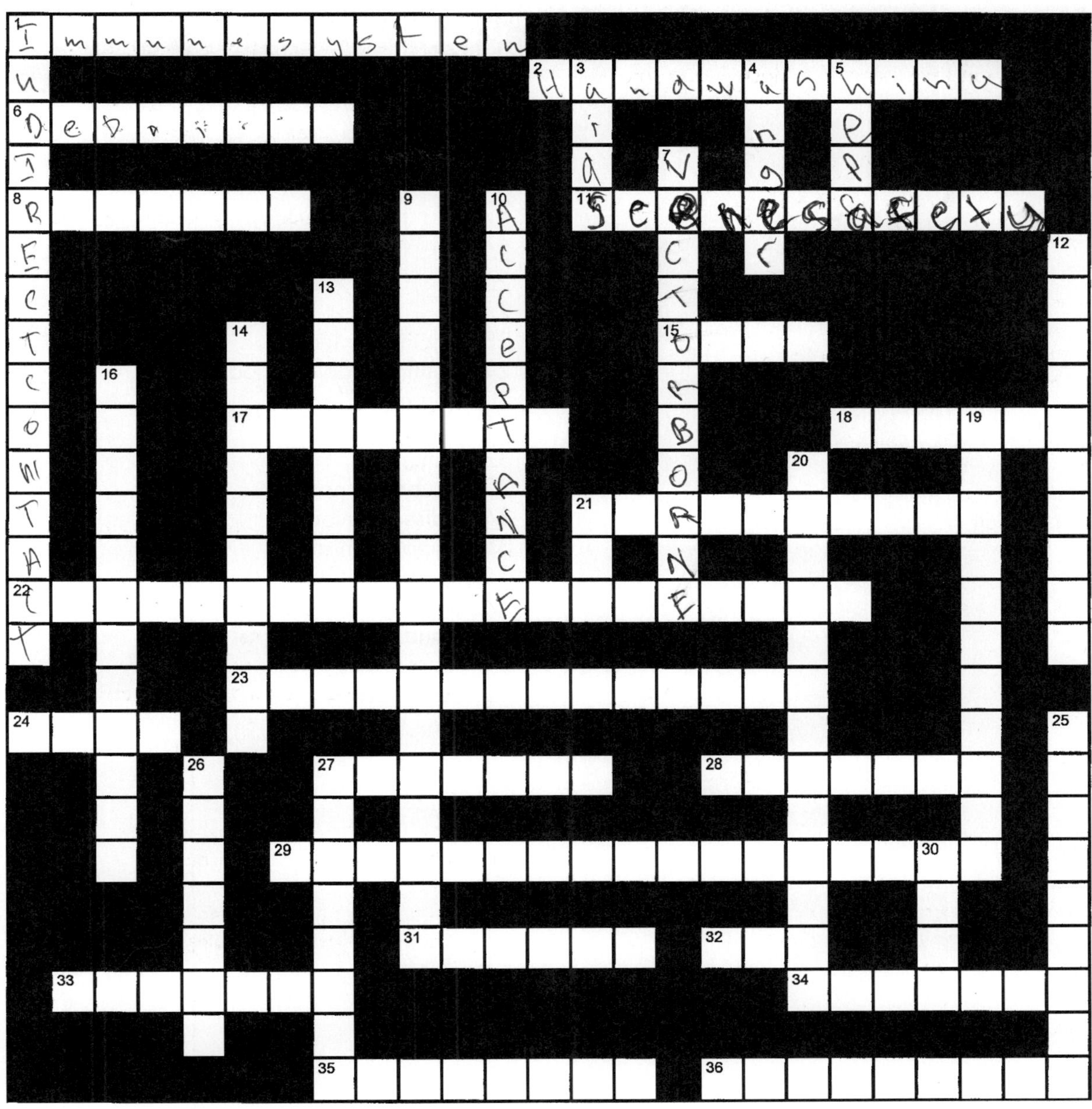

ANSWER KEY

1. a
2. c
3. c
4. b
5. b
6. d
7. b
8. a
9. d
10. a
11. d
12. c
13. d
14. a
15. c
16. b
17. d
18. c
19. a
20. a
21. b
22. d
23. c
24. a
25. d
26. b
27. c
28. Chain of evidence
29. Communicable period
30. Depression
31. Dying declaration
32. Immune
33. Incubation period
34. Indirect contact
35. Microorganisms
36. Sharps container
37. Staging area
38. Standard precautions
39. Tuberculosis
40. Vector borne

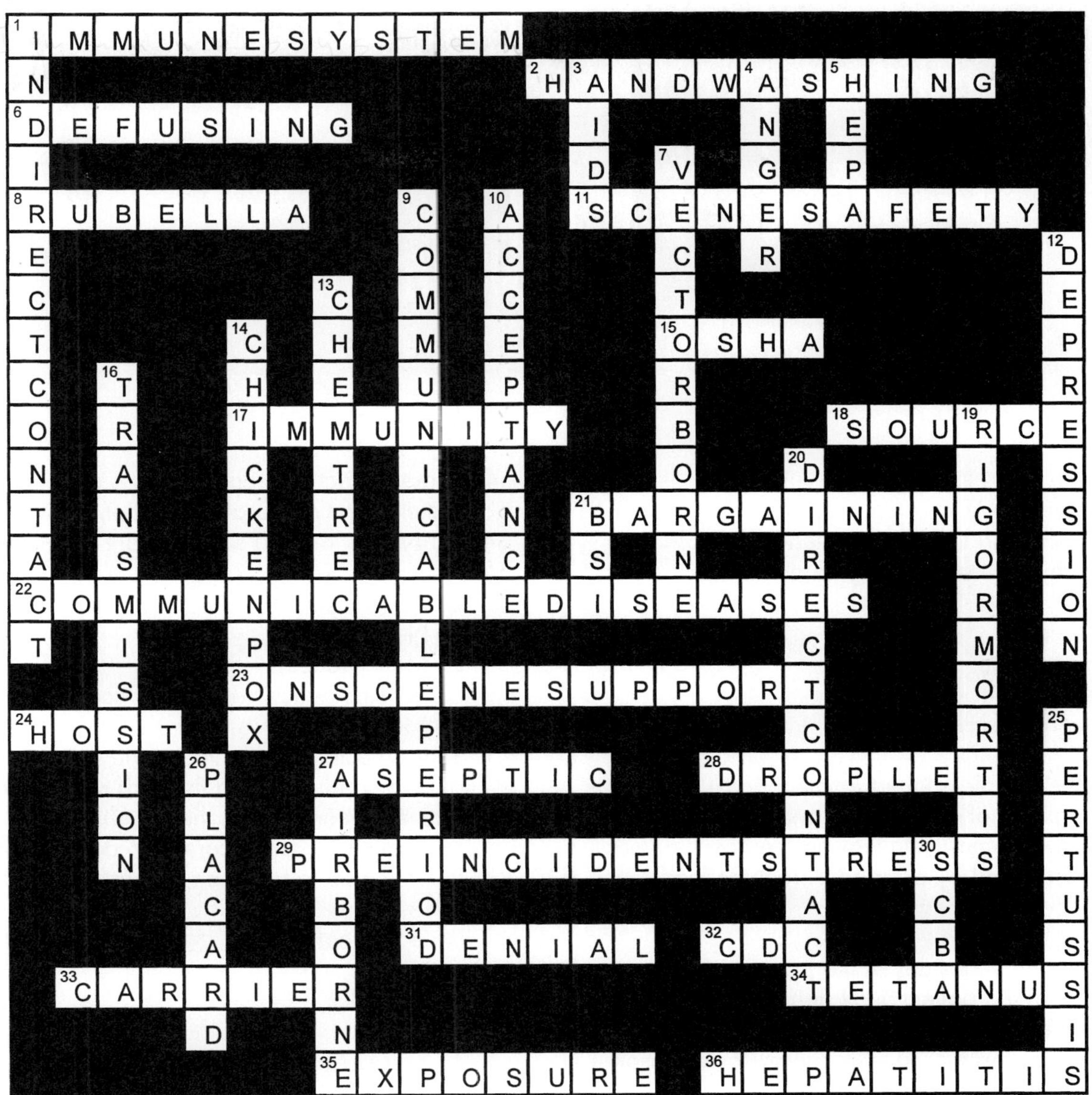
1 IMMUNESYSTEM
2 HANDWASHING
6 DEFUSING
8 RUBELLA
11 SCENESAFETY
15 OSHA
17 IMMUNITY
18 SOURCE
21 BARGAINING
22 COMMUNICABLEDISEASES
23 ONSCENESUPPORT
24 HOST
27 ASEPTIC
28 DROPLET
29 PREINCIDENTSTRESS
31 DENIAL
32 CDC
33 CARRIER
34 TETANUS
35 EXPOSURE
36 HEPATITIS
1 INDIRECTCONTACT
3 AIDS
4 ANGER
5 HEP
7 VECTORBORNE
9 COMMUNICABLEPERIOD
10 ACCEPTANCE
12 DEPRESSION
13 CHEMTREC
14 CHICKENPOX
16 TRANSMISSION
19 RIGORMORTIS
20 DIRECTCONTACT
25 PERTUSSIS
26 PLACARD
27 AIRBORNE
30 SCBA

Chapter 3 Medicolegal and Ethical Issues

1. A serious effort to acquire the requisite skills taught in the initial EMT training program, as well as a continued effort to prevent deterioration of knowledge, is the best way to maintain:

   a. Respect
   b. Competence
   c. Certification
   d. Analytical skills

2. You have completed the treatment and transportation of a patient who sustained a gunshot wound to the chest. On leaving the hospital you are approached by a reporter from the local newspaper. You may:

   a. Share the vital signs of the patient
   b. Say that the patient is all right and give the reporter a copy of the ambulance call report
   c. Refer the reporter to your supervisor or hospital officials for comment
   d. Tell the past medical history as told to you by the patient

3. The body of knowledge, laws, policies, standards, and guidelines set forth by various standard-setting organizations that provides the basis of prehospital care, along with the everyday practice of other providers, best describes:

   a. Values of practice
   b. The standard of care
   c. Emergency laws
   d. Competence

4. A duty to act, a breach of duty, an injury to the patient, and a causal connection between the injury and the EMT's actions are all ingredients of:

   a. Abandonment
   b. Negligence
   c. Malfeasance
   d. An emergency medical services system

5. Your ambulance is on the scene where a 72-year-old woman tripped on the curb and injured her hip. You inform her of the benefits and consequences of the care provided and she agrees to allow you to treat her. She is being treated

   under the concept of ___________ consent.

   a. Implied
   b. Applied
   c. Expressed (informed)
   d. Presumed

6. Your ambulance is on the scene of a 54-year-old woman who is having a heart attack. During treatment of this patient, you hear another call for a child who is choking approximately 1 mile away. If you leave your patient and respond to the child who is choking, you may be guilty of:

   a. Malfeasance
   b. Abandonment
   c. Negligence
   d. Breach of duty

7. Your ambulance is dispatched to the scene of a "man down." On arrival you find a 52-year-old unconscious patient. Treatment may be rendered

   under the concept of ___________ consent.

   a. Informed
   b. Expressed
   c. Implied
   d. Surrogate

8. An emancipated minor is a(n):

   a. Individual who is younger than the legal adult age but who is living independently of the parent
   b. Child who is injured at school and the parent is at work
   c. Patient who has been judged mentally incompetent by the court
   d. Individual who is younger than the legal adult age but who is injured while working

9. Good Samaritan laws are designed to protect the:

   a. EMT against legal action from abandonment of the patient
   b. EMT against legal action from gross negligence when driving the ambulance
   c. EMT against legal action if cardiopulmonary resuscitation (CPR) is not started on a patient in witnessed cardiac arrest and who is pronounced dead at the scene
   d. Any person who is functioning in a nonprofessional capacity and without an expectation of remuneration

10. Rigor mortis, decapitation, and extreme dependent lividity are acceptable criteria for:

    a. Rapid transport to the hospital
    b. Requesting a physician to the scene to assist in patient care
    c. Withholding CPR
    d. Bypassing the local community hospital and transporting the patient to the nearest trauma center

11. All the following are true regarding do not resuscitate (DNR) orders *except*:

    a. A DNR order requires a written physician order (generally signed by the physician) to be legally acceptable.
    b. When in doubt regarding DNR orders, the EMT should attempt resuscitation.
    c. They do not direct stopping treatment for other conditions, such as administration of oxygen for shortness of breath.
    d. The spouse of a patient can refuse resuscitation efforts without a written DNR order.

12. If an EMT observes a person removing evidence from a crime scene, he or she should:

    a. Report it to police and document the event
    b. Ignore it because that is the role of the police, not the EMT
    c. Investigate the issue carefully before making a decision
    d. Retrieve the object from the individual and place it in its original location

13. A patient's willingness to donate his or her organs is commonly documented on a:

    a. Passport
    b. DNR order
    c. Driver's license
    d. Social Security card

14. Deviation from the accepted standard of care that results in the injury of a patient best describes:

    a. Malpractice
    b. An ethical breach
    c. Nonfeasance
    d. Battery

15. An alert, adult patient complaining of chest pain is refusing medical care. You should first:

    a. Have the patient sign a release form
    b. Try to convince the patient to go to the hospital
    c. Place the patient on the stretcher and transport
    d. Advise the patient to call again if the pain becomes worse

16. You are called to the scene of a cardiac arrest. The patient is a 72-year-old man who the family states collapsed in bed approximately 15 minutes before your arrival. The family tells you that the patient has terminal cancer and does not want to be resuscitated. The family does not have a DNR. There is no dependent lividity or rigor mortis evident. Based on this information you should:

    a. Abide by the family's wishes and do not resuscitate the patient
    b. Begin CPR and transport the patient
    c. Not begin CPR until your supervisor responds to the scene
    d. Run a short (abbreviated) code and then pronounce the patient

17. You are called to the scene of a restaurant, where you encounter a 54-year-old female patient. According to her companion, the patient became very pale and then had a syncopal episode that lasted for about 2 minutes. The patient is now alert and is refusing any further care. Although the patient tells you her demographic information she refuses your attempts to assess her condition, including taking vital signs. Her companion tells you that you should take the patient to the hospital but the patient refuses. You should:

    a. Restrain the patient and transport her to the hospital
    b. Tell the companion that there is nothing more that you can do and leave
    c. Explain to the patient your concerns for her welfare and state that her condition may be life threatening. If she still refuses care, contact online medical control, if available, and have your patient sign a refusal of medical advice
    d. Wait with the patient for 15 to 30 minutes to see if any symptoms recur; if they do not recur, leave the scene

18. The guiding standard of effective medical practice is referred to as the ____________.

19. List the four elements that must be proven for negligence to exist.

    ____

    ____

    ____

    ____

20. Physical contact with a person without his or her consent and without legal justification is known as ____________.

21. Good Samaritan legislation:

    a. Is only applicable in approximately 25% of the country
    b. Alleviates the need for the EMT to be concerned about his or her actions
    c. Is intended to encourage people to help others without fear of litigation when emergencies arise
    d. Only protects you when you are a paid emergency medical services professional while at work

22. You are treating a 27-year-old man who was the target of a drive-by shooting. The patient sustained a gunshot wound to the left upper leg. The police are concerned that all evidence be optimally preserved. You:

    a. Do not remove the patient's pants because the bullet hole is evidence
    b. Remove or cut the pants but try to avoid cutting through the bullet hole
    c. Should not be concerned with the patient's clothing because this is not considered evidence
    d. Only transport the patient after the police crime scene unit has photographed the patient's wounds

Questions 23 to 25 refer to the following scenario.

> You respond to the shopping mall and encounter an 18-year-old woman who tripped on a loose piece of carpeting and twisted her ankle. Your evaluation reveals a swollen left ankle without any other trauma. The patient is alert and oriented and tells you that she wants to sue the store. You advise the patient that you want to take her to the hospital for further evaluation.

23. The type of consent that is required before treating this patient is:

    a. Implied consent
    b. Informed consent
    c. No consent is required because the patient is an emancipated minor
    d. Consent can only be granted by the police because the patient intends to sue

24. The patient agrees to be transported to the hospital and you help her walk to the ambulance. While walking, the patient stumbles and falls to the ground, injuring her wrist. Having this patient walk, rather than immobilizing her ankle and transporting her on a stretcher, is a deviation from:

    a. The Good Samaritan laws
    b. The level of consent that the patient agreed to
    c. The standard of care
    d. Quality care (abandonment)

25. You are now en route to the hospital and have an estimated arrival time of 25 minutes. The patient is in severe pain, both in her ankle and her wrist. While you are working as an EMT, you have the keys to the advanced life support cabinet in the ambulance and you administer a pain reliever to the patient from the advanced life support equipment. Use of this equipment by an EMT is:

    a. Outside of the scope of practice
    b. Allowable under the "golden rule" concept
    c. Outside the level of consent that the patient agreed to
    d. Allowable for a volunteer EMT but not for a paid EMT

Questions 26 and 27 refer to the following scenario.

> You respond to the local nursing home and encounter an 87-year-old woman in her bed in severe respiratory distress. The nursing home tells you that the local community hospital, approximately 12 minutes away, is expecting the patient in the emergency department. In addition to a lengthy medical history, the nursing home gives you a copy of a valid DNR order that was signed by all appropriate parties 2 weeks ago. The patient is currently receiving low-flow oxygen by a nasal cannula. The patient is not able to answer any questions at this time.

26. Care for this patient en route to the hospital consists of:

    a. Removing the supplemental oxygen and providing psychological first aid and transport; no interventions can be performed because of the DNR
    b. Maintaining the oxygen as established by the personnel from the nursing home at its current level but making no adjustments because of the DNR
    c. Providing any needed interventions to properly treat this patient's respiratory distress, including adjusting the oxygen delivery system as required
    d. Only providing specific care if the patient has a health care proxy present

27. You are approximately 3 minutes from the hospital when the patient stops breathing. You should:

    a. Begin positive-pressure ventilation by mouth to mouth or some other adjunct
    b. Continue to monitor the patient but do not provide any positive-pressure ventilations
    c. Return the patient to the nursing home because no care can be rendered
    d. Begin CPR

Across

2. Committee that approves research studies
4. A person who is legally able to make medical decisions for a patient who is incapacitated
5. Permission to medically treat
6. Maintaining a patient's right to privacy
10. Process by which an emotionally disturbed or incompetent patient who is a danger to self or others is moved to a medical facility by police and emergency personnel
13. The legal requirement to evaluate and treat a patient
14. Deviation from the accepted standard of care resulting in injury to the patient
16. Consent to medically treat an unconscious patient
17. Orders directing health care providers not to provide CPR
18. The process of securing items of potential importance at a crime scene
20. A bracelet or necklace that indicates a preexisting medical condition
21. Negligent act or omission that violates the standards of care expected
23. Practices by health care providers that reduce the possibility of a lawsuit
24. Guiding rule of effective medical practice

Down

1. Individual who is younger than the legal adult age but who is legally allowed to give consent because he or she is married
3. Offensive touching or use of force on a person
7. Specific statements of instruction regarding care that a patient does or does not want performed, should he or she become incapacitated
8. Parameters and limitations of a medical provider
9. Laws designed to protect the private citizen who is functioning in a nonprofessional capacity and without an expectation of remuneration
11. A clear connection between the patient's injury and actions taken or omitted by the EMT (an element that must be present to prove negligence)
12. "Do onto others as you would have them do onto you"
15. Consent to medically treat, after providing the patient with knowledge of the steps of procedures and related risks
19. An EMT who prematurely leaves a patient in need of emergency care and transportation to a hospital is subject to a charge of ____
22. A threat or attempt to inflict bodily harm on a person

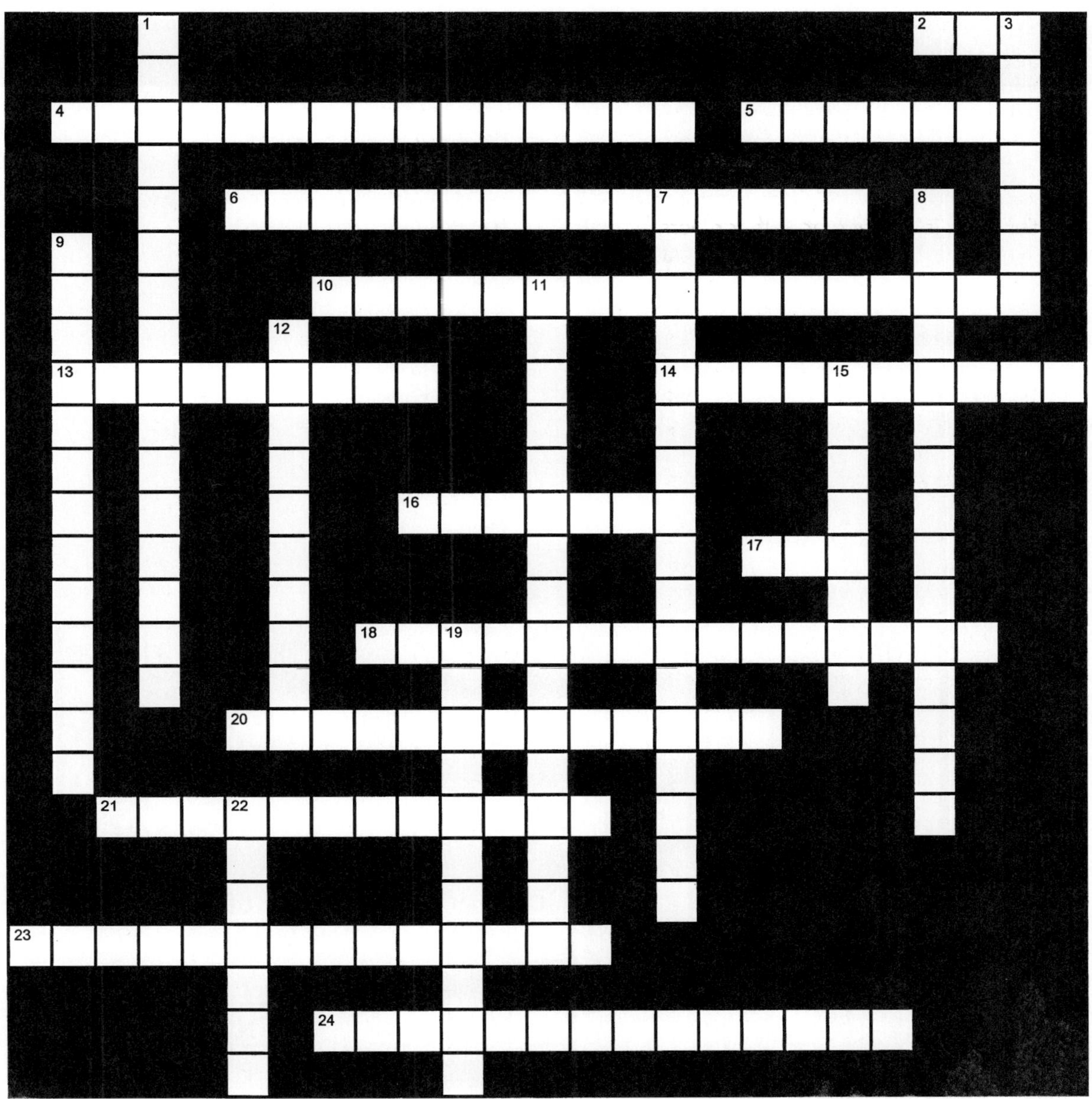
1
2
3
4
5
6
7
8
9
10
11
12
13
14
15
16
17
18
19
20
21
22
23
24

ANSWER KEY

1. b
2. c
3. b
4. b
5. c
6. b
7. c
8. a
9. d
10. c
11. d
12. a
13. c
14. a
15. b
16. b
17. c
18. Standard of care
19. Duty to act
    Breach of duty
    Injury
    Causal connection
20. Battery
21. c
22. b
23. b
24. c
25. a
26. c
27. b

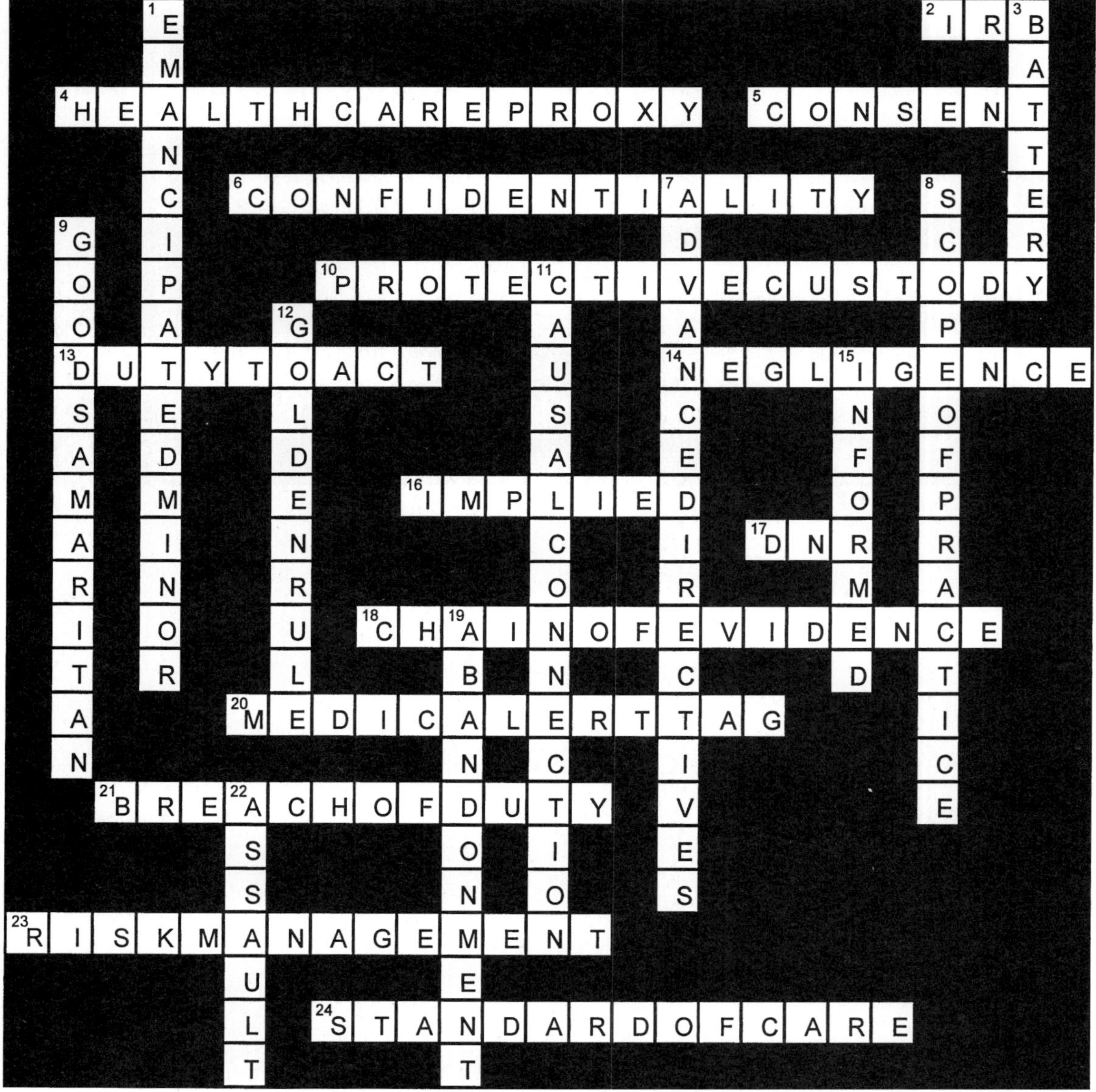

Chapter 4 The Human Body

Match the definition in column B to the correct term in column A.

Column A	Column B
1. _____ Medial	a. Toward the rear of the body
	b. Toward midline
2. _____ Proximal	c. Lying face down
	d. Movement away from the body
3. _____ Superior	e. Toward the point of origin
4. _____ Posterior	f. Toward the head
5. _____ Prone	
6. _____ Abduction	

7. The study of the structure or form of living things is called:

   a. Anatomy
   b. Physics
   c. Biology
   d. Physiology

8. Which of the following is a function of the skeletal system?

   a. Gives structure and support
   b. Produces plasma
   c. Destroys red blood cells
   d. Initiates respiration

9. In the normal anatomic position, the body is erect with feet together and parallel, arms extended, and palms and head facing:

   a. Medially
   b. Posteriorly
   c. Anteriorly
   d. Laterally

10. The heart, great vessels, esophagus, and trachea are located in which of the following body spaces?

    a. Pleura
    b. Peritoneal cavity
    c. Mediastinum
    d. Pelvic cavity

Match the type of spinal vertebrae in column A to the correct number found in the human spine in column B.

Column A	Column B
11. _____ Cervical vertebrae	a. Twelve mobile
	b. Five fused
12. _____ Thoracic vertebrae	c. Seven mobile
	d. Four fused
13. _____ Lumbar vertebrae	e. Five mobile
14. _____ Sacrum	
15. _____ Coccyx	

16. The ilium, ischium, and pubis collectively form the:

    a. Shoulder girdle
    b. Pelvic girdle
    c. Thoracic cage
    d. Metacarpal bones

17. The abdominal quadrants are created by two intersecting lines that meet at the:

    a. Xiphoid process
    b. Epigastric region
    c. Umbilicus
    d. Pubic bone

Match the type of muscle in column A to its function in column B.

Column A	Column B
18. ____ Voluntary or skeletal muscle	a. Movement of arms
19. ____ Involuntary or smooth muscle	b. Pumping of blood
20. ____ Cardiac muscle	c. Digestion

21. The respiratory structure responsible for preventing aspiration of food and other materials into the airway is called the:

    a. Bronchiole
    b. Carina
    c. Pharynx
    d. Epiglottis

22. The movement of oxygen from the lungs to the blood occurs at the level of the:

    a. Bronchi
    b. Alveoli
    c. Trachea
    d. Larynx

23. The pumping chambers of the heart that deliver blood to the lungs and body tissues are called the:

    a. Septums
    b. Sinuses
    c. Atria
    d. Ventricles

24. The major artery that delivers blood to the body or systemic circulation is called the:

    a. Aorta
    b. Pulmonary artery
    c. Coronary artery
    d. Vena cava

25. The type of vessel that permits diffusion to take place and that is one cell thick is called a(n):

    a. Capillary
    b. Vein
    c. Arteriole
    d. Artery

26. The type of blood cell that is responsible for combating infection is called:

    a. Red blood cell
    b. White blood cell
    c. Platelet
    d. Plasma

27. The protein that is responsible for the transport of oxygen and carbon dioxide is called:

    a. Plasma
    b. Thrombin
    c. Hemoglobin
    d. Fibrinogen

28. Which of the following is part of the central nervous system?

    a. Spinal cord
    b. Brain
    c. Peripheral nerves
    d. Both a and b

29. The part of the brain responsible for balance and coordination is called the:

    a. Cerebrum
    b. Pons
    c. Medulla
    d. Cerebellum

30. The body system concerned with maintaining homeostasis and influencing growth, reproduction, and response to stress through the release of hormones is called the:

    a. Digestive system
    b. Circulatory system
    c. Endocrine system
    d. Lymphatic system

31. The organ responsible for the release of insulin, which allows the metabolism of glucose, is the:

    a. Liver
    b. Gallbladder
    c. Pancreas
    d. Spleen

32. The largest part of the digestive tract, where absorption of nutrients occurs, is called the:

    a. Esophagus
    b. Liver
    c. Small intestine
    d. Rectum

33. The urinary system tube responsible for transporting urine from the bladder to the external opening of both the male and female genitalia is called the:

    a. Ureter
    b. Urethra
    c. Common bile duct
    d. Prostate

34. The tube that connects the ovary to the uterus is called the:

    a. Fallopian tube
    b. Cervix
    c. Ovarian tubule
    d. Uterine duct

35. The heart, lung, and brain depend on one another to maintain vital functions. Which of the following reasons best explains why a patient stops breathing after a cardiac arrest?

    a. Lack of oxygen to the brainstem
    b. Loss of voluntary breathing control
    c. Damage to the cerebrum
    d. Toxicity of blood

36. ___________ is the anatomic term for "toward the front of the body."

37. ___________ are vessels that direct blood flow away from the heart.

38. ___________ is the anatomic term that means "on both sides."

39. ___________ is the substance that connects the ribs to the sternum.

40. ___________ is the layer of skin that houses the nerves.

41. The ___________ is the respiratory muscle that separates the chest and abdomen.

42. Organs known as ___________ filter liquid waste from the body.

43. ___________ is another term for the voice box.

44. ___________ attaches bone to bone.

45. The ___________ is the large artery of the wrist and is used to check the pulse.

46. ___________ attaches muscle to bone.

47. ___________ is another term for the chest.

48. ___________ is another term for the windpipe.

49. ___________ are vessels that direct blood flow toward the heart.

Questions 50 to 53 refer to the following scenario.

> You respond to a call at a construction site, where you find a 32-year-old woman who fell approximately 15 feet while working on the roof, landing on her right side. She is found lying on her back. As you evaluate the patient you discover that she complains of pain to the back of her neck. You also discover that there is some swelling on the patient's left forearm, just below her elbow. The patient's left thigh is deformed approximately halfway between the hip and the knee. There is no break in the skin at the injury sites.

50. The position that you find the patient in is called:

    a. Prone
    b. Supine
    c. Trendelenburg
    d. Left lateral recumbent

51. When you make your radio presentation to the hospital, you describe the injury to the patient's forearm as:

    a. An injury to the humerus, proximal to the elbow
    b. An injury to the humerus, distal to the elbow
    c. An injury to the radius/ulna, proximal to the elbow
    d. An injury to the radius/ulna, distal to the elbow

52. The injury to the thigh halfway between the hip and knee would best be described as:

    a. An injury to the proximal femur
    b. An injury to the mid femur
    c. An injury to the proximal humerus
    d. An injury to the mid humerus

53. After delivering the patient to the hospital, the physician compliments you on the way you treated this patient. The physician tells you that the x-ray film reveals that she sustained a fracture to her thoracic spine. You remember that the thoracic spine is composed of:

    a. Four vertebrae
    b. Five vertebrae
    c. Seven vertebrae
    d. Twelve vertebrae

Questions 54 to 57 refer to the following scenario.

> You respond to a call for a 54-year-old man complaining of dizziness. During your evaluation the patient tells you that he was eating dinner when he began to choke on a piece of meat and could not breathe. His wife administered the Heimlich maneuver, which cleared the piece of meat, but the patient is now dizzy. When you further examine the patient you notice that he has a very weak pulse and that his lips appear to be slightly blue in color.

54. You suspect that when the patient was choking, the piece of meat was lodged in his:

    a. Esophagus
    b. Trachea
    c. Bronchus
    d. Stomach

55. In documenting the patient's skin color on your prehospital care report, you would indicate that the patient appeared:

    a. Pale
    b. Flushed
    c. Jaundiced
    d. Cyanotic

56. Each beat of this patient's heart results in the pulse that you feel when you evaluate the patient. The pulse is generated when the:

    a. Atria contract
    b. Atria relax
    c. Ventricles contract
    d. Ventricles relax

57. The component of blood that when bound to oxygen gives skin its pink color and when not bound to oxygen gives skin a blue appearance is (are):

    a. White blood cells
    b. Plasma
    c. Platelets
    d. Hemoglobin

Questions 58 and 59 refer to the following scenario.

> You respond to an act of violence at a bar. As you approach the scene you notice that it is safe and the police are on the scene. You are directed to evaluate a 23-year-old man who was punched in the left eye and kicked in the chest. The patient is found sitting at the curb and tells you that he is very upset. When you evaluate the patient you determine that his pulse rate is 120 beats/min and that he is breathing rapidly.

58. As you continue your evaluation of this patient you

    remember that the hormone ___________
    is released in times of stress.

59. During your evaluation of the patient, you look for signs of inadequate breathing. All the following are signs of inadequate breathing *except*:

    a. Diminished breath sounds
    b. Unequal chest expansion
    c. Clear (present and equal) breath sounds
    d. Accessory muscle use

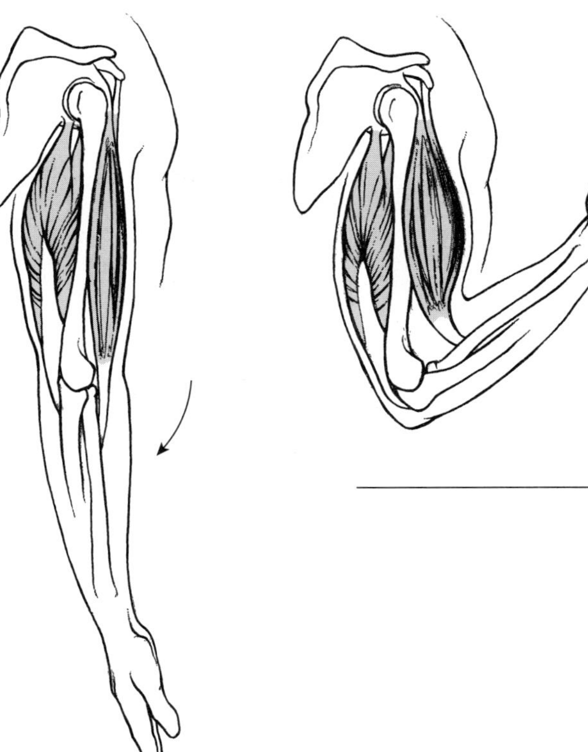

Fig. 4-1

Match the movement with the correct diagram in Fig. 4-1.

Flexion

Extension

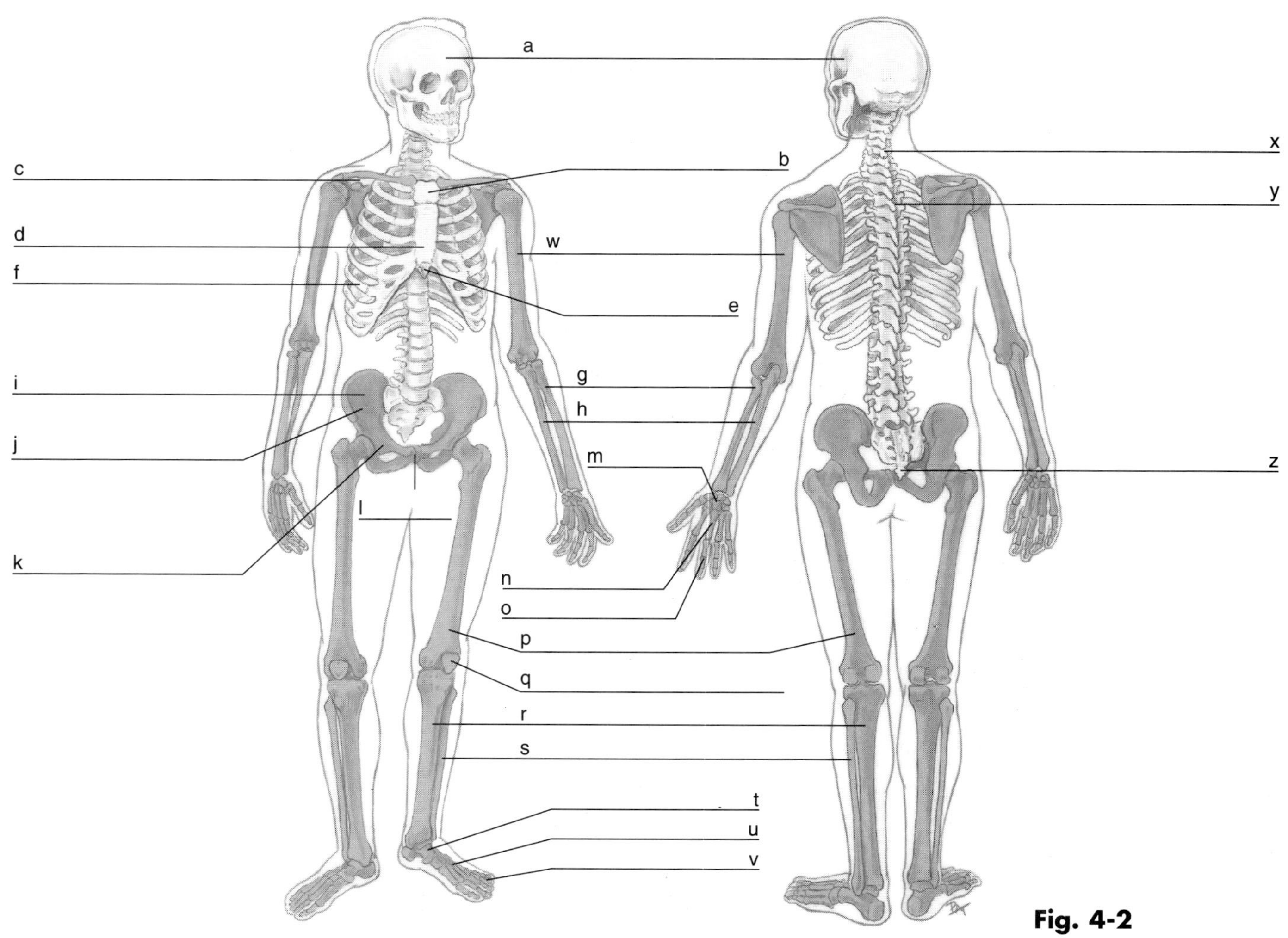

Fig. 4-2

Match the name of the bone with the correct location in Fig. 4-2.

Question	Choices
a. _____	Carpals
b. _____	Cervical vertebrae
c. _____	Clavicle
d. _____	Coccyx
e. _____	Femur
f. _____	Fibula
g. _____	Humerus
h. _____	Iliac crest
i. _____	Ischium
j. _____	Manubrium
k. _____	Metacarpals
l. _____	Metatarsals
m. _____	Patella
n. _____	Pelvis
o. _____	Phalanges
p. _____	Phalanges
q. _____	Pubis
r. _____	Radius
s. _____	Ribs
t. _____	Skull
u. _____	Sternum
v. _____	Tarsals
w. _____	Thoracic vertebrae
x. _____	Tibia
y. _____	Ulna
z. _____	Xiphoid process

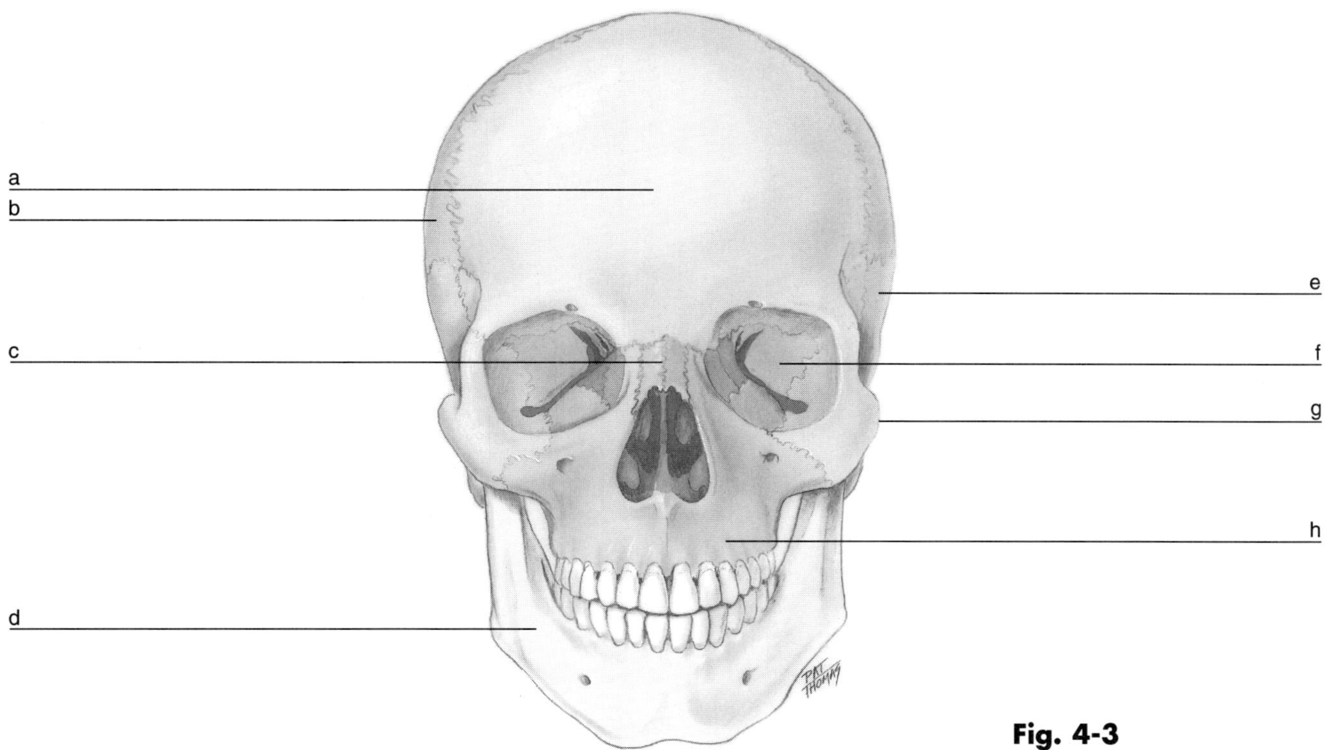

Fig. 4-3

Match the name of the bone with the correct location in Fig. 4-3.

Question	Choices
a. _____	Frontal bone
b. _____	Mandible
c. _____	Maxilla
d. _____	Nasal bone
e. _____	Orbital bones
f. _____	Parietal bone
g. _____	Temporal bone
h. _____	Zygomatic bone

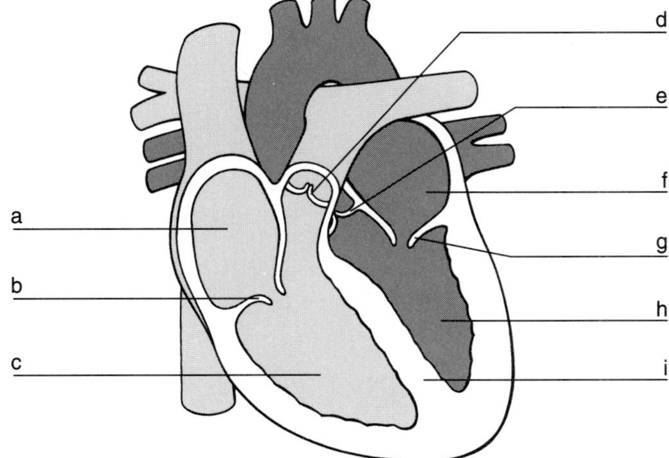

Fig. 4-4

Match the name of the structure with the correct location in Fig. 4-4.

Question	Choices
a. _____	Aortic valve
b. _____	Left atrium
c. _____	Left ventricle
d. _____	Mitral valve
e. _____	Pulmonary valve
f. _____	Right atrium
g. _____	Right ventricle
h. _____	Tricuspid valve
i. _____	Ventricular septum

Across

1. Eight bones of the wrist
3. Large artery of the arm used in measuring blood pressure
7. Thigh bone
10. Seven bones of the ankle
11. Artery palpable in the thigh
12. The fluid in which oxygen and nutrients are transported
13. Nostrils
14. Armpit
16. Bones that surround the eye
19. Organ that filters blood
20. An imaginary plane separating the body into right and left halves
22. Artery found in the neck used for pulse check
23. Navel
25. Collectively, the bones of the cranium and the face
27. A body standing erect with feet together and parallel, arms at the sides, palms and head facing forward
30. _____ ribs are not attached to the sternum
31. The larger bone of the lower leg
33. Outermost layer of the skin
35. Breastbone
36. Flap of cartilage that covers the larynx during swallowing
39. The primary artery of the circulatory system
40. Nerve impulses travel from the brain to the peripheral nervous system via the _____ _____
41. Collarbone
42. Section of the spinal column that contains 12 vertebrae
43. Windpipe
44. The main organ of respiration

Down

1. Outpocketing of the brain located behind the brainstem
2. Section of the spinal column that contains five fused bones
4. Cavity that contains the stomach, intestines, liver, spleen, gallbladder, pancreas, kidneys, and ureters
5. Space between the ribs
6. Lower part of the brain that exits the skull
8. An imaginary line that passes through the middle of the clavicles parallel to the midline
9. Bone on the medial side of the forearm
15. Bones of the spinal column
17. Respiratory tubes that branch off just after the trachea
18. Protective covering that separates the heart from the other organs
21. Food pipe
24. Primary site for absorption in the digestive system
26. Toward the rear
28. The upper jaw
29. Largest organ of the body
32. Further from the trunk
34. Sole of the foot
35. The system that gives support and structure to the body
37. Position of the body lying on its face
38. Position of the body lying on its back

Puzzle 4A

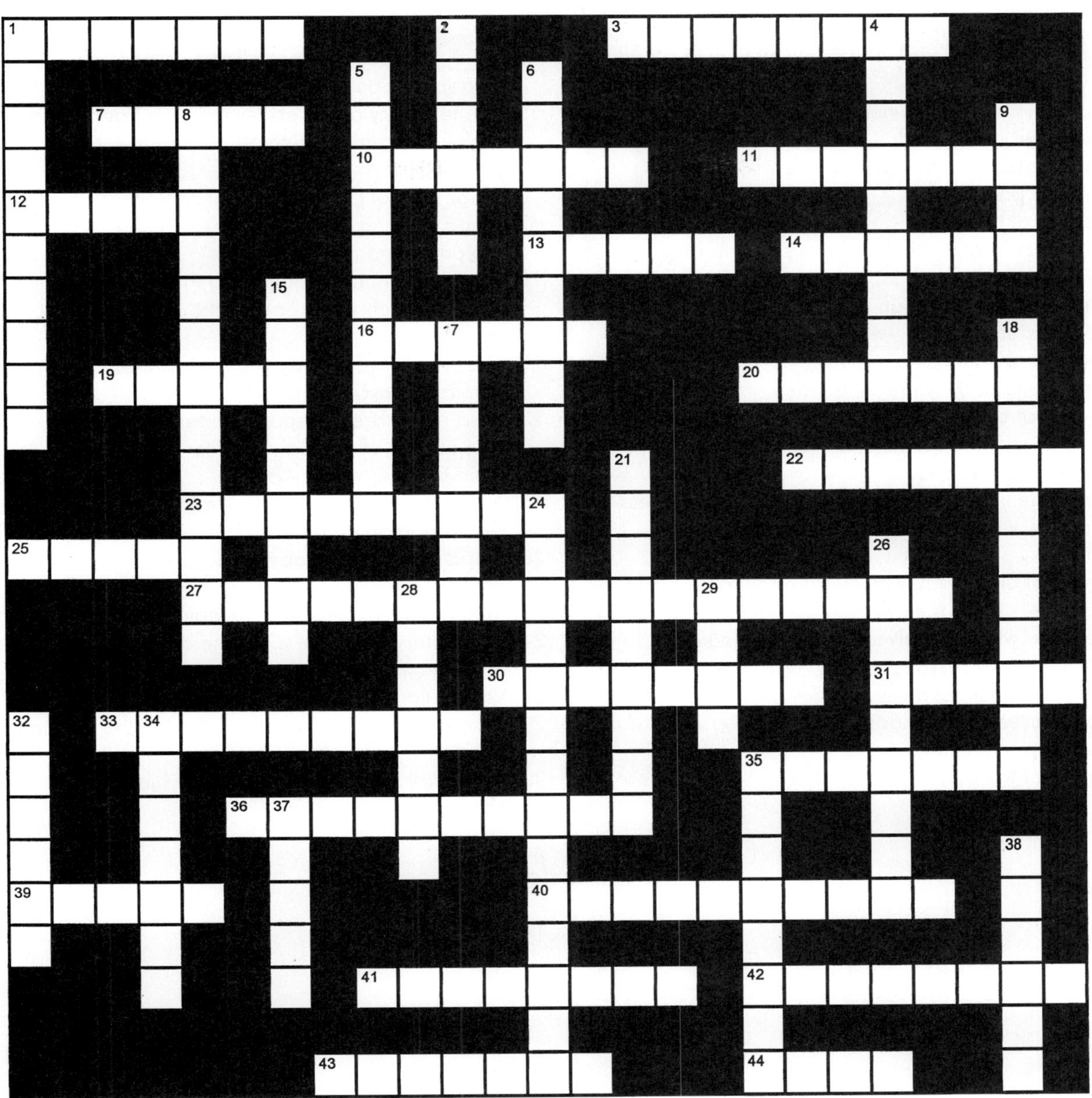

Puzzle 4A

Across

1. Structures that maintain the one-way flow of blood in the vessels
3. Respiratory response when the diaphragm contracts and pushes downward
9. Muscle's ability to contract on its own
11. Sitting up position
14. Stopping of the heart
15. Bluish discoloration of the mucous membranes or skin
16. The waste product of respiration
19. Redness of the skin in an area of infection or inflammation
21. Air sacs in the lungs
22. Position of a body lying on its side
25. The sum of cellular activity
27. The relative acidity or alkalinity of a fluid
28. Partially digested food
31. Membrane that is surgically opened to gain access to the airway when an obstruction exists above the larynx
32. Turning of an extremity away from the midline of the body
33. Disease in which the alveoli are damaged or destroyed
34. Ventricular contraction
35. Force exerted by the blood volume on the walls of the vessels
36. Pigment of the skin

Down

2. _____ muscles are controlled by a person's will
4. Hypoperfusion
5. The tendency of molecules to move from an area of higher concentration to an area of lower concentration
6. Fragments of cells necessary for clotting
7. Blood clot
8. No pulse and no respirations
10. Fundamental unit of all living things
11. Movement of a joint so that the two parts are closer together
12. The amount of air inspired and expired during one respiratory cycle
13. Area of the brain responsible for intellectual function and control of skeletal muscles
15. Fluid that protects the brain
17. Amount of air breathed in 1 minute
18. Liquid portion of the blood
20. Blood disorder characterized by a deficiency of the proteins used for clotting
23. Inflammatory disease of the epiglottis
24. Respiratory response when the diaphragm relaxes and rises within the chest
26. Ventricular relaxation
29. Movement of the elbow from the bent to the straight position
30. Substance, secreted in the liver, which aids fat absorption

Puzzle 4B

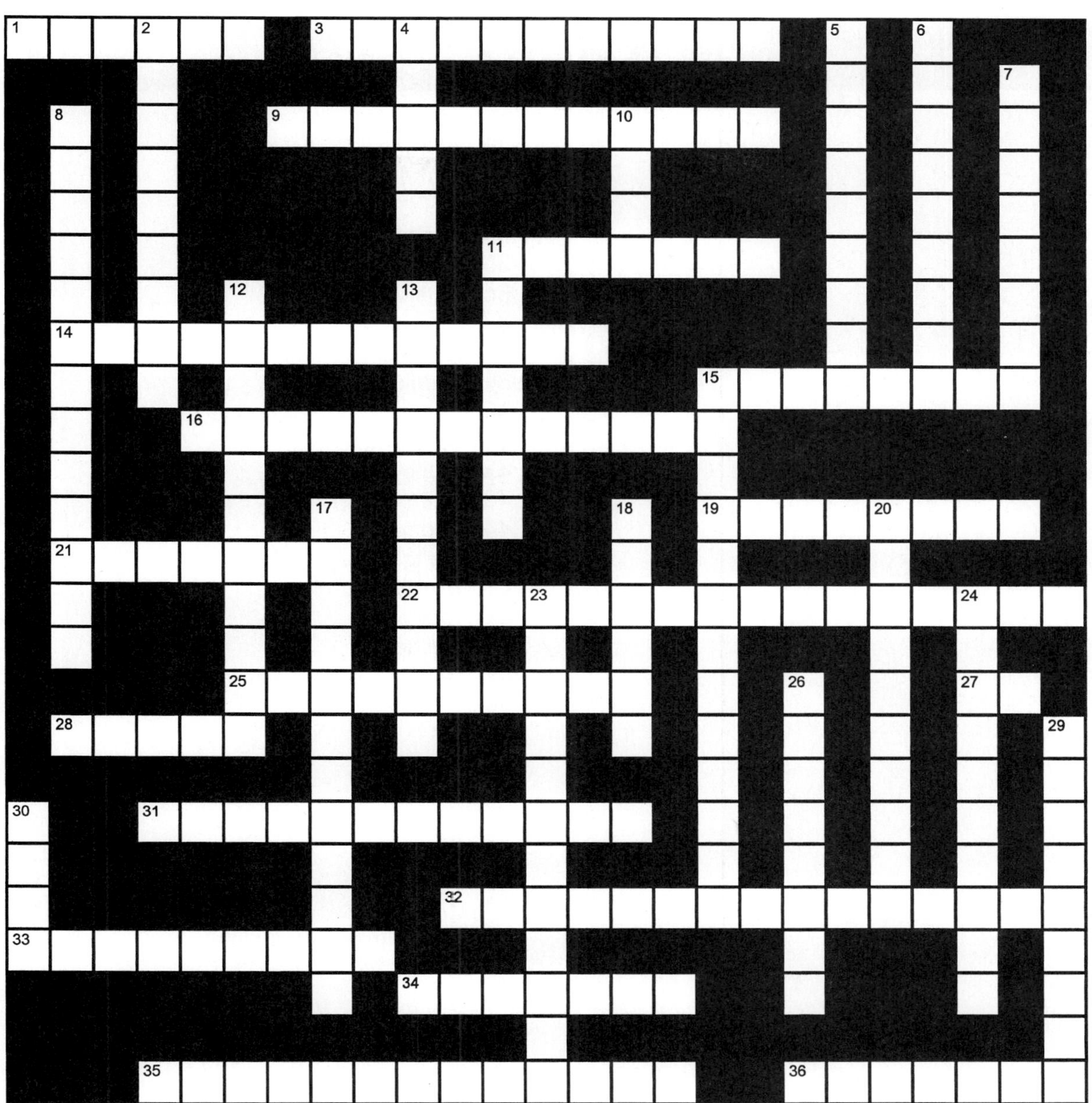
1
2
3
4
5
6
7
8
9
10
11
12
13
14
15
16
17
18
19
20
21
22
23
24
25
26
27
28
29
30
31
32
33
34
35
36

Puzzle 4B

ANSWER KEY

1. b
2. e
3. f
4. a
5. c
6. d
7. a
8. a
9. c
10. c
11. c
12. a
13. e
14. b
15. d
16. b
17. c
18. a
19. c
20. b
21. d
22. b
23. d
24. a
25. a
26. b
27. c
28. d
29. d
30. c
31. c
32. c
33. b
34. a
35. a
36. Anterior
37. Arteries
38. Bilateral
39. Cartilage
40. Dermis
41. Diaphragm
42. Kidneys
43. Larynx
44. Ligaments
45. Radial artery
46. Tendons
47. Thorax
48. Trachea
49. Veins
50. b
51. d
52. b
53. d
54. b
55. d
56. c
57. d
58. Epinephrine (adrenaline)
59. c

Answers to Fig. 4-1

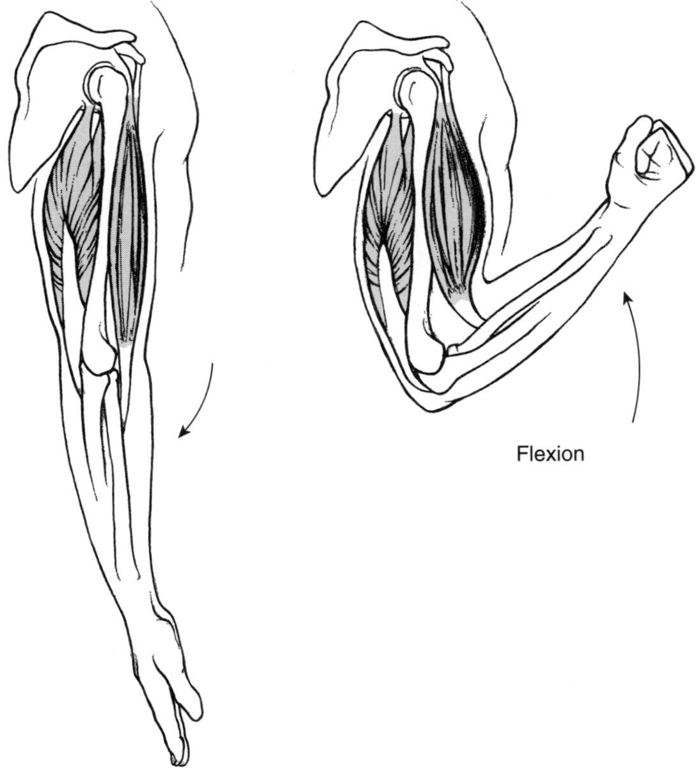

Answers to Fig. 4-2

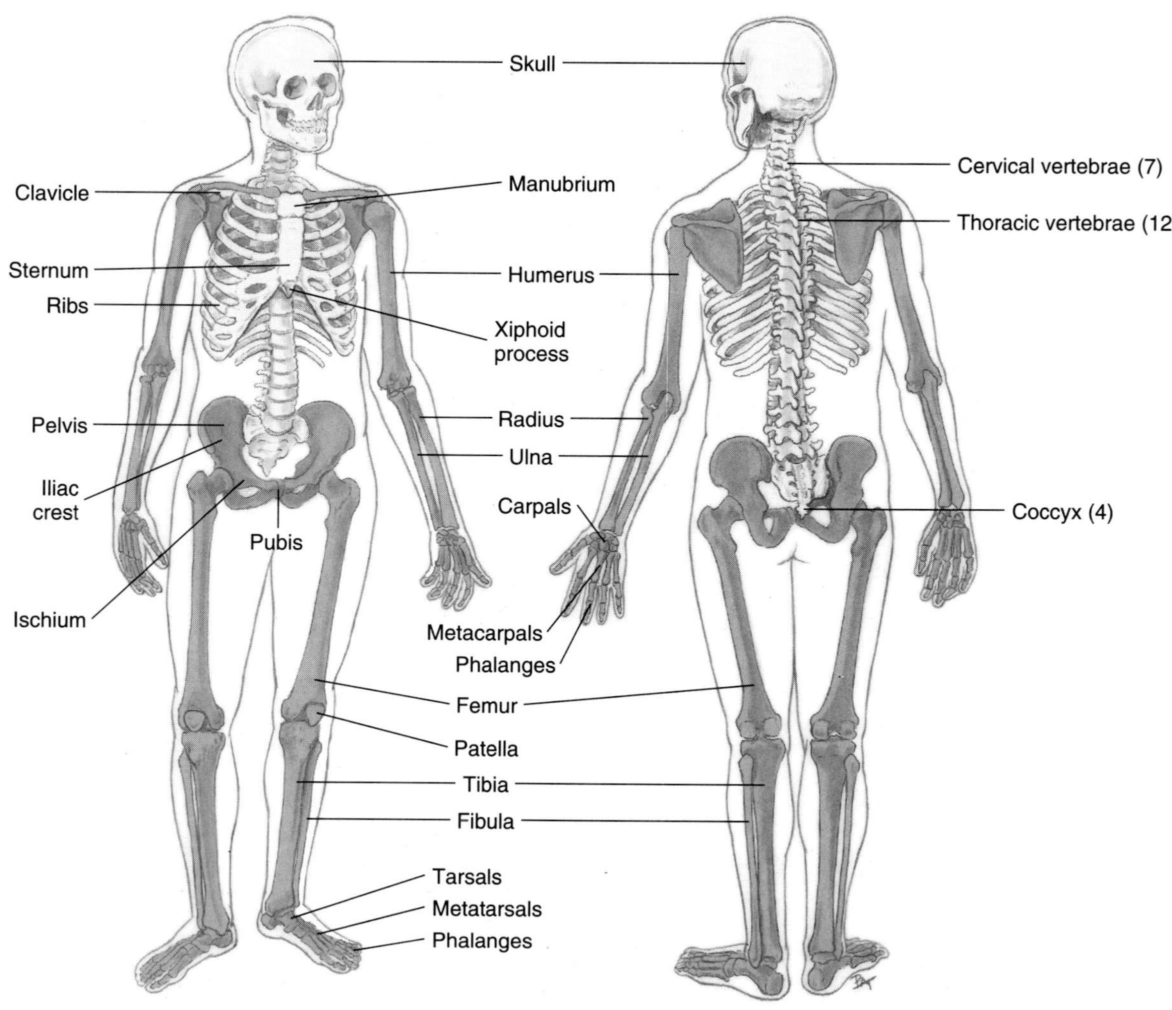

a. Skull
b. Manubrium
c. Clavicle
d. Sternum
e. Xiphoid process
f. Ribs
g. Radius
h. Ulna
i. Pelvis
j. Iliac crest
k. Ischium
l. Pubis
m. Carpals
n. Metacarpals
o. Phalanges
p. Femur
q. Patella
r. Tibia
s. Fibula
t. Tarsals
u. Metatarsals
v. Phalanges
w. Humerus
x. Cervical vertebrae
y. Thoracic vertebrae
z. Coccyx

Answers to Fig. 4-3

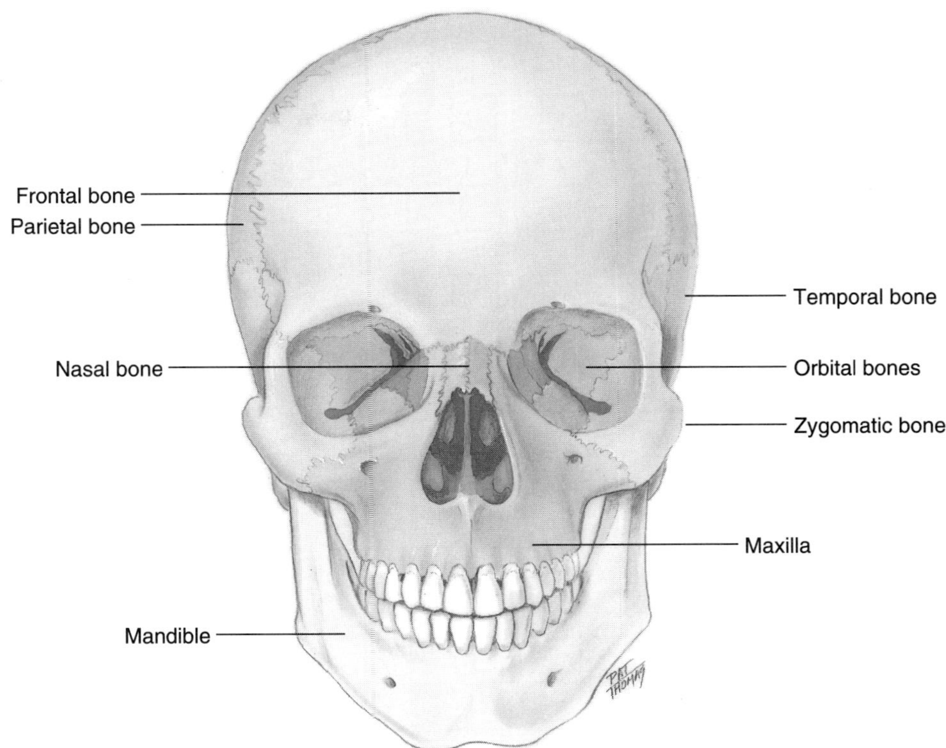

a. Frontal bone
b. Parietal bone
c. Nasal bone
d. Mandible
e. Temporal bone
f. Orbital bones
g. Zygomatic bone
h. Maxilla

Answers to Fig. 4-4

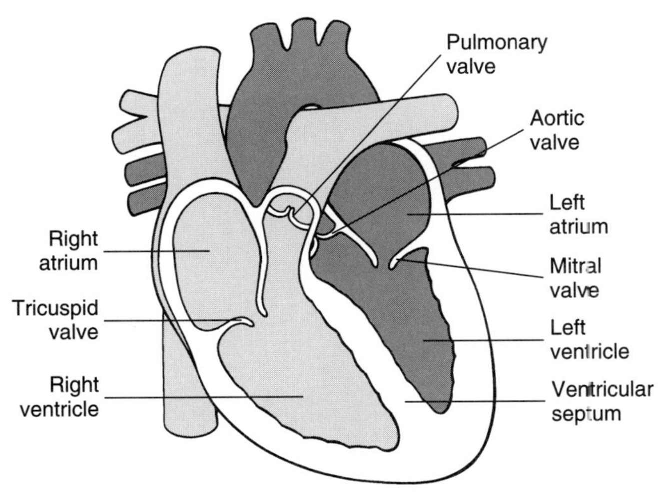

a. Right atrium
b. Tricuspid valve
c. Right ventricle
d. Pulmonary valve
e. Aortic valve
f. Left atrium
g. Mitral valve
h. Left ventricle
i. Ventricular septum

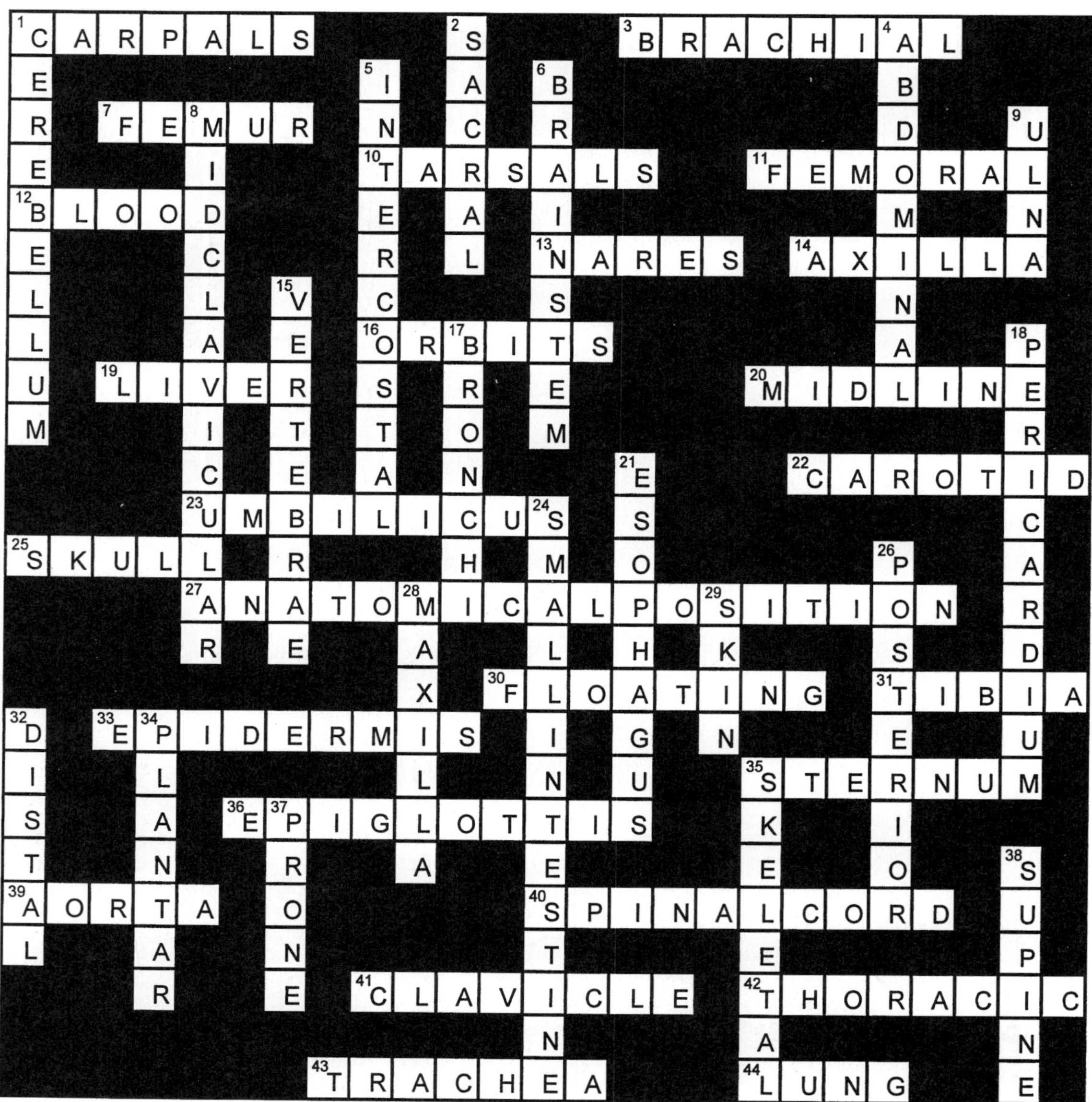

Puzzle 4A

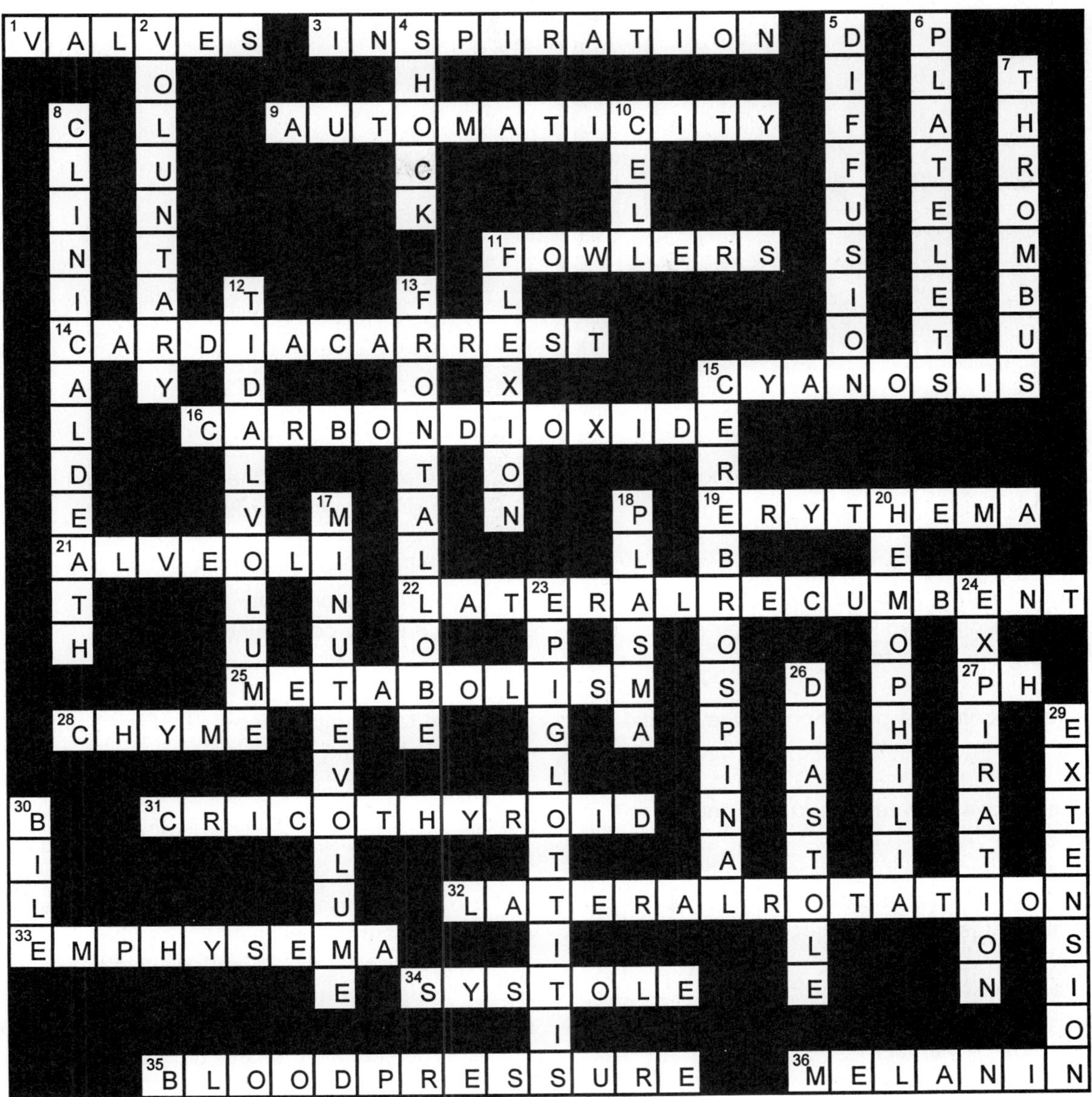
1 VALVES
2 VOLUNTARY
3 INSPIRATION
4 SHOCK
5 DIFFUSION
6 PLATELET
7 THROMBUS
8 CLINICALDEATH
9 AUTOMATICITY
10 CELL
11 FOWLERS
11 FLEXION
12 TIDALVOLUME
13 FRONTALLOBE
14 CARDIACARREST
15 CYANOSIS
15 CEREBROSPINAL
16 CARBONDIOXIDE
17 MINUTEVOLUME
18 PLASMA
19 ERYTHEMA
20 HEMOPHILIA
21 ALVEOLI
22 LATERALRECUMBENT
23 EPIGLOTTIS
24 EXPIRATION
25 METABOLISM
26 DIASTOLE
27 PH
28 CHYME
29 EXTENSION
30 BILE
31 CRICOTHYROID
32 LATERALROTATION
33 EMPHYSEMA
34 SYSTOLE
35 BLOODPRESSURE
36 MELANIN

Puzzle 4B

Chapter 5 Baseline Vital Signs and SAMPLE History

1. The best method for evaluating the adequacy of ventilation is by:

   a. Observing chest rise
   b. Placing a mirror near the mouth and nose
   c. Feeling the chest wall for expansion
   d. Checking the pulse rate

2. The correct location of palpation for the carotid pulse is:

   a. At the groove between the larynx and muscle in the neck
   b. At the angle of the jaw adjacent to the muscle
   c. Just above the suprasternal notch
   d. Just above the clavicle, adjacent to the trachea

3. The carotid pulse should be palpated on:

   a. Either side of the neck
   b. The side opposite the rescuer
   c. The same side as the rescuer
   d. Both sides of the neck each time

4. The carotid pulse should be initially palpated for:

   a. 2 to 3 seconds
   b. 3 to 5 seconds
   c. 5 to 10 seconds
   d. 10 to 20 seconds

5. Which of the following questions reflects the best way to inquire about a chest pain complaint in a medical history?

   a. Was your chest pain squeezing in nature?
   b. How would you describe the pain in your own words?
   c. Did it feel like someone was standing on your chest?
   d. Was the pain viselike in nature?

6. The expression of the patient's main complaint in his or her own words is called the:

   a. History of present illness
   b. Primary problem
   c. Primary complaint
   d. Chief complaint

7. The four major diseases that are routinely inquired about during the past medical history with older adult patients are:

   a. Heart disease, epilepsy, chronic obstructive pulmonary disease, high blood pressure
   b. Heart disease, diabetes, cancer, high blood pressure
   c. Diabetes, chronic obstructive pulmonary disease, high blood pressure, stroke
   d. Heart disease, diabetes, chronic obstructive pulmonary disease, high blood pressure

8. The normal range of respiratory rate in the adult is approximately ______ breaths/min.

   a. 5 to 15
   b. 10 to 15
   c. 12 to 20
   d. 15 to 25

Match the respiratory sound in column A with the likely underlying problem in column B.

Column A	Column B
9. _____ Gurgling	a. Obstruction by the tongue
	b. Fluid in the airway
10. _____ Snoring	c. Narrowed lower airway
	d. Narrowed upper airway

11. _____ Wheezing

12. _____ Stridor

---

13. The artery routinely used to monitor the pulse in the conscious adult patient is the:

    a. Radial
    b. Femoral
    c. Brachial
    d. Ulnar

14. The normal range of pulse rate for an adult at rest is approximately __________ beats/min.

    a. 40 to 60
    b. 50 to 70
    c. 60 to 80
    d. 80 to 120

15. The diastolic blood pressure is recorded on the basis of when:

    a. Auscultated sounds diminish or disappear
    b. Auscultated sounds first appear
    c. Palpated pulses disappear
    d. Palpated pulses are first felt

16. Blood pressure determined by listening through a stethoscope is called blood pressure by:

    a. Auscultation
    b. Palpation
    c. Oscillation
    d. Vibration

17. Which artery is routinely monitored while auscultating a blood pressure?

    a. Radial
    b. Brachial
    c. Ulnar
    d. Femoral

18. What is the name for the component of blood pressure associated with the first sound heard through the stethoscope?

    a. Diastolic
    b. Systolic
    c. Pulse
    d. Contractile

19. Which component of blood pressure is obtained when using the palpation technique?

    a. Diastolic
    b. Systolic
    c. Pulse
    d. Contractile

20. The pulse that can be palpated in the anterolateral aspect of the wrist, just below the thumb is the:

    a. Brachial
    b. Ulnar
    c. Radial
    d. Humeral

21. Vital signs include all the following *except*:

    a. Respirations
    b. Pulse
    c. Temperature
    d. Breath sounds

22. What is the main reason why baseline vital signs are so important to the care of the patient?

    a. Patients expect their vital signs to be taken and would be suspicious of care if you did not take their vital signs
    b. They provide a baseline value by which the effectiveness of therapy can be measured
    c. To prevent legal problems related to the care of the patient if you are sued at a later time
    d. To compare one patient with another for quality assurance studies related to vital sign changes

23. All the following are abnormal blood pressures in an adult patient *except:*

    a. 190/100 mm Hg
    b. 150/98 mm Hg
    c. 124/82 mm Hg
    d. 84/54 mm Hg

24. What is the pulse of a patient in severe shock likely to feel like?

    a. Strong and slow
    b. Weak and rapid
    c. Strong and irregular
    d. Weak and irregular

25. Capillary refill in a child is considered delayed when the refilling time is:

    a. Less than 1 second
    b. 1 second
    c. 2 seconds
    d. Greater than 2 seconds

26. Which of the following skin colors are associated with impaired blood flow and poor perfusion?

    a. Pale
    b. Flushed
    c. Jaundiced
    d. Cherry red

27. Which skin color is often associated with abnormalities with the liver?

    a. Cyanotic
    b. Pale
    c. Flushed
    d. Jaundiced

28. Which of the following descriptions best describes normal pupils?

    a. Midpositional, equal, and reactive
    b. Dilated, equal, and reactive
    c. Constricted, equal, and nonreactive
    d. Dilated, equal, and nonreactive

29. Which of the following pupils would you describe as normally reactive?

    a. A pupil that becomes larger when a light is projected into the eye
    b. A pupil that becomes smaller when a light is projected into the eye
    c. A pupil that is unchanged when a light is projected into the eye
    d. A pupil that becomes larger, then smaller when a light is projected into the eye

30. Which of the following pupils is most constricted?

    a. ● b. ● c. ● d. ●

31. What is the skin temperature and moisture of a patient in shock likely to reveal?

    a. Cool, moist skin
    b. Warm, moist skin
    c. Cool, dry skin
    d. Warm, dry skin

32. Which of the following is a sign?

    a. Chest pain
    b. Nausea
    c. Swollen ankles
    d. Dizziness

33. All the following problems can occur if vital signs are not accurately taken and recorded by a prehospital provider *except*:

    a. The hospital staff could misinterpret changes in the patient's condition
    b. The EMT can inappropriately treat the patient in the field
    c. The patient may be inappropriately prioritized in the emergency department
    d. The provider could be criminally prosecuted for failure to make an accurate record

34. Medical identification cards, bracelets, and necklaces will usually provide all of the following valuable information about the patient *except*:

    a. Medications
    b. Allergies
    c. Family history
    d. Past medical history

35. The measure of the force that blood exerts on the walls of the arteries is called ___________.

36. The membrane of the interior surface of the eyelids, used to assess skin color, is the ___________.

37. A blood pressure should be taken in children above ___________ years of age.

38. ___________ is the mnemonic used to stay organized during your history taking.

39. An exaggerated opening of the nostrils on inspiration, which is a sign of respiratory distress seen in infants and children, is called ___________.

40. ___________ are inward depressions of muscular areas between the ribs, above the clavicles, and below the sternum seen in a patient in respiratory distress.

Across

1. The P in SAMPLE
4. Description of large pupil size
6. Harsh, low-pitched sound caused by the tongue partially blocking the airway
11. Point at which the sound disappears when the pressure in a blood pressure cuff is released and represents the point at which the ventricle relaxes
12. General range of vital signs that are considered normal
13. Listening to the sounds made by the internal organs of the body
18. Normal skin temperature
20. Clue to the patient's condition that you can see, hear, smell, or feel
21. The patient's description of the main problem
23. The M in SAMPLE
24. Artery found in the groin
27. A pupil that does not respond to light
31. Examine by feel or touch
33. The A in SAMPLE
34. Pulse used to assess unresponsive patients
35. Term used to describe breathing that requires increased respiratory effort
36. Opening in the iris of the eye that normally reacts to light
37. Pulse found at the wrist
38. Yellowish skin color

Down

1. Skin color indicating poor perfusion or impaired blood flow
2. Number of breaths per minute
3. Sound created by air moving through a fluid
5. Pulse found at the elbow
7. Abnormal rhythmic whining sound sometimes heard at the end of exhalation
8. The E in SAMPLE
9. High blood pressure
10. Description of small pupil size
14. Diagnostic test in which the nailbed is compressed and released
15. The L in SAMPLE
16. Voicebox
17. Blood pressure machine
18. High-pitched, whistling sound often heard in patients with asthma
19. Crowing sound usually heard on inspiration
22. Felt by palpating an artery close to the skin
25. Skin temperature indicating fever
26. Something felt by the patient and communicated to the EMT
28. Bluish skin color
29. First sound heard when the pressure in the blood pressure cuff is released, which represents the pressure of ventricular contraction
30. Skin color indicating possible exposure to heat or carbon monoxide
32. A child sitting and perched on both hands with the head and neck thrust forward is said to be in the _____ position
34. Skin temperature indicating poor perfusion

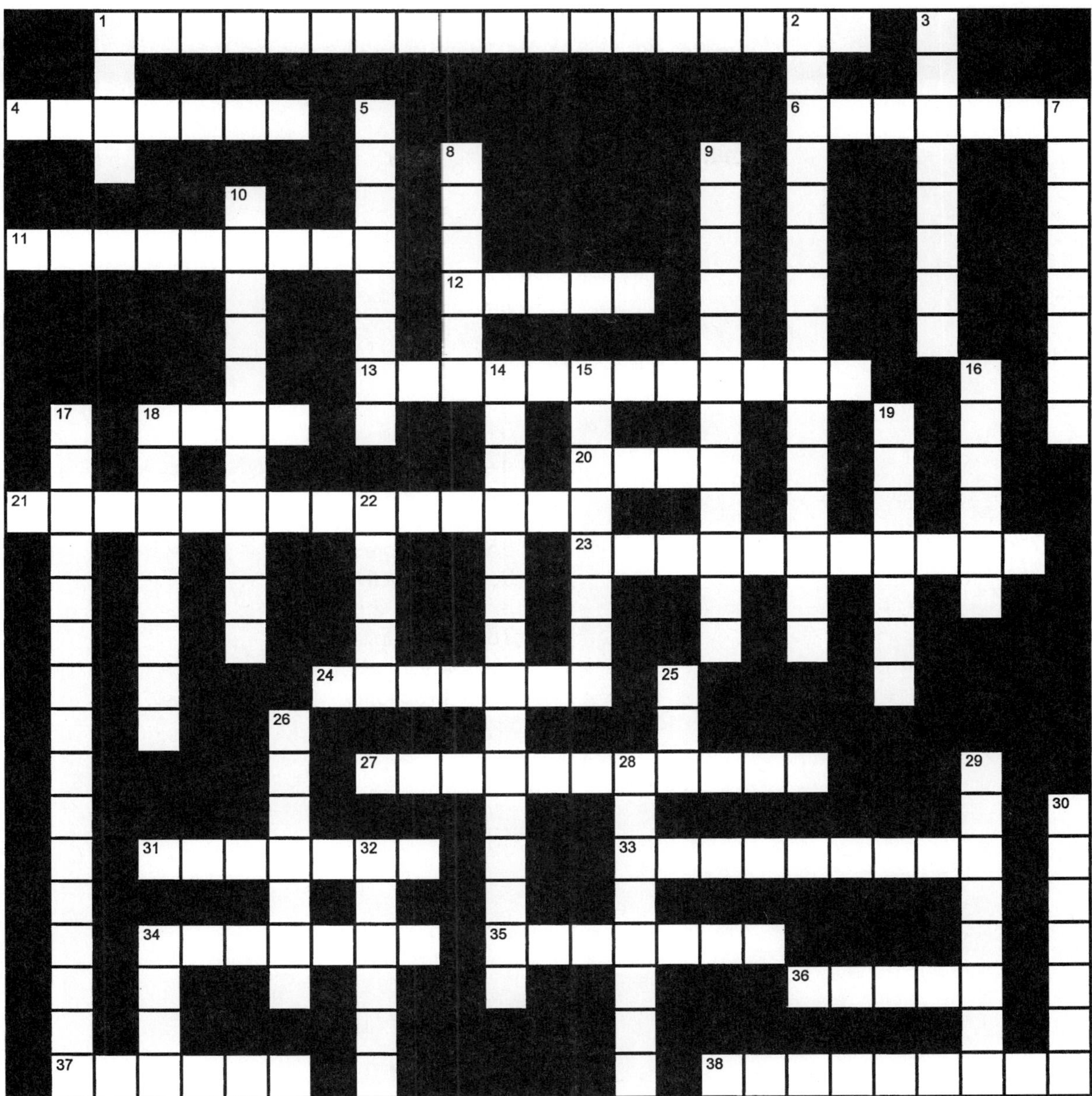
1
2
3
4
5
6
7
8
9
10
11
12
13
14
15
16
17
18
19
20
21
22
23
24
25
26
27
28
29
30
31
32
33
34
35
36
37
38

ANSWER KEY

1. a
2. a
3. c
4. c
5. b
6. d
7. d
8. c
9. b
10. a
11. c
12. d
13. a
14. c
15. a
16. a
17. b
18. b
19. b
20. c
21. d
22. b
23. c
24. b
25. d
26. a
27. d
28. a
29. b
30. a
31. a
32. c
33. d
34. c
35. Blood pressure
36. Conjunctiva
37. Three
38. SAMPLE
39. Nasal flaring
40. Retractions

		[1]P	A	S	T	M	E	D	I	C	A	L	H	I	S	T	O	[2]R	Y		[3]G			
		A																E			U			
[4]D	I	L	A	T	E	D		[5]B										[6]S	N	O	R	I	N	[7]G
		E						R		[8]E						[9]H		P			G			R
					[10]C			A		V						Y		I			L			U
[11]D	I	A	S	T	O	L	I	C		E						P		R			I			N
					N			H		[12]N	O	R	M	S		E		A			N			T
					S			I		T						R		T			G			I
					T			[13]A	U	S	[14]C	U	[15]L	T	A	T	I	O	N			[16]L		N
	[17]S		[18]W	A	R	M		L			A		A			E		R		[19]S		A		G
	P		H		I						P		[20]S	I	G	N		Y		T		R		
[21]C	H	I	E	F	C	O	M	[22]P	L	A	I	N	T			S		R		R		Y		
	Y		E		T			U			L		[23]M	E	D	I	C	A	T	I	O	N	S	
	G		Z		E			L			L		E			O		T		D		X		
	M		I		D			S			A		A			N		E		O				
	O		N				[24]F	E	M	O	R	A	L		[25]H					R				
	M		G			[26]S					Y				O									
	A					Y		[27]N	O	N	R	E	A	[28]C	T	I	V	E				[29]S		
	N					M					E			Y								Y		[30]F
	O		[31]P	A	L	P	A	[32]T	E		F			[33]A	L	L	E	R	G	I	E	S		L
	M					T		R			I			N								T		U
	E		[34]C	A	R	O	T	I	D		[35]L	A	B	O	R	E	D					O		S
	T		O			M		P			L			T				[36]P	U	P	I	L		H
	E		L					O						I								I		E
	[37]R	A	D	I	A	L		D						C		[38]J	A	U	N	D	I	C	E	D

Chapter 6 Lifting and Moving Patients

1. The scientific method of efficiently lifting large weights so as not to injure oneself is best described as:

   a. Ergonomics
   b. Body mechanics
   c. Body preservation
   d. Longevity

2. When lifting a patient, you should use the muscles in your:

   a. Lower back
   b. Upper back
   c. Legs
   d. Pelvis

3. When carrying a stretcher with a patient on it, your back should be:

   a. Flexed
   b. Hyperextended
   c. Held straight
   d. Curved

4. When performing a patient lift, your arms should be:

   a. As close to your body as possible
   b. As far apart as possible
   c. Flexed at the elbow
   d. With palms facing downward

5. All the following illustrate the best way to avoid injury while moving a patient *except*:

   a. Moving slowly
   b. Moving in unison with your partner
   c. Maintaining a firm grip on the stretcher
   d. Using twisting or sharp movements

6. While moving a patient, it is important to do all the following *except:*

   a. Communicate with your partner
   b. Keep your muscles contracted for long periods of time
   c. Maintain your footing
   d. Keep your back straight

7. Before lifting or carrying a patient, the EMT should do all the following *except*:

   a. Determine the weight to be lifted
   b. Know the abilities of yourself and your partner
   c. Keep the weight as close to your body as possible
   d. Flex at the waist during the lifting process

8. The most commonly used and most effective method for placing a wheeled stretcher into an ambulance is the:

   a. Side carry method
   b. Front and back carry method
   c. Sitting position method
   d. Vertical lift method

9. A one-handed carry with a stretcher can be used when:

   a. There are only two people available for the carry
   b. You need to compensate for an imbalance
   c. There are multiple people available for the carry
   d. You cannot maintain a straight posture

10. When using the one-handed carry technique, the EMT should:

    a. Keep the back in a locked position
    b. Keep the back in the flexed position
    c. Compensate for the imbalance
    d. Flex at the waist when picking up the object with one hand

11. Which of the following statements is correct when carrying a patient down a flight of stairs?

    a. The EMT at the bottom of the device will have most of the weight
    b. The EMT at the top of the device will have most of the weight
    c. Each EMT shares the weight distribution equally
    d. The incline has no bearing on the distribution of the weight

12. Back injuries to the EMT commonly occur:

    a. When using the one-handed carry
    b. When carrying a patient down the stairs
    c. When reaching or stretching during the lifting process
    d. When lifting a patient into the ambulance

13. When reaching or stretching, the EMT should reach no more than:

    a. 5 to 10 inches from the body
    b. 15 to 20 inches from the body
    c. 20 to 25 inches from the body
    d. 30 to 35 inches from the body

14. When performing a log roll, the EMT positioned at the patient's ___________ should supervise the movements.

    a. Head
    b. Shoulder
    c. Hip
    d. Lower leg

15. Before performing a log roll on a patient who fell 30 feet, the EMT should:

    a. Tie the patient's hands and legs together
    b. Immobilize the cervical spine
    c. Obtain written consent
    d. Ask the patient if he or she can move the head from side to side

16. When pushing or pulling a patient to the ambulance, it is important to:

    a. Pull, because it is safer than pushing
    b. Push, because it is safer than pulling
    c. Carry the patient whenever possible, because it is more stable than pushing or pulling
    d. Keep elbows locked while pushing or pulling

17. Proper technique for pushing and pulling patients includes all the following *except*:

    a. Keeping your back locked straight
    b. Keeping the patient's weight close to your body
    c. Keeping your elbows bent with arms close to your body
    d. Keeping your elbows locked with arms close to your body

18. Patient movement considerations can be classified as all the following *except*:

    a. Emergency moves
    b. Urgent moves
    c. Semiurgent moves
    d. Nonurgent moves

19. Patients should be moved first, then treated, in all the following situations *except:*

    a. When the patient has inadequate breathing
    b. There is serious threat of fire or explosion
    c. When life-saving care cannot be given because of the patient's location
    d. When the patient and the scene are stable

20. The method for quickly removing a patient in respiratory arrest from a car is called:

    a. Load and go
    b. Rapid extrication
    c. Scoop and run
    d. Triage

21. Patients in the late stages of pregnancy should be transported in the ___________ position.

22. The simplest technique for moving a patient who is in immediate danger from a fire or an explosion is the ___________.

23. The primary concern for unconscious patients is ___________ management.

Match the device in column A with its primary use in column B.

Column A	**Primary Use of Device**
24. _____ Wheeled cot	a. Used to move patients over rough terrain or during high-angle rescues
25. _____ Stair chair	

26. _____ Vest-type device	b. The primary device for immobilizing the supine patient
27. _____ Long spine board	c. Aluminum device that splits lengthwise to facilitate moving the patient off the ground
28. _____ Scoop stretcher	d. The primary device to move the conscious medical patient up or down stairs
29. _____ Stokes basket	e. Used for carrying a patient through narrow corridors
30. _____ Flexible (Reeve's) stretcher	f. The preferred device for transporting a patient along smooth terrain
	g. Used to immobilize and extricate the seated patient from an automobile

Questions 31 to 33 refer to the following scenario.

You respond to a motor vehicle incident and find a woman walking around outside the car. She informs you that she was driving the car when it was hit in the rear by another car. Another EMS crew is caring for the patient in the second car. Your patient is complaining of neck pain.

31. The best device that you can use to immobilize this patient is a:

    a. Long spine board
    b. Stokes basket
    c. Scoop stretcher
    d. Vest-type device

32. As you immobilize this patient to the appropriate device, you use:

    a. A cervical collar with a head immobilization device; the torso and legs do not need to be secured to the device
    b. A cervical collar with a head immobilization device, securing the torso and the legs to the device
    c. Straps to secure the head, torso, and legs to the device; a cervical collar is not needed once the patient is on the device
    d. A head immobilization device along with straps to secure the torso and legs to the device

33. You notice that the second EMS crew is caring for their patient, who is lying supine on the pavement. You would expect the EMS crew to move the patient by:

    a. Using an extremity carry and placing the patient on a long spine board
    b. Using an extremity carry and placing the patient directly on the ambulance stretcher
    c. Using the log roll to place the patient on a long spine board
    d. Using the vest-type device to move the patient to the ambulance stretcher

Questions 34 and 35 refer to the following scenario.

> You respond to a call and find a 43-year-old man on the second floor of a house complaining of abdominal pain. The patient tells you that he has a history of gallbladder disease and he thinks he is having another gallbladder attack. Because of the pain the patient tells you that he can't walk down the stairs.

34. The best device to move this patient down the stairs is the:

    a. Ambulance stretcher
    b. Long spine board
    c. Scoop stretcher
    d. Stair chair

35. The position of comfort for most patients complaining of abdominal pain is:

    a. Supine
    b. Prone
    c. Supine with the knees bent
    d. Supine with the head elevated

Across

2. Shortness of breath
4. Strongest bones of the body
7. A technique to quickly move a patient is to use his clothes, foot, or a blanket to _____ the patient along the long axis of the body
8. Device ideal for removing patients on rough terrain or high-angle rescues
10. An _____ _____ is necessary if there is an immediate threat of death to the patient or the rescuer
14. When performing a log roll, the EMT positioned at the patient's _____ should supervise the movements
15. Stretcher that permits height adjustment
17. Preferred device for transporting a patient along smooth terrain
19. Procedure used to quickly remove a patient from an automobile wreck with minimal movement of the spinal column
21. Color code of oxygen tanks
22. Never lift using your _____
23. Largest long bone of the body
25. Patients with abdominal pain are more comfortable positioned with their _____ _____
26. Position where the patient is lying supine on a surface inclined 45 degrees with the head lower than the feet

Down

1. Patients in late stages of pregnancy should not be placed supine because this causes the fetus to compress the _____ _____
3. To maximize the effectiveness of the hands during a lift, use the _____ _____
5. Method for raising a heavy device
6. Method used for lifting large weights without injuring one's self
9. Stretcher that splits into two sections
11. Preferred method for loading a patient into the stair chair
12. Best method for transporting a conscious patient, with no suspicion of neck or spinal injury, down steps
13. Used to immobilize and extricate victims of automobile accidents found in a sitting position
16. Method used to safely transfer a patient with a suspected spinal injury onto a backboard
18. Procedure for immobilizing patients from the standing position to a long spine board
20. Left lateral recumbent position
24. Patients not in immediate environmental danger, but who are seriously ill or injured, may require an _____ move
25. Kendrick extrication device

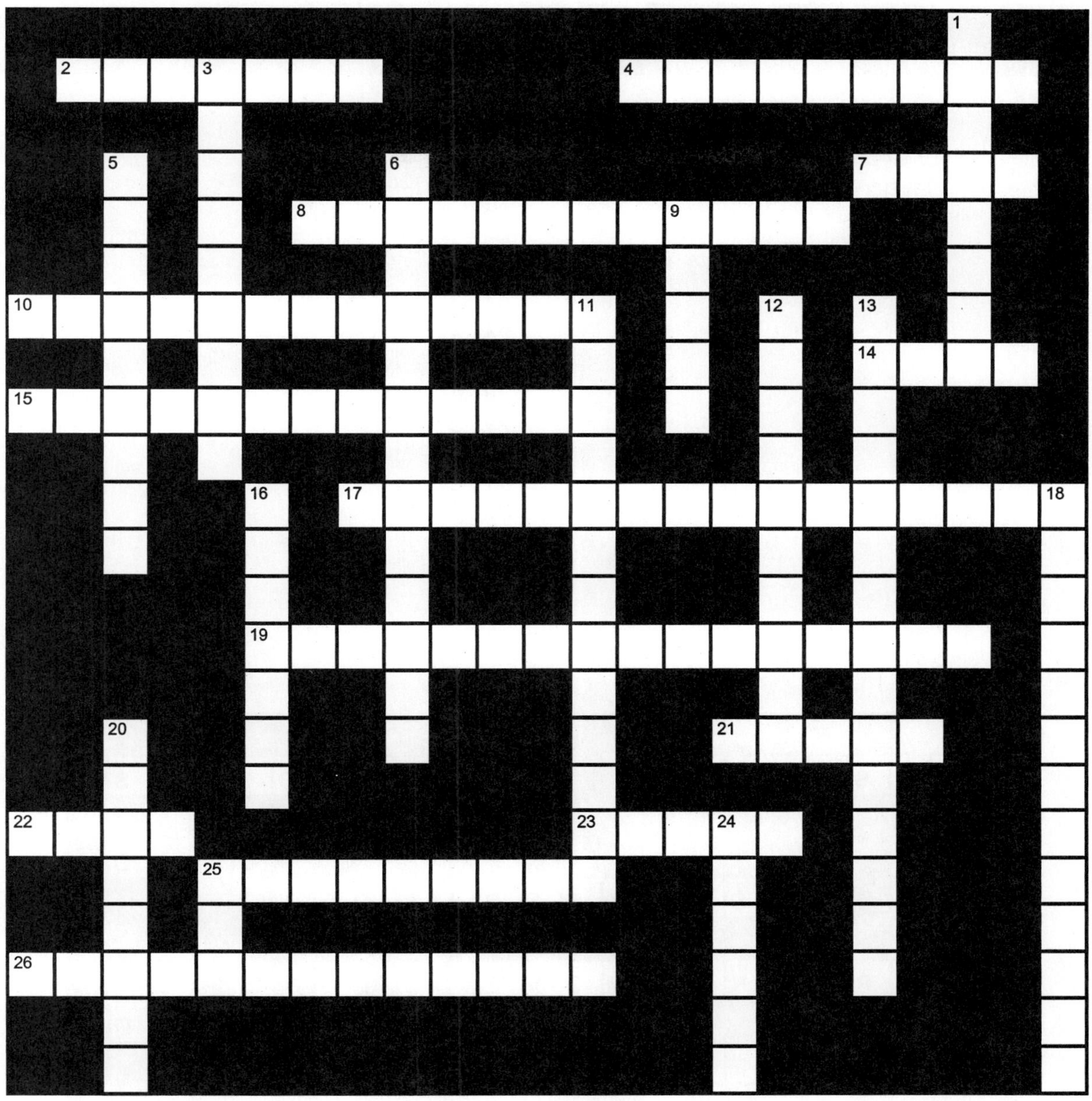
1
2
3
4
5
6
7
8
9
10
11
12
13
14
15
16
17
18
19
20
21
22
23
24
25
26

ANSWER KEY

1. b
2. c
3. c
4. a
5. d
6. b
7. d
8. a
9. c
10. a
11. a
12. c
13. b
14. a
15. b
16. b
17. d
18. c
19. d
20. b
21. Left lateral recumbent
22. Clothes drag
23. Airway
24. f
25. d
26. g
27. b
28. c
29. a
30. e
31. a
32. b
33. c
34. d
35. c

Across

2 DYSPNEA
4 LONGBONES
7 DRAG
8 STOKESBASKET
10 EMERGENCYMOVE
14 HEAD
15 MULTILEVELCOT
17 WHEELEDSTRETCHER
19 RAPIDEXTRICATION
21 GREEN
22 BACK
23 FEMUR
25 KNEESBENT
26 TRENDELENBURG

Down

1 VENACAVA
3 POWERGRIP
5 POWERLIFT
6 BODYMECHANICS
9 SCOOP
11 EXTREMITYLIFT
12 STAIRCHAIR
13 SHORTSPINEBOARD
16 LOGROLL
18 RAPIDTAKEDOWN
20 RECOVERY
24 URGENT

Chapter 7 Airway

1. The structure that covers the trachea during swallowing to prevent aspiration is called the:

   a. Pharynx
   b. Epiglottis
   c. Thyroid cartilage
   d. Cricoid cartilage

2. The respiratory structure that is palpable just above the sternum is the:

   a. Bronchus
   b. Trachea
   c. Carina
   d. Bronchiole

3. The muscle that separates the chest and abdomen is called the:

   a. Diaphragm
   b. Intercostal
   c. Abdominis recti
   d. None of the above

4. The normal resting tidal volume for an adult is approximately:

   a. 500 mL
   b. 800 mL
   c. 1000 mL
   d. 2000 mL

5. The process by which gases move from an area of higher concentration to an area of lower concentration is called:

   a. Ventilation
   b. Respiration
   c. Diffusion
   d. Transportation

6. The portion of the lung where diffusion takes place is called the:

   a. Bronchi
   b. Pleura
   c. Bronchiole
   d. Alveoli

7. When the brainstem sends messages to the intercostals and diaphragm, they contract and increase the size of the thoracic cavity. At that point, the pressure within the thoracic cavity:

   a. Increases
   b. Decreases
   c. Remains the same
   d. None of the above

8. The amount of air inhaled and exhaled during a given breath is called the:

   a. Residual volume
   b. Expiratory reserve
   c. Total volume
   d. Tidal volume

9. What percentage of oxygen does normal atmospheric air contain?

   a. 15%
   b. 21%
   c. 28%
   d. 50%

10. The portion of the brain responsible for regulation of breathing is called the:

    a. Cerebrum
    b. Cerebellum
    c. Hypothalamus
    d. Brainstem

11. During positive-pressure ventilation, adequate tidal volume is evaluated primarily on the basis of:

a. Chest rise
b. Skin color
c. Pupil response
d. None of the above

12. The most common complication of excessive or forceful ventilation is:

a. Pneumothorax
b. Gastric distention
c. Oxygen toxicity
d. Air embolism

13. Which of the following administration devices results in the highest oxygen delivery to the patient?

a. Nasal cannula
b. Venturi mask
c. Nonrebreather mask
d. Simple face mask

14. The most common cause of airway obstruction is:

a. Allergic reactions
b. Food
c. The tongue
d. Trauma to the airway

15. In patients with suspected spinal trauma, the manual airway maneuver of choice is the:

a. Jaw thrust without head tilt
b. Head tilt/neck lift
c. Head tilt/chin lift
d. Tongue pull

16. The correct ventilation rate for a nonbreathing adult patient is one breath every:

a. 3 seconds
b. 4 seconds
c. 5 seconds
d. 6 seconds

17. In the absence of spinal injury, the airway maneuver of choice is the:

a. Modified jaw thrust
b. Head tilt/neck lift
c. Head tilt/chin lift
d. Tongue pull

18. When inserting an oropharyngeal airway, the patient begins to gag and choke. Your next action should be to:

a. Remove the airway
b. Use a smaller airway
c. Lubricate the airway
d. Tape the airway in place

19. To ensure proper sizing, an oropharyngeal airway is measured from the corner of the patient's mouth to the:

a. Angle of the jaw
b. Top of the ear
c. Cheekbone
d. Trachea

20. The pocket mask used in conjunction with 15 L of oxygen per minute can result in maximum oxygen concentrations of approximately:

a. 16%
b. 21%
c. 30%
d. 50%

21. The major complication of a bag-valve-mask resuscitator is:

a. Overventilation and pneumothorax
b. Low tidal volumes caused by errors in technique
c. Rupture of the bag during exhalation
d. Valve failure from clogging

22. What is the maximum percentage of oxygen delivery for a bag-valve-mask used with an oxygen reservoir?

a. 25% to 35%
b. 50% to 60%
c. 75% to 80%
d. 90% to 100%

23. To avoid confusion with other gases, an oxygen tank is painted:

a. Blue
b. Purple
c. Red
d. Green

24. The tank pressure of a full oxygen cylinder is usually:

a. 700 lb per square inch
b. 1000 lb per square inch
c. 2000 lb per square inch
d. 4000 lb per square inch

25. The system used to avoid misplacement of a regulator on portable oxygen cylinders is called the:

    a. Oxygen cylinder safety system
    b. Pin index safety system
    c. Gas delivery safety system
    d. Regulator safety system

26. Which of the following oxygen cylinders is the most portable?

    a. D cylinder
    b. G cylinder
    c. H cylinder
    d. M cylinder

27. Regulators are designed to provide a safe pressure to the delivery device of approximately:

    a. 10 to 20 psi
    b. 20 to 30 psi
    c. 40 to 70 psi
    d. 100 to 120 psi

28. A flowmeter that uses a gravity-controlled ball to measure the liter flow rates to the delivery device is called a:

    a. Bourdon gauge
    b. Pressure-compensated flowmeter
    c. Constant flow selector
    d. Double-staged flowmeter

Match the delivery device in column B to the appropriate oxygen concentrations in column A.

Column A	Column B
29. 90% at 10 to 15 L	a. Nasal cannula
	b. Nonrebreather mask
30. 24% to 40% at 2 to 6 L	

31. When suctioning the upper airway, you should activate the negative pressure:

    a. When the tip is in the oropharynx
    b. Before insertion
    c. At the entrance of the mouth
    d. Halfway between the teeth and the pharynx

32. All the following are signs of inadequate breathing *except:*

    a. Altered mental status
    b. Nasal flaring
    c. Flushed skin
    d. Retractions

33. Lifting at the angles of the jaw while maintaining the head in the neutral inline position best describes the:

    a. Modified jaw thrust
    b. Head tilt/chin lift
    c. Chin pull
    d. Tongue jaw lift

34. The best way to remove liquid secretions from the airway in the field is by:

    a. Finger sweeps
    b. Back blows
    c. Portable suction
    d. Abdominal thrusts

35. When using a jaw thrust in conjunction with bag-valve-mask device, you can lift the mandible at the:

    a. Center of the chin
    b. Angle of the jaw
    c. Lower portion of the cheekbones
    d. Soft tissues of the mandible

36. When using the bag-valve-mask, the major advantage of two rescuers is that this method:

    a. Decreases leakage of air from a two-handed mask seal
    b. Decreases fatigue of the rescuers involved in the resuscitation
    c. Ensures a smoother bag squeeze during the breath
    d. Positions the rescuers at the head of the patient

37. To ensure proper delivery of volume when using a flow-restricted, oxygen-powered ventilation device, you should release the lever (or button) when:

    a. A whistling sound occurs
    b. You observe adequate chest rise
    c. Resistance is encountered
    d. The cheeks are distended

38. To ensure proper sizing, a nasopharyngeal airway is measured from the tip of the nose to the:

    a. Angle of the jaw
    b. Middle of the ear
    c. Cheekbone
    d. Larynx

39. When a patient cannot tolerate a nonrebreather mask, you should:

    a. Place it over the nose or corner of the mouth
    b. Switch to a nasal cannula
    c. Hold the mask firmly in place
    d. Lay the patient supine to decrease anxiety

40. The tidal volume multiplied by the respiratory rate is called the ___________.

41. When using mouth-to-mask ventilation in the adult patient without supplemental oxygen, volumes of approximately ___________ to ___________ mL should be delivered.

42. When using mouth-to-mask or bag-valve-mask ventilation in an adult patient with supplemental oxygen, volumes of approximately ___________ to ___________ mL should be delivered.

43. The nose is divided into two compartments by the ___________.

44. Blue-gray skin color is called ___________.

45. Low oxygen content in the blood is called ___________.

46. When delivering positive-pressure ventilation, ___________ can be used to compress the esophagus, thereby reducing the chances of gastric distention.

47. The narrowest part of the pediatric airway is at the ring formed by the ___________.

Questions 48 to 52 refer to the following scenario.

> You respond to a call at a shopping center and encounter an approximately 3-year-old boy who is having a seizure. Bystanders tell you that the patient has been seizing for the past 5 minutes. The patient exhibits signs of seizure activity, his teeth are clenched closed, and his lips appear to be blue.

48. The best way to establish an airway in this patient is to:

    a. Force the patient's teeth apart and insert an oropharyngeal airway
    b. Insert a nasopharyngeal airway
    c. There is no need to establish an airway; wait until seizure activity stops and then assess the patient's respiratory status
    d. Apply a nasal cannula at 2 L/min

49. The procedures needed to insert an airway device in this patient require that:

    a. The bevel is facing toward the septum
    b. The bevel is facing away from the septum
    c. Whatever pressure is needed to insert the device is used
    d. Another airway device is used if the airway cannot successfully be inserted in one nostril

50. Once the child's seizure activity stops, you determine that the patient is not breathing. The best device to use to ventilate this patient is:

    a. Mouth-to-mouth ventilations
    b. A bag-valve-mask device without supplemental oxygen
    c. A flow-restricted, oxygen-powered ventilator
    d. A bag-valve-mask device connected to 15 L/min of oxygen

51. The volume of air that you use to ventilate this patient with each breath is called the:

    a. Minute volume
    b. Residual volume
    c. Tidal volume
    d. Stroke volume

52. The rate at which you will ventilate this patient is:

    a. 10 times per minute
    b. 12 times per minute
    c. 15 times per minute
    d. 20 times per minute

Questions 53 to 56 refer to the following scenario.

> You respond to a restaurant where you find a 67-year-old woman unconscious and unresponsive on the floor. The patient has a pulse but is not breathing. When you evaluate the patient's airway you notice large quantities of partially chewed food in the patient's mouth.

53. The best way to clear this patient's airway is to:

    a. Insert an oropharyngeal airway
    b. Insert a nasopharyngeal airway
    c. Use your gloved fingers to sweep out as much debris as possible
    d. Use a suction device with a soft catheter

54. After you clear the patient's airway you begin to provide positive-pressure ventilations. The rate at which you will ventilate this patient is:

    a. 10 times per minute
    b. 12 times per minute
    c. 15 times per minute
    d. 20 times per minute

55. En route to the hospital the patient begins to vomit, resulting in large quantities of liquid vomitus in the patient's mouth. You should:

    a. Suction continuously until you arrive at the hospital
    b. Use the suction device for no more than 15 seconds
    c. Insert an oropharyngeal airway, which will allow for uninterrupted ventilations
    d. Use a flow-restricted, oxygen-powered ventilator to clear the airway

56. While you provide positive-pressure ventilation to your patient, you instruct your partner to apply downward pressure to the patient's neck in an effort to close the esophagus and reduce the amount of air entering the patient's stomach. This is called:

    a. Cricoid pressure
    b. Tracheal pressure
    c. Esophageal pressure
    d. Tracheal deviation

Questions 57 to 61 refer to the following scenario.

> You respond to a call for a patient that was struck by a car. The scene has been secured by the police and fire department before your arrival. You find a 42-year-old man lying on his face in the roadway. The patient does not respond to verbal or painful stimuli.

57. The position that you find this patient in is called:

    a. Supine
    b. Trendelenburg
    c. Prone
    d. Left lateral recumbent

58. Your first steps in treating this patient include:

    a. Immobilizing the patient in the position you find him and transporting him rapidly to the hospital
    b. Performing a log roll to position the patient on his back while maintaining cervical spinal immobilization
    c. Placing the patient in the left lateral recumbent position to maintain an open airway
    d. Applying nasal cannula oxygen to the patient while you begin to immobilize him in the position that you found him

59. Once you have properly immobilized your patient, you open the airway by using:

    a. The head tilt/chin lift method
    b. The head tilt/jaw lift maneuver
    c. The jaw thrust maneuver
    d. A blanket roll under the patient's neck

60. You begin to transport your patient to the hospital. You are alone with the patient in the back of the ambulance when the patient stops breathing. The best way for you, as a single rescuer, to ventilate this patient is by:

    a. Performing mouth-to-mouth ventilations
    b. Performing a head tilt to open the airway while ventilating with a bag-valve-mask device
    c. Performing a jaw thrust to open the airway while ventilating with a pocket mask
    d. Using a nonrebreather oxygen mask

61. On arrival at the hospital, you continue to support your patient's respirations while providing supplemental oxygen. Your portable oxygen tank, which you bring with you into the hospital, is a:

    a. D cylinder
    b. G cylinder
    c. H cylinder
    d. M cylinder

Across

1. Smallest type of airway tubes
5. Safety system that allows only a regulator designed for oxygen to be attached to an oxygen tank
9. A series of tubes that extend from the mouth and nose down into the lungs
11. Tube that connects the stomach to the mouth
12. Disease marked by damage of the alveoli
14. In normal breathing the diaphragm is assisted by the _____ _____
15. Abnormal rhythmic sound heard at the end of exhalation
17. Accessory muscles of respiration in the neck that elevate the upper ribs
21. Technique used to open the airway of a patient without suspected cervical spine injury
22. Pain resulting from inflammation or scarring of the linings of the chest cavity and lungs
23. Voice box
24. Covering of the outer surface of the lungs
27. In children and infants, this organ is large in relation to the airway and has a greater potential for obstruction
29. Emphysema and bronchitis are two forms of _____
31. Technique used to open the airway of a patient with a suspected cervical spine injury
32. Precaution designed to reduce the risk of transmission of pathogens from moist body substances
33. Laryngectomy
34. The major stimulus of ventilation
36. Space occupied by the heart, great vessels, trachea, main stem bronchi, esophagus, and nerves
37. Breastbone
38. An oxygen delivery device that delivers a precise percentage of oxygen often used for patients with COPD
39. Cone-shaped organs of respiration

Down

2. Nostrils
3. Pigment found in the red blood cell
4. Throat
6. Primary muscle of respiration
7. Whistling noise associated with narrowed bronchioles that may be heard without a stethoscope
8. Airway used in an unconscious patient without a gag reflex
10. Expanding of the stomach by an accumulation of air
13. Exaggerated opening of the nostrils on inspiration
16. Lining of the inner surface of the chest cavity
18. Sleepy appearance
19. Disease causing rapid swelling of the epiglottis
20. The primary stimulus to breathe in some patients with COPD
25. Bluish discoloration of the mucous membranes or skin
26. Drawing in of the spaces between the ribs to aid in breathing
28. Flap of cartilage that covers the larynx during swallowing
30. Difficulty breathing
32. Singular term for bronchi
33. The high-pitched breath sound heard with narrowing of the upper respiratory tract
35. Color code of oxygen tanks

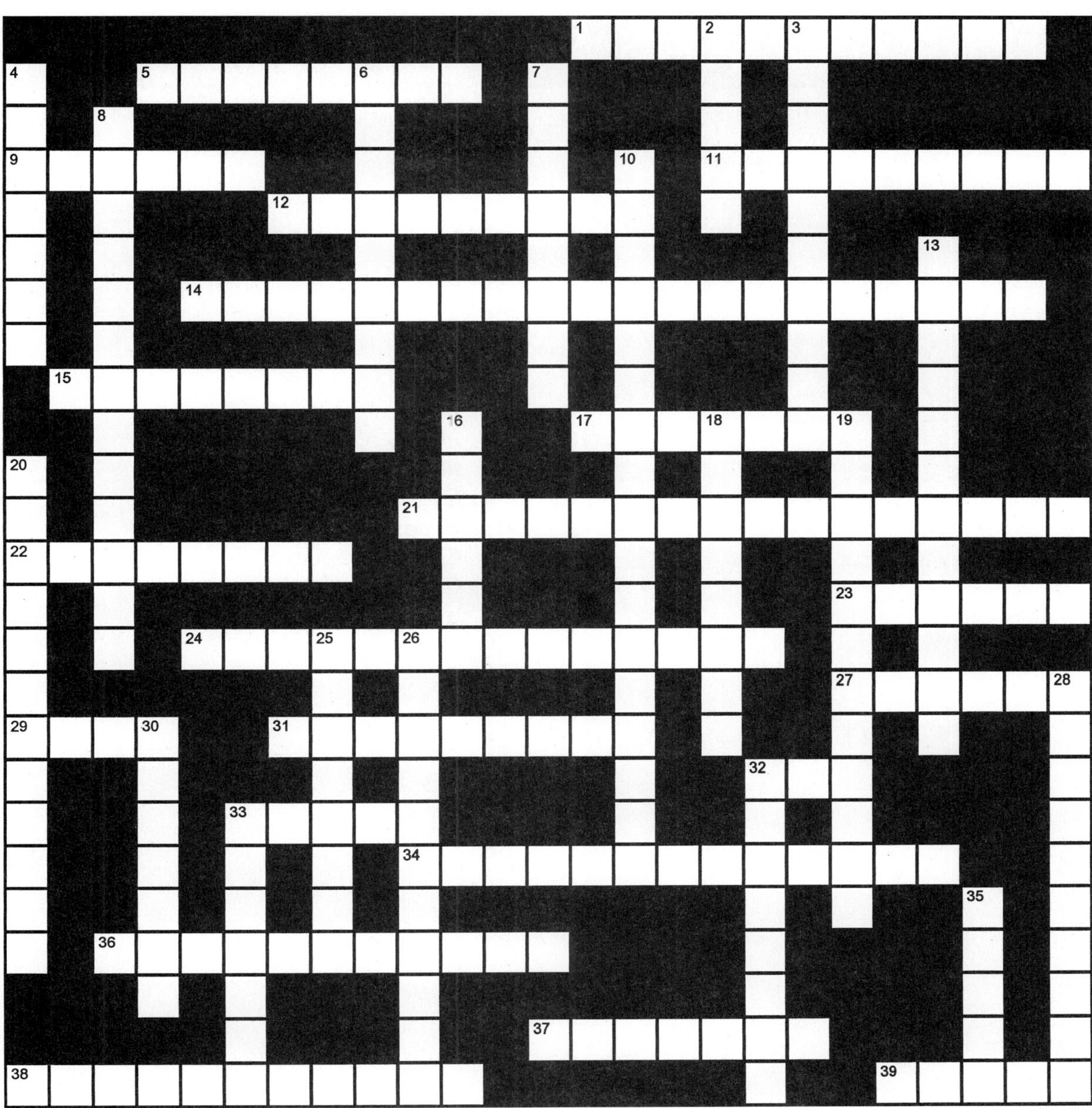

ANSWER KEY

1. b
2. b
3. a
4. a
5. c
6. d
7. b
8. d
9. b
10. d
11. a
12. b
13. c
14. c
15. a
16. c
17. c
18. a
19. a
20. d
21. b
22. d
23. d
24. c
25. b
26. a
27. c
28. b
29. b
30. a
31. a
32. c
33. a
34. c
35. b
36. a
37. b
38. a
39. b
40. Minute volume
41. 700 to 1000
42. 400 to 600
43. Nasal septum
44. Cyanosis
45. Hypoxia
46. Cricoid pressure
47. Cricoid cartilage
48. b
49. a
50. d
51. c
52. d
53. c
54. b
55. b
56. a
57. c
58. b
59. c
60. c
61. a

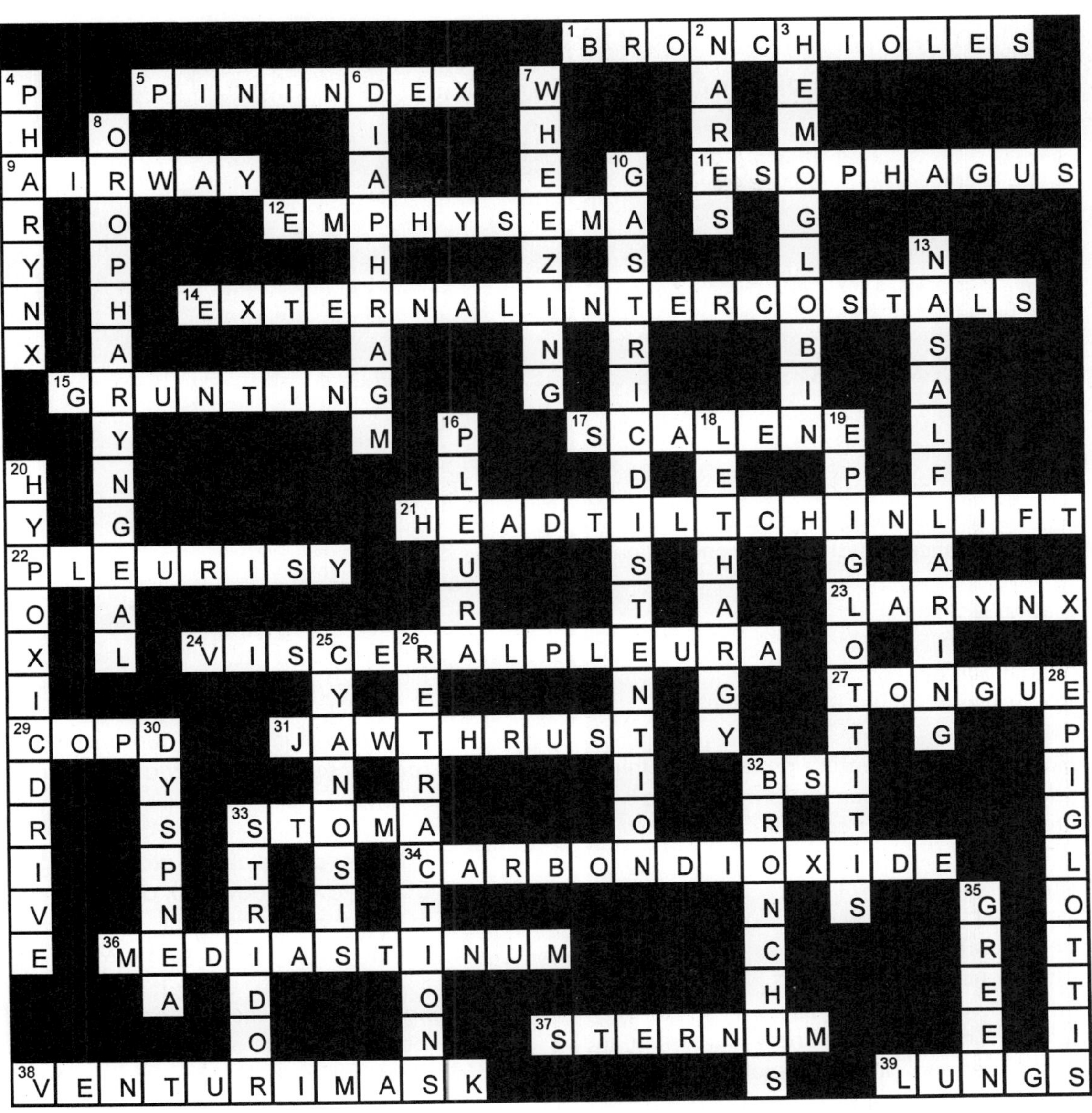
BRONCHIOLES
PININDEX
AIRWAY
ESOPHAGUS
EMPHYSEMA
EXTERNALINTERCOSTALS
GRUNTING
SCALENE
HEADTILTCHINLIFT
PLEURISY
LARYNX
VISCERALPLEURA
TONGUE
COPD
JAWTHRUST
BSI
STOMA
CARBONDIOXIDE
MEDIASTINUM
STERNUM
VENTURIMASK
LUNGS
PHARYNX
DIAPHRAGM
WHEEZING
NARES
HEMOGLOBIN
OROPHARYNGEAL
GASTRICDISTENTION
NASALFALLIAING
PLEURA
LETHARGY
EPIGLOTTITIS
HYPOXICDRIVE
CYANOSIS
RETRACTION
EPIGLOTTI
DYSPNEA
BRONCHUS
STRIDOR
GREEN

Chapter 8 Scene Size-up

1. Gathering information from bystanders, identifying hazards, securing the scene, and calling for specialized assistance are all components of the:

   a. Focused assessment
   b. Scene size-up
   c. Secondary survey
   d. Dispatch review

2. The routine practice of wearing protective clothing (e.g., gloves, goggles) when performing certain procedures (e.g., bleeding control) is called:

   a. General infection prevention
   b. Barrier protection model
   c. Immunization techniques
   d. Body substance isolation

3. When splash from a bleeding artery is possible, the recommended personal protective equipment includes:

   a. Mask, goggles, gown, and gloves
   b. Mask only
   c. Gloves only
   d. Gown and goggles only

4. When delivering a baby, the recommended personal protective equipment is the wearing of:

   a. Mask, goggles, gown, and gloves
   b. Mask only
   c. Gloves only
   d. Gown and goggles only

5. When bandaging a minor abrasion where splash of blood is not likely, the recommended personal protective equipment is the wearing of:

   a. Mask, goggles, and gown
   b. Mask only
   c. Gloves only
   d. Gown and goggles only

6. Traffic delineation devices used at a crash scene include all the following *except*:

   a. Traffic cones
   b. Flood lights directed at traffic
   c. Lights on the ambulance
   d. Flares

7. A good rule of thumb for approaching a potentially hazardous scene is to stop and evaluate from a position:

   a. 100 feet away, uphill, and upwind
   b. 50 feet away, downhill, and downwind
   c. 100 feet away, downhill, and downwind
   b. 50 feet away, uphill, and upwind

8. Using the "rule of thumb" for placing traffic delineation devices on a highway, what is the minimum distance they should be placed from an incident on a 50 mph road?

   a. 50 feet
   b. 100 feet
   c. 150 feet
   d. 200 feet

9. After ensuring that the scene is safe, it is important to identify the mechanism of injury and determine the total number of patients at the scene so that the:

   a. Initial assessment is more organized
   b. Need for additional resources is identified
   c. Workload can be distributed between you and your partner
   d. Appropriate lifting equipment can be secured

10. You arrive at a scene where there are 12 injured patients. After ensuring scene safety, what should you do first?

    a. Call for additional units
    b. Begin triage
    c. Begin your initial assessment
    d. Begin treating the most serious patients

11. The process of identifying the underlying cause of an illness or injury is called identifying the:

    a. Initial pathology
    b. Detailed assessment finding
    c. Focused physical cause
    d. Mechanism of injury or illness

TRUE OR FALSE

12. _____ Requesting additional resources to the scene of the incident is part of the scene size-up.

13. _____ The detailed physical assessment should be completed during the scene size-up.

14. _____ The most common hazard encountered by the EMT is the traffic surrounding auto incidents.

15. _____ The use of flares as a traffic delineation device is most beneficial in the daytime.

16. _____ When responding to a violent call, such as a shooting, you should approach the scene as soon as possible and initiate care while awaiting police arrival.

17. _____ Reconstructing the forces of injury helps the EMT to anticipate potential injuries.

18. _____ Patient triage and initial assessment of the patient should be instituted before ensuring scene safety.

19. _____ Self-contained breathing apparatus should be worn when treating a patient with suspected tuberculosis.

20. _____ A multiple casualty incident plan should only be initiated after an emergency medical services supervisor has responded to the scene and assessed the situation.

Questions 21 and 22 refer to the following scenario.

> You respond to a motor vehicle incident on a country road outside town. Your initial scene size-up reveals that two cars have been involved in a head-on collision at a high rate of speed. There are 5 patients in one car and 3 patients in the other car. One vehicle is leaking gasoline out of the rear of the car and a puddle of gasoline is spreading down the roadway.

21. While your partner quickly evaluates the patients you attempt to provide scene safety. All the following traffic delineation devices are appropriate for use in this scenario *except*:

    a. Cones
    b. Reflectors
    c. Flares
    d. Barricades

22. Based on the number of patients involved in this incident you would initiate your department's

    ___________ plan.

Across

1. The manner in which an injury was incurred is called the _____ _____ _____
4. Universal precautions and body substance isolation
9. Sorting calls by priority
10. Precautions taken by health care professionals to prevent transmission of pathogens by touching the surface of infected materials
12. These traffic delineation devices are especially helpful at night but should not be used in an area where gasoline has spilled
14. Precaution designed to reduce the risk of transmission of pathogens from moist body substances
18. Approach the scene of a hazardous materials incident uphill and _____
19. Any situation in which the rescuers are risking serious injury as the result of entering the area
21. Standard precautions apply to all body fluids except _____

Down

2. Precautions designed to reduce the risk of transmission of blood-borne pathogens
3. An assessment of the surroundings that will provide information to aid patients and ensure the well-being of the EMT
5. Transmission of microorganisms carried in the air and inhaled by a susceptible host
6. EMTs can determine the _____ _____ _____ through patient history
7. _____ _____ precautions are used for patients with documented or suspected infection with highly transmissible pathogens
8. Reflectors, flares, traffic cones, and battery-operated lights are examples of _____ _____ devices
11. A term used to describe a hazardous materials incident
13. These traffic delineation devices are helpful in alerting the sleepy driver because of the sound they make if they are driven over
15. Type of disease transmission that occurs when an infected person coughs or sneezes
16. Specialized mask and regulator with portable air supply used by rescue personnel in environments that might contain hazardous materials
17. When approaching a scene, stop _____ and upwind
20. Traffic devices should be placed at least _____ times the distance of the posted speed limit

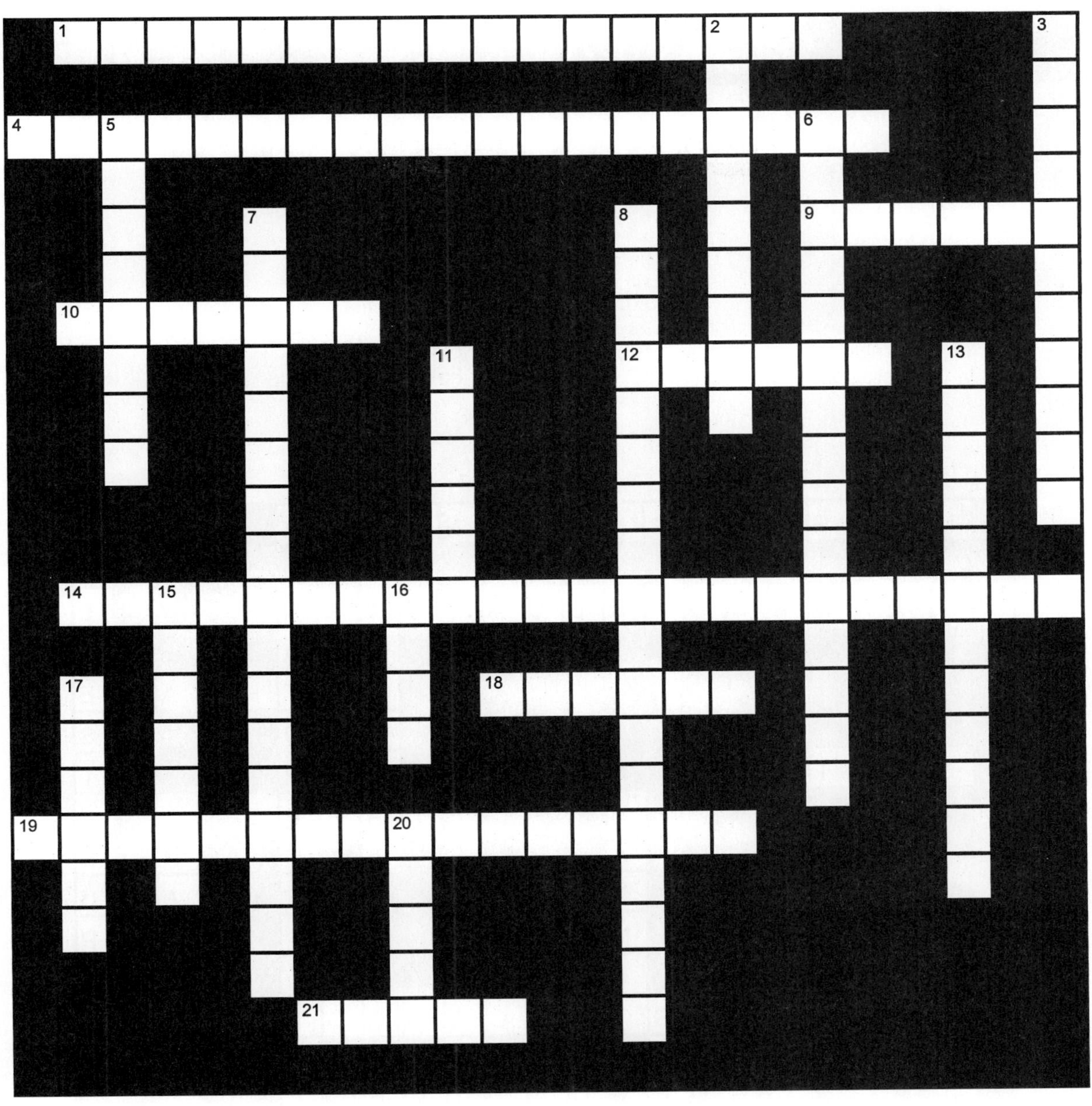

ANSWER KEY

1. b
2. d
3. a
4. a
5. c
6. b
7. a
8. c
9. b
10. a
11. d
12. True
13. False
14. True
15. False
16. False
17. True
18. False
19. False
20. False
21. c
22. Mass casualty

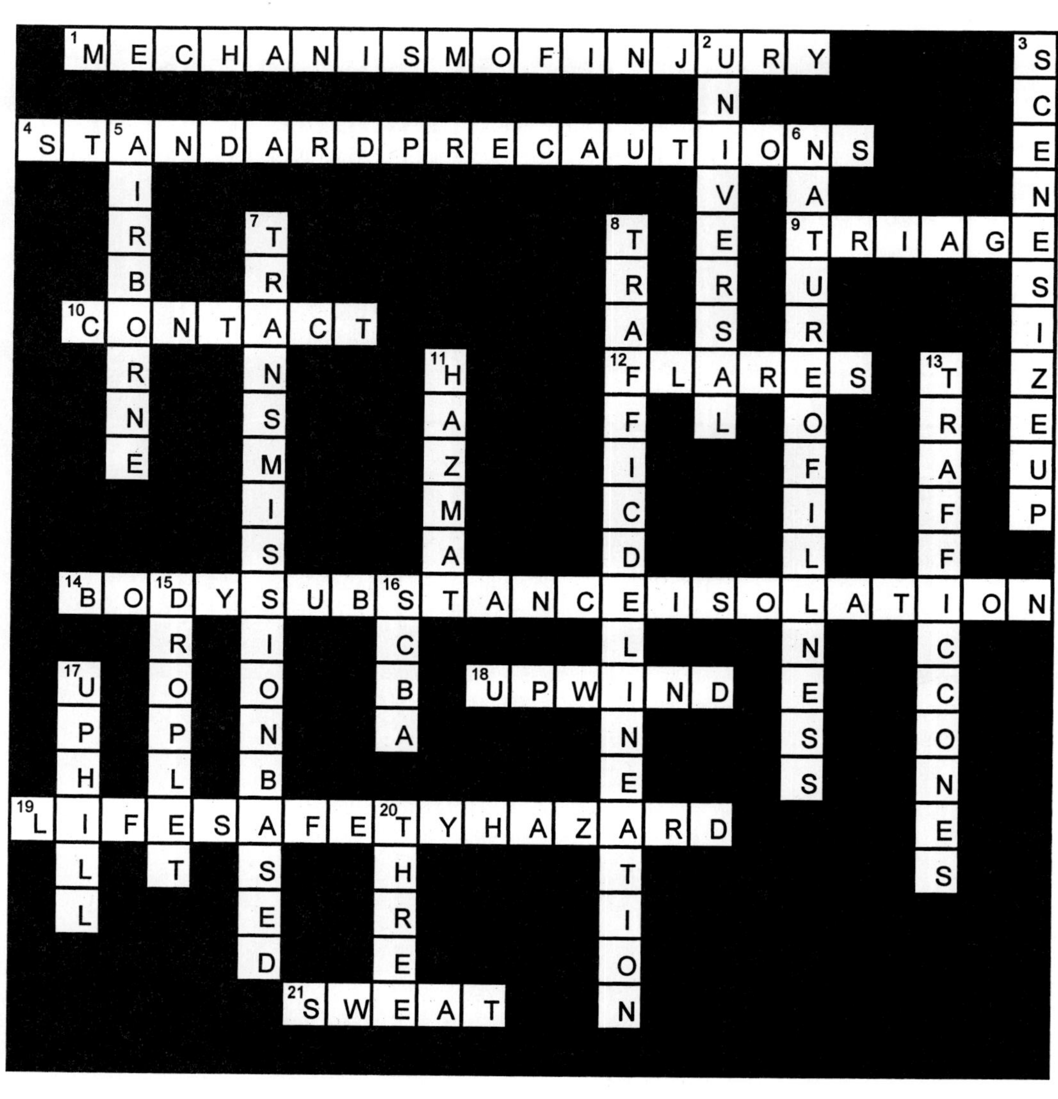

Chapter 9 Initial Assessment

1. The general impression is a series of initial questions and observations regarding the patient's condition, age, sex, and chief complaint and is designed to identify:

   a. Scene safety
   b. Life-threatening conditions
   c. A diagnosis
   d. Underlying pathophysiology

2. After establishing unresponsiveness in a prone trauma patient you should:

   a. Leave the patient in the prone position and continue with your survey
   b. Log-roll the patient to the lateral recumben- position and continue with your survey
   c. Log-roll the patient to the supine position and continue with your survey
   d. Leave the patient in the prone position and transport immediately

3. The **V** of the AVPU evaluation of mental state refers to a patient's ability to respond to:

   a. Vigorous stimuli
   b. Verbal stimuli
   c. Visual stimuli
   d. Vivid stimuli

4. When opening the airway of an infant to assess breathing, you should place the head in the:

   a. Neutral or sniffing position
   b. Hyperextended position
   c. Slightly flexed position
   d. Elevated position

5. Tilting the head back with one hand while lifting the lower margin of the jaw with the index and middle fingers of the other hand best describes the:

   a. Jaw thrust without head tilt
   b. Chin pull maneuver
   c. Head tilt/neck lift
   d. Head tilt/chin lift

6. The best method for evaluating the adequacy of ventilation is by:

   a. Observing chest rise
   b. Placing a mirror near the mouth and nose
   c. Feeling the chest wall for expansion
   d. Checking the pulse rate

7. The correct location of palpation for the carotid pulse is:

   a. A groove between the larynx and muscle in the neck
   b. At the angle of the jaw adjacent to the muscle
   c. Just above the suprasternal notch
   d. Just above the clavicle, adjacent to the trachea

8. In general, the carotid pulse should be palpated on:

   a. Either side of the neck
   b. The side opposite the rescuer
   c. The same side as the rescuer
   d. Both sides of the neck each time

9. The carotid pulse should be initially palpated for approximately:

   a. 2 to 3 seconds
   b. 3 to 5 seconds
   c. 5 to 10 seconds
   d. 10 to 20 seconds

10. Capillary refill in the child is considered delayed when refill takes more than:

    a. 0.5 seconds
    b. 1.0 seconds
    c. 1.5 seconds
    d. 2.0 seconds

11. Inline immobilization of the cervical spine is essential in trauma patients to avoid injury to the:

    a. Brain
    b. Soft tissues of the neck
    c. Bony structures
    d. Spinal cord

12. When a patient has adequate breathing but is short of breath, he or she should be treated with:

    a. Oxygen
    b. A bag-valve-mask
    c. Psychological care only
    d. A flow-restricted, oxygen-powered ventilation device

13. A patient who is unresponsive and breathing at a rate of 5 breaths/min, should be treated with:

    a. Nonrebreather mask
    b. A bag-valve-mask with supplemental oxygen
    c. Psychological care only
    d. A Venturi mask

14. Which of the following signs are common to infants and small children but not adults?

    a. Nasal flaring
    b. Accessory muscle use
    c. Cyanosis
    d. Decreased breath sounds

15. When opening the airway of a child when no trauma is suspected, the head should be:

    a. Slightly tilted
    b. Hyperextended
    c. Flexed
    d. Neutral

16. A 6-month-old infant's pulse should initially be palpated at which artery?

    a. Carotid
    b. Radial
    c. Femoral
    d. Brachial

17. Which of the following should be assessed during the initial assessment?

    a. Contusions on the head
    b. External bleeding
    c. Instability of the pelvic bone
    d. Abdominal distention

18. Skin color that is cyanotic usually reflects:

    a. Poorly oxygenated red blood cells
    b. Hypothermia of tissues
    c. Hyperthermia
    d. Liver disease

19. Which of the following skin findings are commonly associated with shock states?

    a. Pale, cool, and clammy
    b. Flushed, warm, and dry
    c. Cyanotic, warm, and dry
    d. Jaundiced, cool, and dry

20. A patient has a complete airway obstruction. Which of the following skin findings is most likely?

    a. Pale
    b. Flushed
    c. Cyanotic
    d. Jaundiced

Questions 21 to 25 refer to the following scenario.

> You respond to the scene of a patient who fell off a roof. On arrival you find a 27-year-old man lying supine in the driveway. The fire department has secured the scene and the scene is safe. A neighbor advises you that the patient was on the roof, approximately 15 feet high, when he stumbled backward and fell to the driveway, striking the back of his head. You and your partner have taken proper body substance isolation precautions.

21. While you check the patient for responsiveness, you should direct your partner to:

    a. Open the airway with a head tilt/chin lift maneuver
    b. Manually stabilize the cervical spine
    c. Log-roll the patient onto his left side to maintain an open airway
    d. Quickly lift the patient onto your stretcher in preparation for rapid transportation

22. You initially ask the patient if he is all right. There is no response and you ask again, in a loud voice, "Are you OK?" The patient responds by groaning. Based on this response you would place him in which AVPU category?

    a. A
    b. V
    c. P
    d. U

23. Evaluation of your patient reveals that he is breathing at approximately 14 breaths/min without the use of any accessory muscles, and there is adequate chest expansion with each breath. Supplemental oxygen:

    a. Is not required at this time
    b. Should be administered by a bag-valve-mask device
    c. Should be administered by a nasal cannula at 4 to 6 L/min
    d. Should be administered by a nonrebreather mask at 15 L/min

24. After checking for responsiveness, airway, and breathing, you would check for circulation by feeling for a pulse at the:

    a. Carotid artery
    b. Femoral artery
    c. Radial artery
    d. Temporal artery

25. You determine whether this patient requires early transportation and determine that:

    a. Early transportation is not indicated because the patient is not unconscious
    b. Early transportation is not indicated because the patient has a patent airway
    c. Early transportation is indicated because the patient fell approximately 15 feet
    d. Early transportation is indicated because the patient has an altered mental status

Across

4. Any patient who sustained significant blunt trauma should be treated as if he or she has a possible _____ _____
5. Normal skin temperature
8. The A of AVPU
9. Yellowish tinge of the sclera, skin, or both, possibly indicating liver or spleen disease
11. Artery used to check the pulse for any adult patient who is unresponsive
12. Method of opening an airway used for an unconscious patient with a suspected cervical spine injury and a jaw fracture
14. Patients who are _____ should be rapidly transported to an appropriate medical facility with further assessment and treatment occurring while en route to the hospital
15. Respiratory distress as evidenced by inward depression of muscular areas and their attached ribs
19. Trauma-induced ventricular fibrillation, such as being hit in the chest by a baseball
20. Normal capillary refill time
21. Skin color indicating possible exposure to heat or carbon monoxide
22. Skin color indicating poor perfusion or impaired blood flow
23. Hot skin temperature may indicate _____
26. Description of cool and moist skin
28. Respiratory distress characterized by alternate use of chest and abdominal muscles during breathing
29. The P of AVPU
30. Mnemonic used to evaluate mental status
31. During the initial assessment the EMT forms a _____ _____ of the patient from observing the patient and the environment
32. The V of AVPU

Down

1. Method used to open the airway of a patient with a suspected cervical spine injury
2. Decreased blood flow as evidenced by pale, moist, and clammy skin
3. Technique used to open the airway of a patient without suspected cervical spine injury
6. _____ _____ system function is evaluated by quickly assessing the patient's level of consciousness
7. Place the head of an infant in the _____ position to avoid bending and kinking the soft trachea
8. Computerized device that allows EMTs and lay rescuers to deliver electrical energy to the heart
10. Diagnostic test in which the nailbed is compressed and released indicative of perfusion condition
11. Blue-gray skin color
13. The U of AVPU
16. The patient's problem in his or her own words
17. Perform a _____ _____ _____ to note potential danger to rescuers, the public, and the patient
18. A sign of respiratory distress in infants and children
22. Normal skin color
24. Artery used to check for a pulse in a patient younger than 1 year of age
25. An unresponsive patient may have his or her _____ blocking the airway
27. Gasping respirations

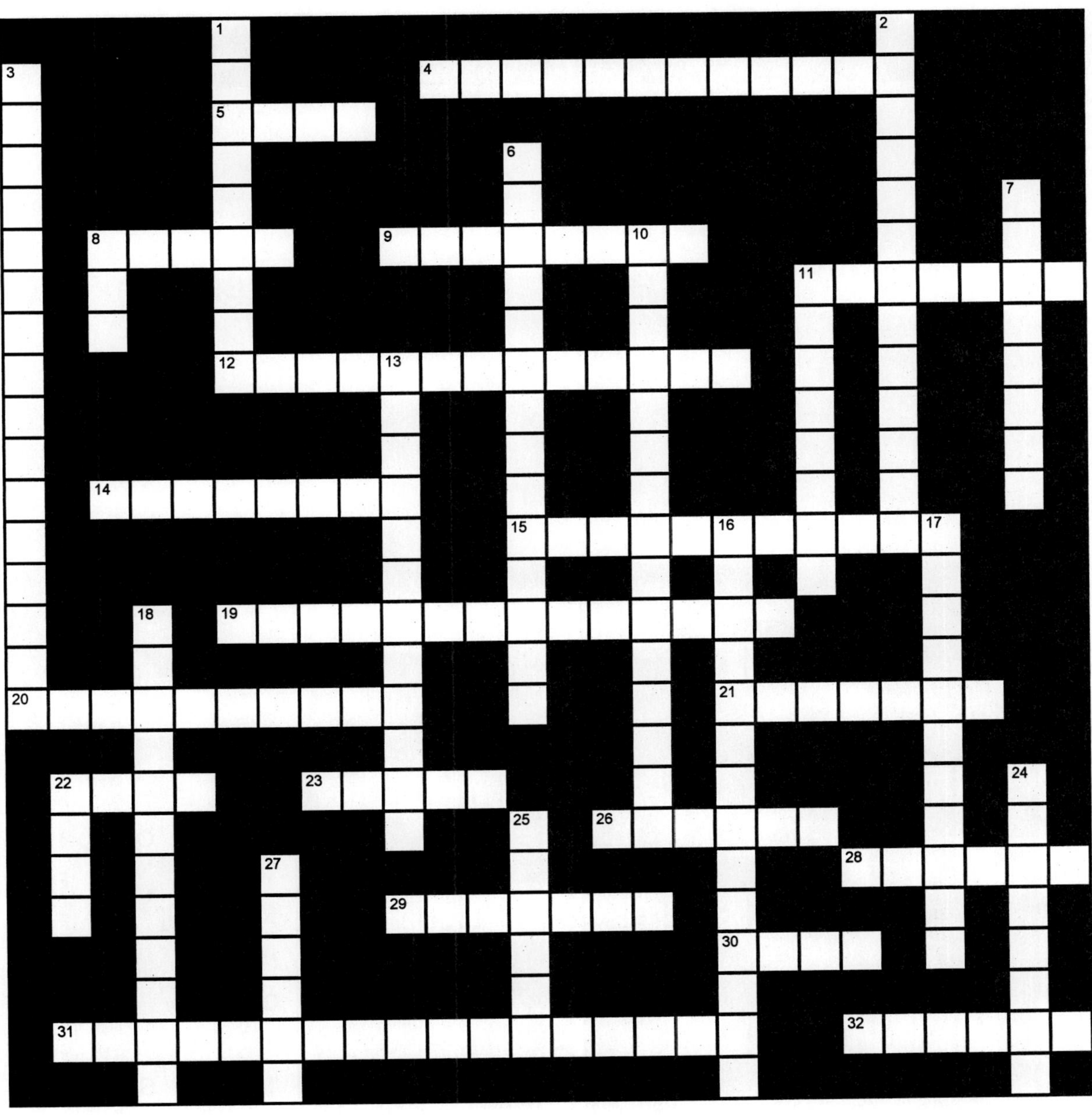
1
2
3
4
5
6
7
8
9
10
11
12
13
14
15
16
17
18
19
20
21
22
23
24
25
26
27
28
29
30
31
32

ANSWER KEY

1. b
2. c
3. b
4. a
5. d
6. a
7. a
8. c
9. c
10. d
11. d
12. a
13. b
14. a
15. a
16. d
17. b
18. a
19. a
20. c
21. b
22. b
23. d
24. c
25. d

Across

4 SPINAL INJURY
5 WARM
8 ALERT
9 JAUNDICE
11 CAROTID
12 TONGUE JAW LIFT
14 UNSTABLE
15 RETRACTIONS
19 COMMOTIO CORDIS
20 TWO SECONDS
21 FLUSHED
22 PALE
23 FEVER
26 CLAMMY
28 SEESAW
29 PAINFUL
30 AVPU
31 GENERAL IMPRESSION
32 VERBAL

1 JAW THRUST
2 HYPOPERFUSION
3 HEAD TILT CHIN LIFT
6 CENTRAL NERVOUS
7 SNIFFING
8 AED
10 CAPILLARY REFILL
11 CYANOTIC
13 UNRESPONSIVE
16 CHIEF COMPLAINT
17 SCENE SIZE UP
18 NASAL FLARING
22 PINK
24 BRACHIAL
25 TONGUE
27 AGONAL

Chapter 10 Focused History and Physical Examination of Trauma Patients

1. Which of the following questions reflects the best way to inquire about a complaint of chest pain or chest discomfort in a history?

   a. Was your chest pain squeezing in nature?
   b. How would you describe the pain or discomfort in your own words?
   c. Did it feel like someone was standing on your chest?
   d. Was the pain viselike in nature?

2. Which of the following statements best explains the reason for performing a rapid trauma assessment?

   a. Internal bleeding must be identified early and controlled at the scene
   b. EMT medications may be lifesaving for serious head injuries
   c. To avoid prolonged discomfort to the patient associated with the examination
   d. To identify serious conditions that were not identified by the initial assessment alone

3. Signs and symptoms, allergies, medications, past medical history, last meal, and events leading up to the problem are components of a:

   a. General impression
   b. Past medical history
   c. SAMPLE history
   d. Chief complaint

4. The four major diseases that are routinely inquired about during the past medical history in older adult patients are:

   a. Heart disease, epilepsy, chronic obstructive pulmonary disease, high blood pressure
   b. Heart disease, diabetes, cancer, high blood pressure
   c. Diabetes, chronic obstructive pulmonary disease, high blood pressure, stroke
   d. Heart disease, diabetes, chronic obstructive pulmonary disease, high blood pressure

5. How many breaths per minute is the normal range of respiratory rate for the adult patient?

   a. 5 to 15
   b. 10 to 15
   c. 12 to 20
   d. 15 to 25

6. The artery routinely used to monitor the rate, regularity, and quality of the pulse in the conscious adult patient is the:

   a. Radial
   b. Femoral
   c. Brachial
   d. Ulnar

7. Blood pressure determined by listening through a stethoscope is called blood pressure by:

   a. Auscultation
   b. Palpation
   c. Oscillation
   d. Vibration

8. The muscles used to determine the presence of respiratory distress are called the:

    a. Deltoid muscles
    b. Pectoral muscles
    c. Diaphragm muscles
    d. Accessory muscles

9. Air beneath the skin that is characterized by a crackling sensation during palpation of the neck and upper chest is called:

    a. Coarse rales
    b. Dermatitis pneumonia
    c. Subcutaneous emphysema
    d. Crepitant rales

10. The structure that can be palpated midline above the sternum is called the:

    a. Esophagus
    b. Pharynx
    c. Glottis
    d. Trachea

11. The rapid trauma assessment is designed to search for:

    a. All possible injuries to the patient
    b. Injuries in the head and trunk area
    c. Injuries that are minor
    d. Life-threatening injuries

12. Breath sound should routinely be auscultated on the upper anterior chest (apexes) and:

    a. Laterally at the bases
    b. Over the xiphoid process
    c. Over the sternum
    d. Over the trachea

13. When palpating a painful abdomen you should begin:

    a. At the site of pain
    b. Away from the site of pain
    c. Just lateral to the site
    d. Just medial to the site

14. The iliac crests of the pelvis are palpated by gentle compression posteriorly and:

    a. Anteriorly
    b. Medially
    c. Laterally
    d. Superiorly

15. When examining the lower extremities, you should compare:

    a. One to the other
    b. Upper thigh to lower leg
    c. Them to the upper extremities
    d. Anterior-posterior diameter to the lateral diameter

16. The posterior tibial pulse is located behind the:

    a. Inner ankle bone (medial malleolus)
    b. Mid-thigh region
    c. Hip region
    d. Kneecap

17. The bone that can be palpated on the anterior surface of the lower leg is the:

    a. Humerus
    b. Tibia
    c. Fibula
    d. Femur

18. The pulse that can be palpated in the anterolateral aspect of the wrist just below the thumb is the:

    a. Brachial
    b. Ulnar
    c. Radial
    d. Humeral

19. Which of the following problems is most likely to result in an absent pulse in one arm?

    a. A shock state with decreased perfusion
    b. An obstruction of an artery by a bone end
    c. Hypotension caused by arterial constriction
    d. Failure of the left side of the heart

20. Having the patient flex and extend the foot, lift the leg, and wiggle the toes most directly evaluates:

    a. Sensory function
    b. Mental state
    c. Motor function
    d. Brainstem function

21. A patient with paralysis of the lower but not the upper extremities has most likely injured the:

    a. Cervical spine
    b. Cerebrum
    c. Lumbar spine
    d. Brainstem

22. Which of the following patients might receive a rapid trauma assessment and be immediately transported without further physical examination?

    a. A patient with injuries to the upper arm
    b. A patient with multiple abrasions on the chest and abdomen
    c. A stable patient with fluid exuding from the nose
    d. A patient with a large chest wound and severe shock

23. What is the reason for reconsidering the mechanism of injury during the focused history and physical examination?

    a. To verify your initial assessment findings
    b. The patient may have provided incorrect information
    c. To help anticipate injury patterns during your examination
    d. It should be reconsidered every 3 to 5 minutes

24. ___________ of the posterior hip causes the leg to rotate internally, adduct, and flex at the knee.

25. A physical finding in the neck that may indicate a backup of blood in the venous system returning to the heart is called ___________.

26. The forces that might have injured the trauma patient are called the ___________ ___________.

27. The mnemonic used during the rapid trauma assessment to remember possible physical findings during the head-to-toe survey is ___________.

28. Injured sections of the thorax moving in opposite directions from the uninjured sections is called ___________.

29. Abnormal change in the position of the windpipe, suggesting injury to the airway or chest, is called ___________.

TRUE OR FALSE

30. _______ A rapid trauma assessment must be performed on every trauma patient, no matter how minor or severe the injury appears.

31. _______ A patient who lacerated her thumb while cutting a bagel requires a focused physical exam of the hand; a rapid trauma assessment is not required.

32. _______ A rapid trauma assessment should be performed on the scene before moving the patient.

Questions 33 to 35 refer to the following scenario.

> You are called to the scene of a person who was struck by a car while riding a bicycle. The police have secured the scene and the scene is safe. You and your partner have taken appropriate body substance isolation precautions. You encounter a 16-year-old girl who is sitting on the curb. She is alert, complaining of pain in her back; her airway, breathing, and circulation are all normal.

33. This patient requires:

    a. A rapid trauma assessment, performed on the scene, because of the mechanism of injury
    b. A rapid trauma assessment, performed in the ambulance, because of the mechanism of injury
    c. A focused physical examination of the patient's back because of an isolated chief complaint
    d. A detailed physical examination performed immediately

34. Spinal immobilization of this patient is:

    a. Not needed because the patient reported that she walked after the incident
    b. Only indicated if the assessment reveals neurologic damage
    c. Immediately indicated and should be performed as soon as possible
    d. Indicated but should not be done until all of the assessment steps are completed

35. On evaluation, you determine that the patient complains of pain on palpation of her lower back. Using the DCAP/BTLS mnemonic you would document that the patient has a(n) ___________ to her lower back.

    a. Contusion
    b. Abrasion
    c. Tenderness
    d. Swelling

Across

2. "Black and blue" mark
3. Two or more ribs broken in two or more places
6. Feeling with the hand or fingers during examination
9. Order of the rapid trauma physical examination
11. Decreased movement on one side of the chest during respirations caused by chest injury
12. An EMT should _____ _____ _____ at an airbag and steering wheel after a crash to determine the potential for internal injury
15. Wounds that result from thermal, chemical, or electrical injury
16. Leakage of plasma into an injured area resulting in swelling
18. The grating of one bone fragment against another
19. Air beneath the skin
22. Mnemonic to remember the key questions in a patient history
23. Artery of the foot, located on the top surface
24. Burn involving the upper and lower layers of the skin, characterized by blistering of the skin
26. An abnormal enlargement of a body part or organ caused by fluid
27. Wound that is created by a sharp object penetrating the skin
28. Top portions of the lungs
29. An injury causing tearing of the skin

Down

1. Mnemonic used to remember possible physical findings identified during the head-to-toe survey
4. Collection of blood beneath the skin
5. Burn involving the "full thickness" of the skin, which may appear blackened and charred
7. Artery that passes just behind the ankle bone
8. A systematic review of each body area to be sure that life-threatening conditions are identified early
10. Pain elicted on touch
13. The _____ _____ _____ in a motor vehicle crash is important in assessing the patient's injuries
14. Wound that occurs as a result of traumatic scraping of the skin
17. Protruding bone on the medial side of the ankle
18. A bruise without a break in the skin
20. Burn involving the upper layer of the skin, characterized by a reddened appearance
21. Structural distortion altering the normal appearance of the body or a part
25. Fracture of this causes the leg to externally rotate and shorten

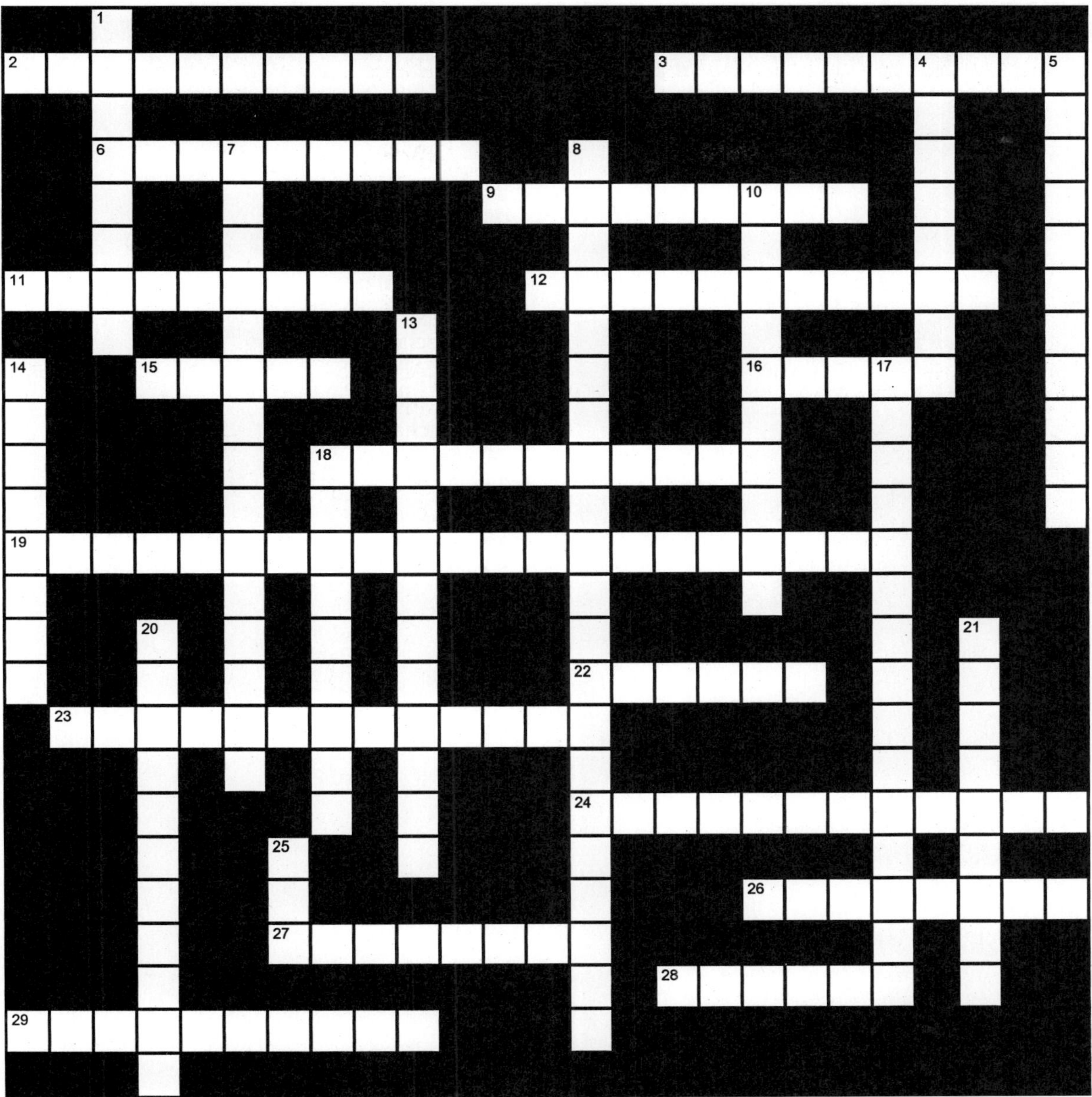
1
2
3
4
5
6
7
8
9
10
11
12
13
14
15
16
17
18
19
20
21
22
23
24
25
26
27
28
29

ANSWER KEY

1. b
2. d
3. c
4. d
5. c
6. a
7. a
8. d
9. c
10. d
11. d
12. a
13. b
14. b
15. a
16. a
17. b
18. c
19. b
20. c
21. c
22. d
23. c
24. Dislocation
25. Jugular vein distention
26. Mechanism of injury
27. DCAP/BTLS
28. Paradoxic motion
29. Tracheal deviation
30. False
31. True
32. True
33. a
34. c
35. c

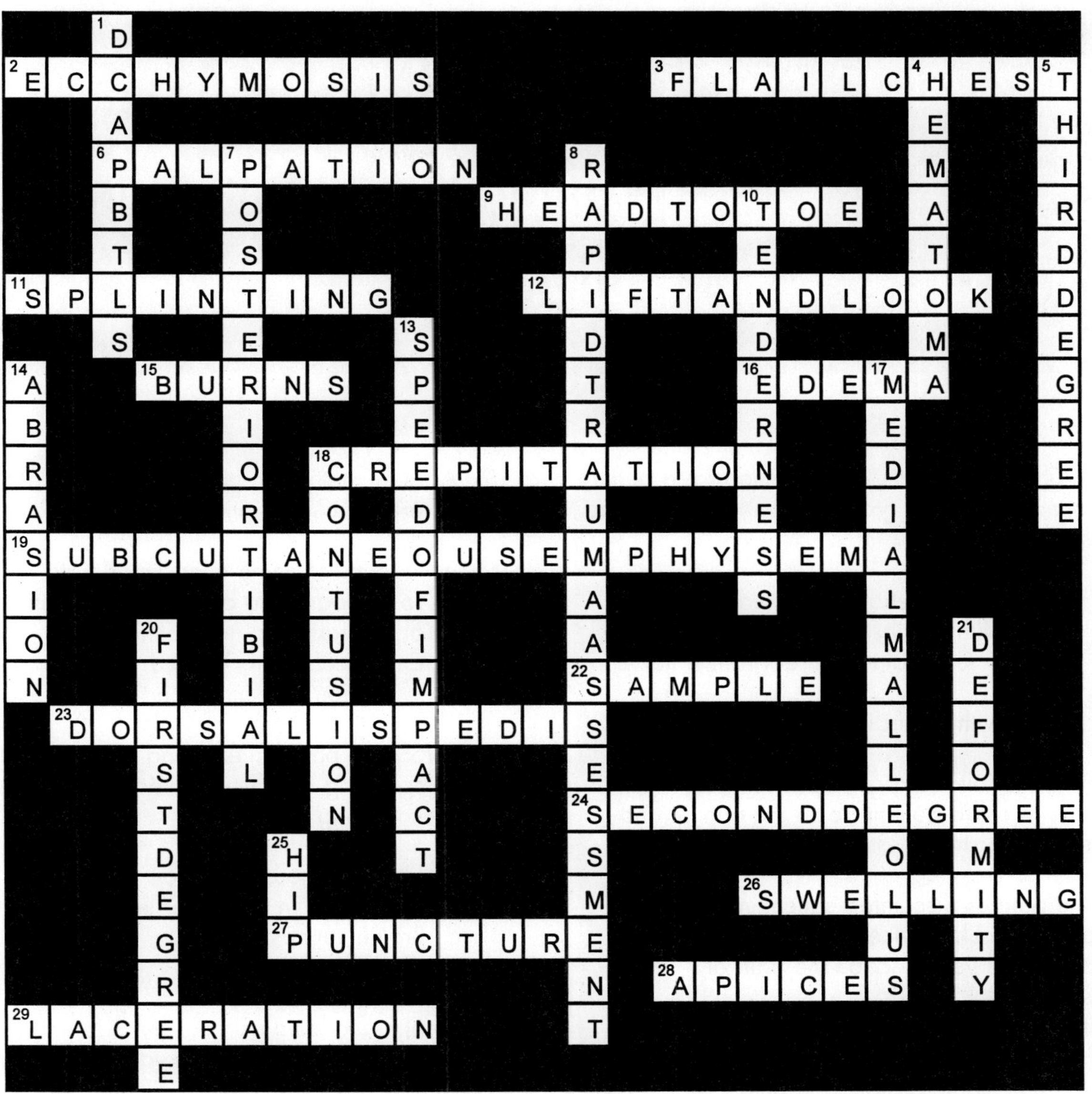
1 D
2 ECCHYMOSIS
3 FLAILCHEST
4 HEMATOMA
5 THIRDDEGREE
6 PALPATION
7 POSTERIORTIBIAL
8 RAPIDTRAUMAASSESSMENT
9 HEADTOTOE
10 TENDERNESS
11 SPLINTING
12 LIFTANDLOOK
13 SPEEDOFIMPACT
14 ABRASION
15 BURNS
16 EDEMA
17 MEDIALMALLEOLUS
18 CREPITATION
19 SUBCUTANEOUSEMPHYSEMA
20 FIRSTDEGREE
21 DEFORMITY
22 SAMPLE
23 DORSALISPEDIS
24 SECONDDEGREE
25 HI
26 SWELLING
27 PUNCTURE
28 APICES
29 LACERATION
DCAPBTLS
CONTUSION

Chapter 11 Focused History and Physical Examination of Medical Patients

1. The OPQRST mnemonic is most suited for a patient presenting with which type of history of presenting illness?

   a. A patient with a behavioral emergency
   b. A patient with an obstetric emergency
   c. A patient who sustained an environmental emergency
   d. A patient with a cardiac emergency

2. Which of the following questions represents the best way to ask a patient about the quality and nature of his or her chest pain or discomfort?

   a. Is the pain or discomfort squeezing in nature?
   b. Does it feel like a vice on your chest wall?
   c. How would you describe the pain or discomfort?
   d. Is the pain or discomfort strong or weak?

OPQRST is a mnemonic designed to help you remember questions that clarify the chief complaint. Fill in the appropriate word next to each letter of the mnemonic.

3. O ________________

4. P ________________

5. Q ________________

6. R ________________

7. S ________________

8. T ________________

9. A useful method to have the patient describe the severity of chest pain or discomfort is:

   a. In terms of being minor, moderate, or severe
   b. To compare it to other types of pain or discomfort (e.g., toothache)
   c. On a scale from 1 to 10
   d. In relation to a pinch on the arm

10. A focused physical examination for a patient complaining of difficulty breathing might include all the following *except:*

    a. Jugular venous distention
    b. Tenderness in the upper legs
    c. Breath sounds
    d. Swelling of the ankles

Match the conditions in column B to the appropriate questions that should be asked for that type of complaint during the focused history in column A (column B conditions can be used more than once):

Column A	Column B
11. ____ Vomiting?	a. Difficulty breathing
	b. Abdominal pain
12. ____ Tongue biting?	c. Seizures
13. ____ Swelling in the ankles or back?	
14. ____ Rectal bleeding?	
15. ____ Productive cough?	

16. While assessing a specific chief complaint (e.g., chest pain), the physical examination can be:

    a. More focused on the type of presenting problem
    b. A comprehensive head-to-toe survey
    c. Eliminated because you already have identified the cause
    d. Limited to the head and neck of the patient

17. While assessing a medical patient who is unresponsive, the physical examination should be:

    a. More focused because the patient cannot respond
    b. A complete head-to-toe survey
    c. Eliminated because you will never identify the cause
    d. Limited to the head and neck

18. When transporting the unconscious patient who is breathing adequately, transport in the

    ___________ position.

19. Asking questions regarding vomiting, antacid use, and rectal bleeding would be most appropriate for a patient presenting with the chief complaint of

    __________________.

20. Asking questions regarding whether the patient has swelling in the ankles or back or has a productive cough would be most appropriate for a patient presenting with the chief complaint of

    __________________.

List the seven questions that you should ask the patient with an obstetric emergency.

21. ______________________________
22. ______________________________
23. ______________________________
24. ______________________________
25. ______________________________
26. ______________________________
27. ______________________________

List the seven key questions to ask the patient with a behavioral emergency.

28. ______________________________
29. ______________________________
30. ______________________________
31. ______________________________
32. ______________________________
33. ______________________________
34. ______________________________

List the seven key questions to ask the patient with a poisoning/overdose.

35. ______________________________
36. ______________________________
37. ______________________________
38. ______________________________
39. ______________________________
40. ______________________________
41. ______________________________

List the eight key questions to ask the patient, or things that you should look for, in a patient with an altered level of consciousness.

42. ______________________________
43. ______________________________
44. ______________________________
45. ______________________________
46. ______________________________
47. ______________________________
48. ______________________________
49. ______________________________

List the six key questions to ask the patient with an allergic reaction.

50. ______________________________

51. ______________________________

52. ______________________________

53. ______________________________

54. ______________________________

55. ______________________________

List the five key questions to ask the patient, or things to look for, in a patient with an environmental emergency.

56. ______________________________

57. ______________________________

58. ______________________________

59. ______________________________

60. ______________________________

Across

2. Assessment performed on a patient who is unresponsive or has an altered mental status
6. Subjective description of the complaint in the patient's own words
8. How long the problem has existed
9. The T in DCAP/BTLS
12. Pain that spreads to another body part or area
14. Respirations, pulse, blood pressure, and mental state
17. The B in DCAP/BTLS
20. The L in DCAP/BTLS
23. The L in SAMPLE
24. The M in SAMPLE
25. Relevant information associated with the chief complaint
26. The E in SAMPLE
27. Frequently the most significant part of patient assessment
28. Information regarding previous illnesses and hospitalizations and current medications

Down

1. The A in DCAP/BTLS
3. The A in SAMPLE
4. The S in SAMPLE
5. The S in DCAP/BTLS
7. The D in DCAP/BTLS
10. Mnemonic to remember the key questions in a patient history
11. Degree of pain
13. Mnemonic used to remember possible physical findings identified during the head-to-toe survey
15. Examination directed toward the chief complaint
16. The P in DCAP/BTLS
18. Behaviors that make the symptoms better or worse
19. When the complaint first occurred
21. The C in DCAP/BTLS
22. Position used for an unresponsive medical patient to protect the airway during transport

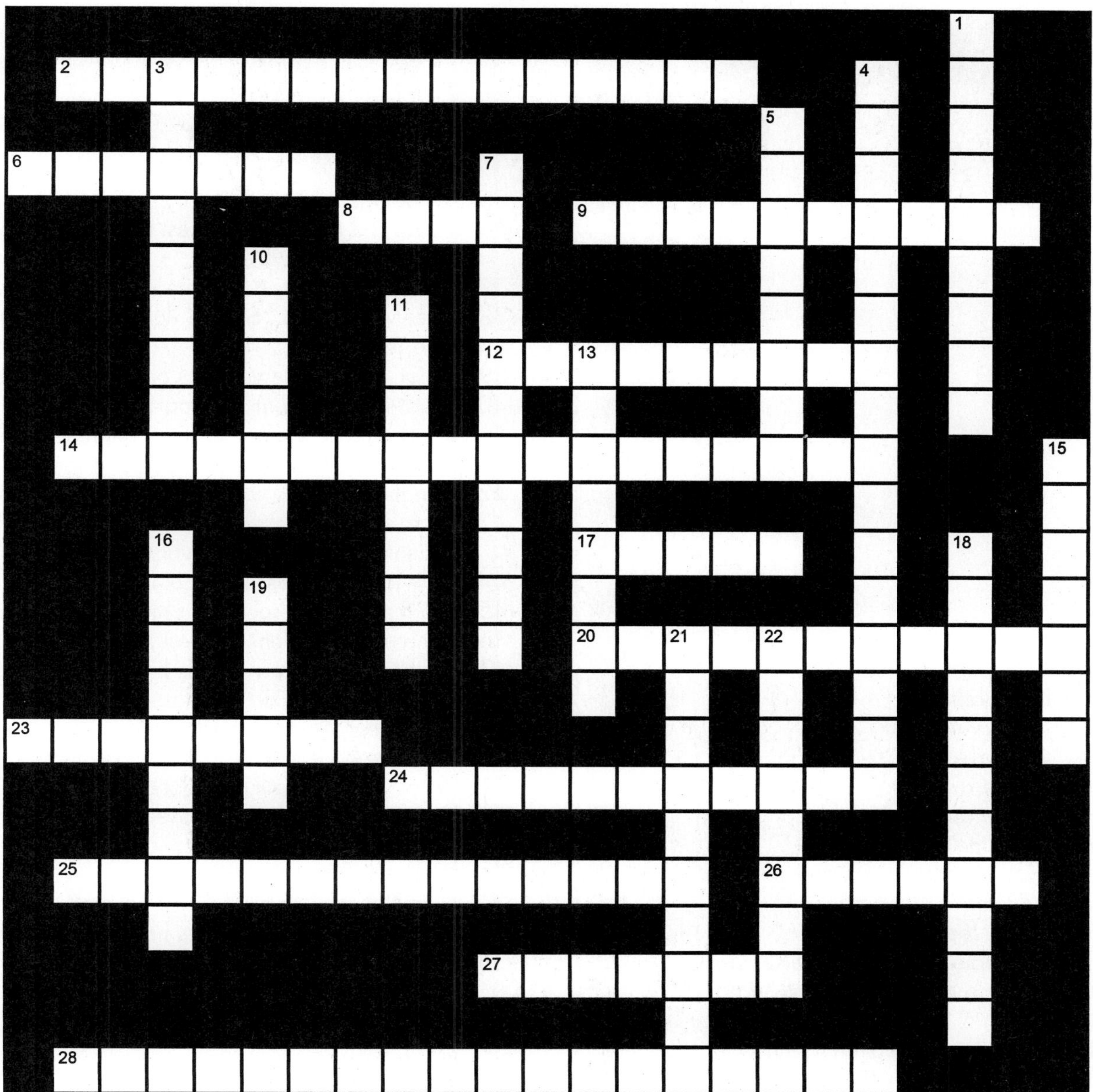

ANSWER KEY

1. d
2. c
3. Onset
4. Provocation
5. Quality
6. Radiation
7. Severity
8. Time
9. c
10. b
11. b
12. c
13. a
14. b
15. a
16. a
17. b
18. Recovery
19. Abdominal pain
20. Difficulty breathing
21. Are you pregnant?
22. How long have you been pregnant?
23. Do you have any pain or contractions?
24. Do you have any vaginal bleeding or discharge?
25. Do you feel the need to push?
26. When was your last menstrual period?
27. Are you (is the baby) crowning?
28. How do you feel?
29. Ask appropriate questions to determine suicidal tendencies (e.g., Do you want to hurt or kill yourself?)
30. Is the patient a threat to self or others?
31. Is there a medical problem along with the behavioral emergency?
32. What is the patient's past medical history?
33. Has the patient/family undertaken any interventions?
34. What medications does the patient take and does he or she take them as prescribed?
35. What was the substance involved?
36. When did the patient ingest the substance or become exposed?
37. How much of the substance was ingested?
38. Over what period of time was the substance ingested?
39. What, if any, interventions have already occurred?
40. What is the patient's estimated weight?
41. What effects, if any, has the patient experienced since the ingestion/exposure?
42. Can the patient or bystander describe the event?
43. What was the onset of the event (what was the patient doing when the event began)?
44. How long has this been going on?
45. Are there any associated symptoms present?
46. Is there any evidence of trauma?
47. What, if any, interventions have already occurred?
48. Has the patient had a seizure?
49. Does the patient have a fever?
50. Does the patient have a history of allergies?
51. What was the patient exposed to?
52. How was the patient exposed?
53. What have been the effects of the exposure?
54. What has been the progression (speed of onset, specific complaints) of the exposure?
55. What, if any, interventions have already occurred?
56. What was the source of the environmental emergency?
57. What was the environment in which the exposure occurred?
58. What was the duration of the exposure?
59. Did the patient lose consciousness?
60. What effects, general or local, has the patient experienced?

Across

2 HEAD TO TOE SURVEY
6 QUALITY
8 TIME
9 TENDERNESS
12 RADIATION
14 BASELINE VITAL SIGNS
17 BURNS
20 LACERATIONS
23 LAST MEAL
24 MEDICATIONS
25 PRESENT ILLNESS
26 EVENTS
27 HISTORY
28 PAST MEDICAL HISTORY

Down

1 ABRASIONS
3 ALLERGIES
4 SIGNS AND SYMPTOMS
5 SWELLING
7 DEFORMITIES
10 SAMPLE
11 SEVERITY
13 DCAPBTLS
15 FOCUSED
16 PUNCTURES
18 PROVOCATION
19 ONSET
21 CONTUSION
22 RECOVERY

Chapter 12 Detailed Physical Examination

1. You respond to a call for a small child who cut her index finger on the sharp edge of a toy. What should the detailed physical examination consist of?

   a. An examination of the finger and hand
   b. An examination of the finger, head, and neck
   c. An examination of the finger, head, neck, and trunk
   d. A comprehensive head-to-toe survey

2. You find a 5-year-old boy who has fallen from a height of 6 feet. The initial assessment and the focused history and physical examination revealed no positive findings. What should the detailed physical examination consist of?

   a. An examination of only the back side of the patient
   b. An examination of only the head and neck
   c. An examination of only the head, neck, and trunk
   d. A complete head-to-toe survey

3. During your detailed history and physical examination of a conscious and alert trauma patient, you note deformity and movement in the mid-face region. Which of the following actions should you consider?

   a. Splinting that region of the face
   b. Inserting an oropharyngeal airway
   c. Reassessing and maintaining an open airway
   d. Inserting a nasopharyngeal airway

4. You note blood drainage from the ear during a detailed physical examination. What actions should you take?

   a. Place the patient's head lower than the torso
   b. Place the patient in the lateral recumbent position
   c. Pack the ear with a soft gauze
   d. Cover the ear with a loose dressing

5. A small particle of debris is noted on the cornea of a trauma patient during your detailed physical examination. The patient is complaining of severe irritation of the eye. What action should you take?

   a. Irrigate the eye with water or saline solution
   b. Cover both eyes with gauze
   c. Apply gentle pressure over the lid
   d. Apply a topical ointment to decrease irritation

6. During the detailed physical examination you note liquid secretions collecting in the airway of an unconscious blunt trauma patient and hear gurgling sounds emitting from the airway. What action should you take?

   a. Transport the patient in the prone position
   b. Suction the patient's airway
   c. Perform a finger sweep
   d. Turn the head to the side

7. You note cyanosis of the lips and nailbeds on a conscious and alert patient during your detailed physical examination. What actions should you take?

   a. Reassess the airway, ventilation, and oxygenation of the patient
   b. Immediately start positive-pressure ventilation with a bag-valve-mask
   c. Administer oxygen by nasal cannula and continue your examination
   d. Elevate the patient's legs to ensure perfusion to the upper body

8. During your detailed physical examination you note an impaled object in the patient's thigh. What action should you take?

   a. Remove the object and apply a dressing to the area
   b. Remove the object and irrigate the area to prevent infection
   c. Leave the object in place and transport immediately
   d. Stabilize the object in place with a bulky dressing

9. Which of the following is an element of the both the detailed physical examination and the focused examination?

   a. Pupil evaluation
   b. Examination of the ears
   c. Jugular venous distention
   d. Examination of the nose

10. Which of the following patients would not receive a detailed physical examination?

    a. A conscious patient who fell from a height of 10 feet
    b. A stable automobile trauma patient
    c. A patient with multiple dog bites
    d. A patient in cardiopulmonary arrest

11. Which of the following physical examination finding might be noted for a trauma patient but not for a medical patient?

    a. Jugular venous distention
    b. Swelling of the ankles
    c. Crepitus of the shoulder
    d. Tenderness in the abdomen

12. Which of the following physical examination components might be performed on a trauma patient but not a medical patient?

    a. Comparison of both pupils for equality and reactivity
    b. Comparison of both thighs for deformity and swelling
    c. A check for breath sound on both sides
    d. Evaluation of jugular venous distention

13. The detailed examination is usually performed:

    a. At the scene before transport
    b. In the ambulance during transport
    c. Just before the initial assessment
    d. At the hospital before transferring the patient

14. During the detailed physical examination a penlight is used to examine the pupils to check to see if the pupils ___________ when exposed to light.

15. A contusion or black and blue discoloration behind the ear may be a sign of a ___________.

16. To control bleeding from the nose, pinch the nose with the patient leaning ___________ if conditions permit.

TRUE OR FALSE

17. _____ Dentures that are stable should be left in place.

18. _____ Injuries identified during the detailed physical examination should be documented on the call report, but emergency department staff should perform treatment of any injuries discovered.

19. _____ The detailed physical examination is performed more rapidly than the initial assessment and focused examination.

20. _____ The scalp is very vascular and small injuries may present with extensive bleeding.

Across

3. The C of DCAP/BTLS
4. Dressings and bandages to control bleeding of the _____ should be applied evenly over a broad area
7. A yellowing of the skin caused by a buildup of bilirubin in the blood
8. The B of DCAP/BTLS
9. A more comprehensive survey than the focused history and physical examination
10. Pupils that are very large in size
12. _____ _____ might be an important finding for a diabetic patient or suspected toxic ingestions
15. The S in DCAP/BTLS
16. A contusion or discoloration _____ _____ _____ may be a sign of a skull injury
19. A patient in diabetic ketoacidosis may have a sweet _____-like odor on their breath
20. The L in DCAP/BTLS
21. Observe the tongue for lacerations after a _____
22. Physical finding that may be present in a patient with a suspected allergic reaction that may result in severe airway compromise and requires rapid treatment and transport

Down

1. The detailed physical examination is typically conducted _____ _____ to the hospital
2. Drainage of blood or blood-tinged spinal fluid from the ear canal should be treated with a _____ _____
5. The P in DCAP/BTLS
6. The white covering of the eye
11. Drainage of blood or blood-tinged spinal fluid from the ear canal could be a sign of a _____ _____
13. The T in DCAP/BTLS
14. The D of DCAP/BTLS
17. The A of DCAP/BTLS
18. The primary concern for the patient with facial injuries is the possibility of _____ compromise

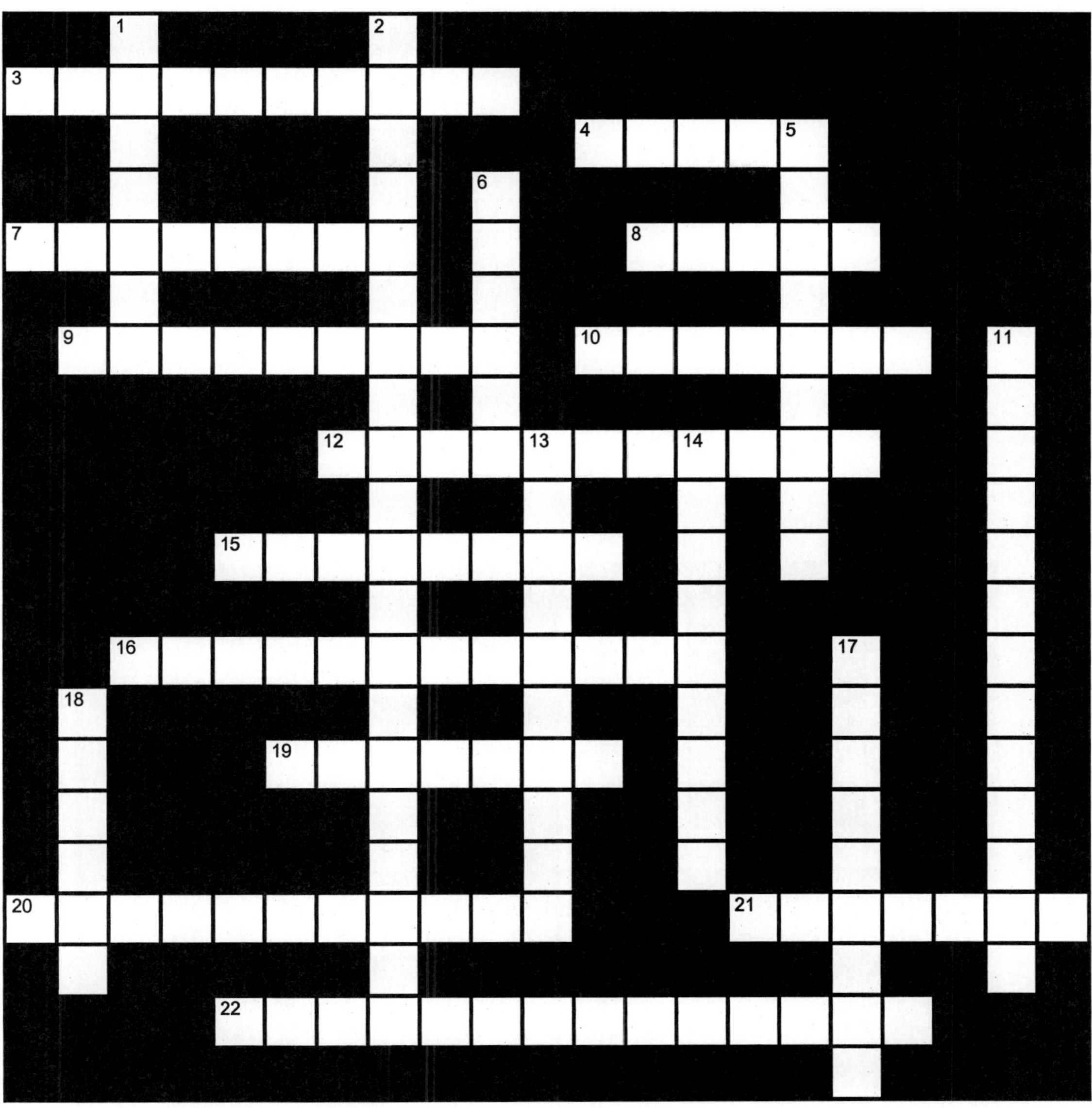
1
2
3
4
5
6
7
8
9
10
11
12
13
14
15
16
17
18
19
20
21
22

ANSWER KEY

1. a
2. d
3. c
4. d
5. a
6. b
7. a
8. d
9. c
10. d
11. c
12. b
13. b
14. Constrict
15. Skull fracture
16. Forward
17. True
18. False
19. False
20. True

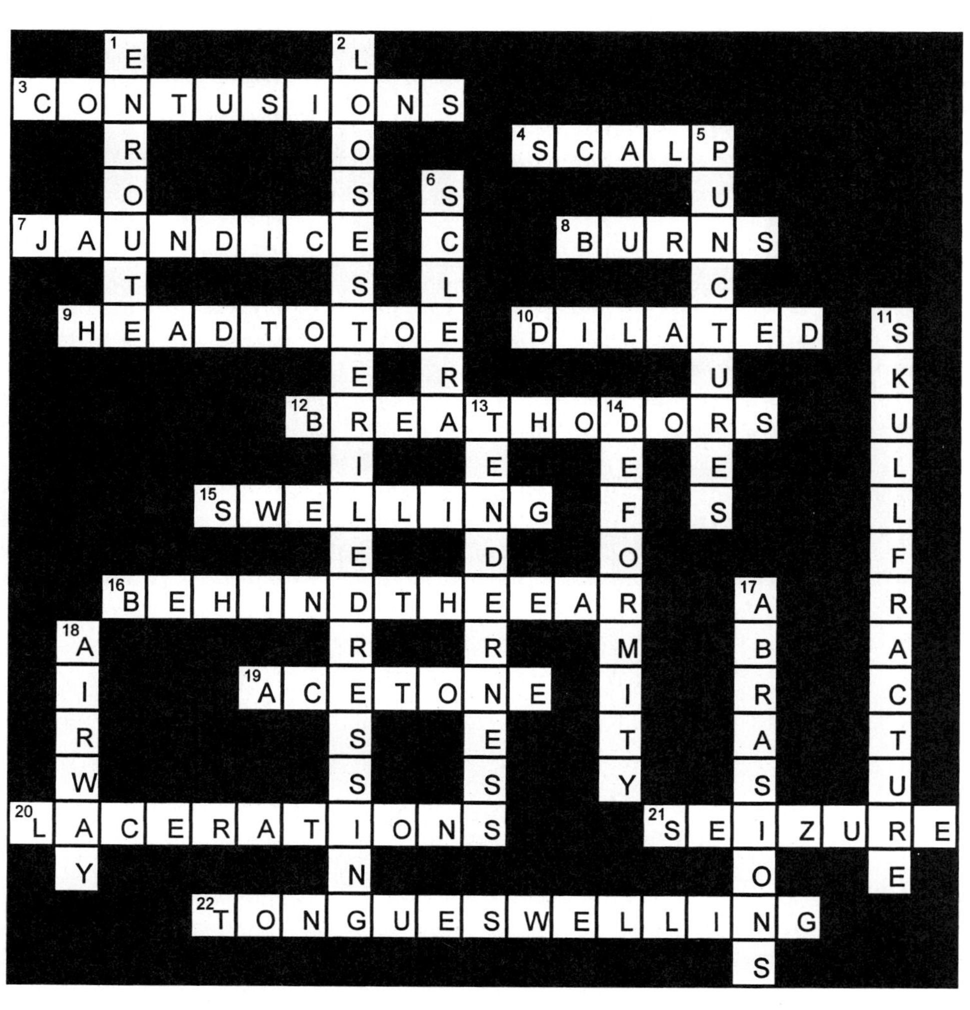

Chapter 13 Ongoing Assessment

1. Which is the most important reason for rechecking vitals signs during the ongoing assessment?

   a. The patient's condition may have deteriorated since your last evaluation
   b. To confirm the accuracy of the reading previously taken by your partner
   c. To ensure effective medical and legal documentation for the record
   d. To reassure the patient that he or she is receiving the best possible treatment

2. Sequential blood pressures of 120/80, 110/76, and 90/60 mm Hg were discovered during your ongoing assessment of a trauma patient. Which of the following would best explain this pattern?

   a. Normal variance in a healthy patient
   b. Changes caused by severe anxiety
   c. Calming of the patient related to oxygen therapy
   d. Trending during uncontrolled internal bleeding

3. You are transporting a 15-year-old boy who was hit by a car and is receiving oxygen by a nonrebreather, has a traction splint on his left leg, and is fully immobilized to a long spine board. All the following are important elements of your ongoing assessment for this patient *except*:

   a. Checking for breath sounds bilaterally
   b. Checking the posterior tibial pulse in the left leg
   c. Rechecking for signs of pelvic injury
   d. Checking his blood pressure

4. During the transport of a patient who was complaining of difficulty breathing, you reassess vital signs and note the following: the patient's mental state changes from alert and oriented to responsive to painful stimuli; his pulse rate increases from 80 to 110 beats/min; and his respiratory rate changes from 12 breaths/min and regular to 24 breaths/min and shallow. What is the value of this information to the physician at the emergency department?

   a. It demonstrates marked improvement in the patient's condition
   b. It indicates that the patient is stable and responding to treatment
   c. It indicates that the patient is getting worse
   d. It indicates that the patient requires minimal additional treatment

5. You are administering oxygen by a nonrebreather to a patient complaining of chest pain and note the following during your ongoing assessment en route to the hospital. The patient becomes cyanotic and unresponsive, respiratory rate is 8 breaths/min and shallow, and pulse is 120 beats/min and thready. What immediate action should you take?

   a. Increase the oxygen concentration
   b. Elevate the patient's head
   c. Administer abdominal thrusts
   d. Administer positive-pressure ventilation

6. You are transporting a patient with a traction splint. What specific evaluation would be most appropriate during your ongoing assessment?

   a. Measure the circumference of the injured extremity
   b. Check for a distal pulse in the injured extremity
   c. Test for tenderness by palpating the injured extremity
   d. Lift the extremity and check for edema in the posterior region

7. An effective method for evaluating changes in the severity of chest pain or discomfort during your ongoing assessment is to:

   a. Have the patient rate the pain or discomfort on a scale of 1 to 10
   b. Have the patient use an appropriate adjective to describe severity
   c. Apply painful stimuli and have the patient compare the two stimuli
   d. Have the patient compare the pain or discomfort to another unrelated event

8. The ongoing assessment is started by:

   a. A review of the initial assessment
   b. Examination of the head
   c. Checking the blood pressure
   d. Checking skin temperature

9. As a general rule, how often should unstable patients be reassessed during your ongoing assessment?

   a. Every 1 minute
   b. Every 5 minutes
   c. Every 10 minutes
   d. Every 15 minutes

10. As a general rule, how often should stable patients be reassessed during your ongoing assessment?

   a. Every 1 minute
   b. Every 5 minutes
   c. Every 10 minutes
   d. Every 15 minutes

List the four key components of the ongoing assessment.

11. ______________________________

12. ______________________________

13. ______________________________

14. ______________________________

15. The reassessment of the patient's mental status should be completed quickly with the mnemonic

   __________.

16. The best visual indicator of an open airway and sufficient breathing is to observe for adequate

   ________________.

List the three abnormal skin colors and a common reason for that physical finding.

17. ______________________________

18. ______________________________

19. ______________________________

20. Empathy and providing emotional support are especially significant in children and which other

   group of patients? __________

Questions 21 to 24 refer to the following scenario.

> You are transporting a 57-year-old man to the hospital. The patient's chief complaint is chest pressure that he describes as constant and rates a 5 on a 10-point pain scale. The patient's skin color looks yellow and the patient tells you that he has liver disease. You have administered oxygen to this patient and your transport time is anticipated to be 12 minutes. After a few minutes receiving oxygen the patient now informs you that the chest pressure is a 3 on a 10-point scale.

21. The reason to reevaluate your patient's pain and rate it on a pain scale is:

   a. To determine your patient's tolerance for pain
   b. To determine when the oxygen can be removed
   c. To determine if your treatment is having any effect
   d. To determine the appropriate position to transport the patient

22. The yellow skin color that you observe in your patient is called:

    a. Cyanosis
    b. Pallor
    c. Mottled
    d. Jaundice

23. Your ongoing assessment of this patient while en route to the hospital includes all the following *except:*

    a. Repeat of the vital signs
    b. A repeat of the initial assessment
    c. A reevaluation of the patient's chest discomfort
    d. A SAMPLE history (signs and symptoms, allergies, medications, past medical problems, last oral intake, events surrounding this illness)

24. Your patient is concerned about his condition and he asks you if he is having a heart attack. You should:

    a. Inform him that he is not having a heart attack and he should remain calm
    b. Inform him that his symptoms indicate that he is having a heart attack but you are here to help him
    c. Inform him that you are not able to diagnose his problem but that you are providing the best possible care for him based on his symptoms
    d. Inform him that you are not allowed to comment on his condition until he is evaluated by a physician at the hospital

Across

2. ALS
5. Pulse, blood pressure, temperature, and respirations
6. Site of a major artery that can be compressed to control bleeding
7. _____ pulse is found in the neck
10. Radios that transmit with low power and limited range
11. The last resort for controlling bleeding
12. _____ _____ should be checked intermittently when a splint is applied to an extremity
13. The patient's problem in his or her own words
14. To control bleeding from the extremities, use _____ in conjunction with direct pressure
15. _____ pulse is found in the wrist
16. _____ _____ is tested by squeezing and releasing the nailbed
17. A reevaluation of the patient

Down

1. When performing _____ _____, it is critical to observe for adequate chest rise
3. _____ patients should be reevaluated every 5 minutes
4. Initial way to control bleeding
8. The _____ pulse is found in the arm near the elbow
9. The inner surface of the eyelids and the anterior part of the sclera

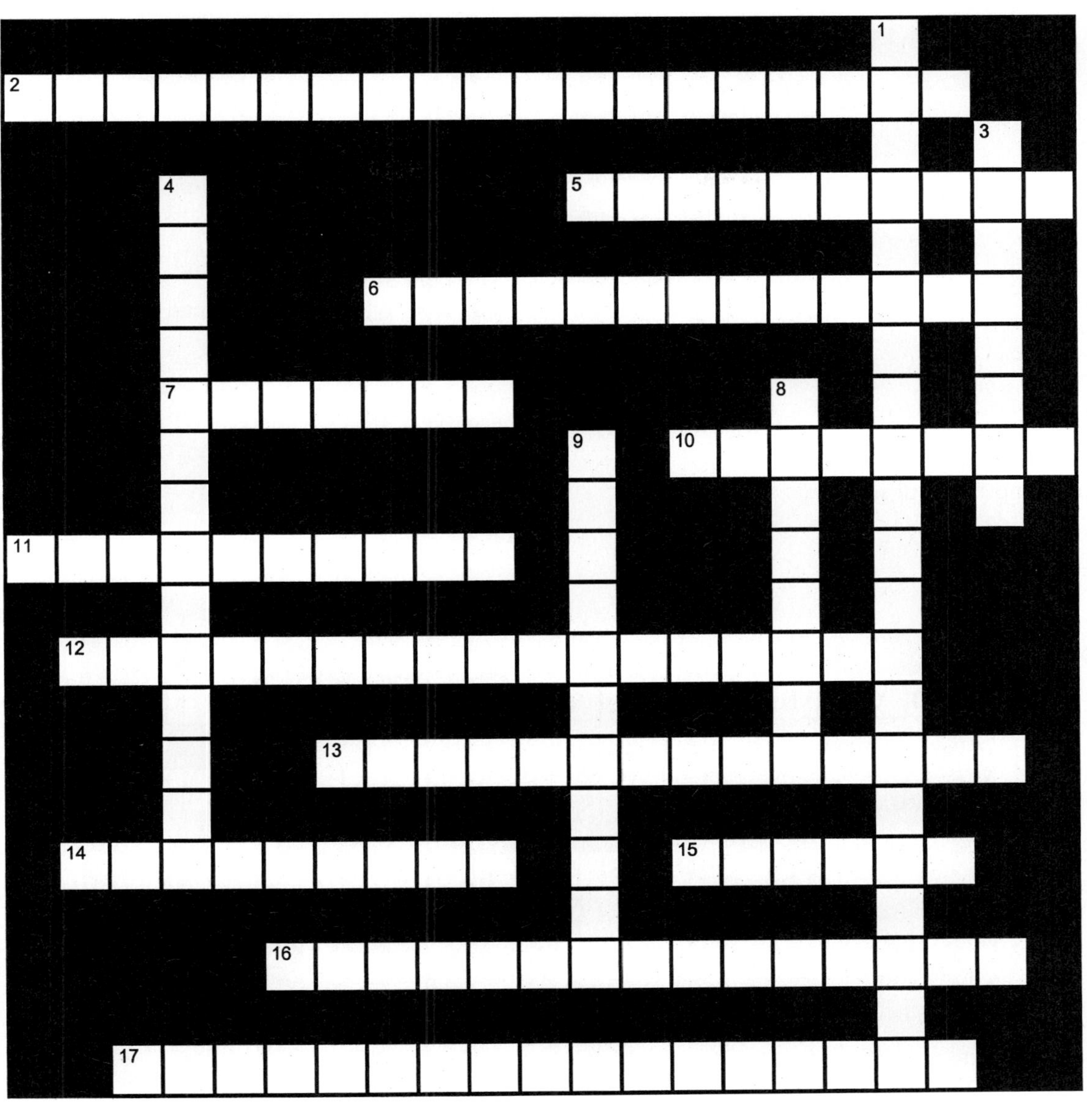
1
2
3
4
5
6
7
8
9
10
11
12
13
14
15
16
17

ANSWER KEY

1. a
2. d
3. c
4. c
5. d
6. b
7. a
8. a
9. b
10. d
11. Repeat the initial assessment
12. Repeat taking the vital signs
13. Repeat the focused assessment
14. Check on all interventions that have been made
15. AVPU
16. Chest expansion
17. Pale skin from shock
18. Cyanotic skin from inadequate oxygenation
19. Flushed skin from fever
20. Older adults
21. c
22. d
23. d
24. c

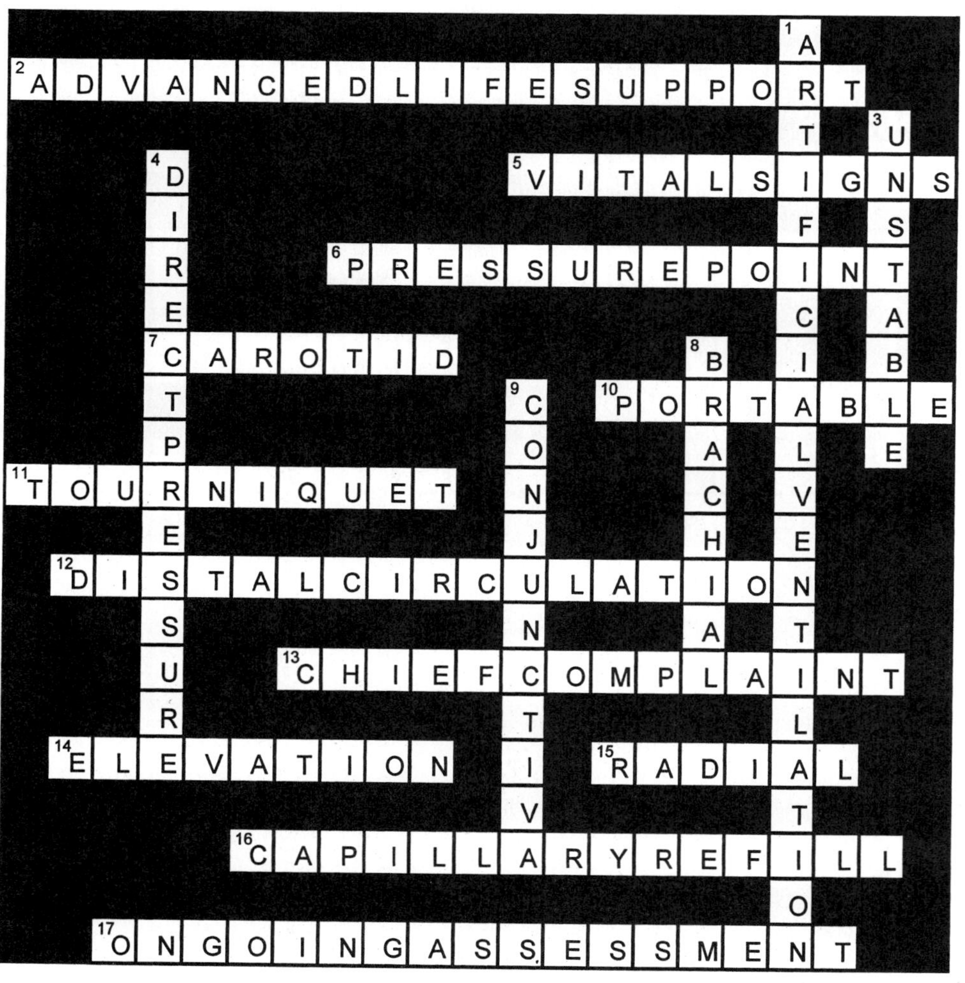

Chapter 14 Communications

1. When initiating a radio call, the EMT should:

   a. Interrupt radio transmission that is in progress
   b. Ask permission to interrupt radio transmission that is in progress
   c. Use the squelch feature on the radio to interrupt any radio transmission in the event of an emergency
   d. Never interrupt a radio transmission

2. The most effective way to begin your radio transmission is to:

   a. Identify yourself and your unit
   b. Present the patient's chief complaint
   c. Present the patient's vital signs
   d. Present the patient's past medical history

3. At the end of each verbal radio exchange, the speaker should end the message with the word(s):

   a. Next
   b. Over
   c. Message complete
   d. Roger

4. When initiating a radio call the EMT should:

   a. Wait for the patient to say "go ahead" before sending your message
   b. Use "yes" and "no" to indicate your acceptance or refusal of the response
   c. Speak in a voice that is louder than normal
   d. Consider using codes to reduce on-air time and summarize communications

5. Which of the following is the typical medical format used for presenting a patient?

   a. Estimated time of arrival, patient's name, and vital signs
   b. Patient's age, sex, and history of present illness (chief complaint)
   c. EMS unit identifier, patient's vital signs, and estimated time of arrival
   d. Patient's physician's name, history of present illness (chief complaint), and estimated time of arrival

6. The typical medical format for presenting a patient should conclude with:

   a. The patient's name, age, and sex
   b. The prehospital treatments rendered and the patient's response thus far
   c. Your EMS identifier, the patient's history of present illness (chief complaint), and past medical history
   d. Your EMS identifier, your estimated time of arrival, and your diagnosis of the patient's condition

7. Which of the following statements is true?

   a. When giving your report, accuracy is essential
   b. When giving your report, accuracy is not essential because the hospital will reassess the patient once you arrive
   c. The EMT is responsible for making a prehospital diagnosis
   d. The EMT should give a lengthy, presumptive report over the radio

8. Which of the following statements is true?

   a. The dispatcher will always notify the receiving hospital
   b. The dispatcher will never notify the receiving hospital
   c. The information you provide is essential in preparing the hospital for your arrival
   d. The information you provide is of no value in preparing the hospital for your arrival

9. Which of the following is *not* an essential component of the verbal report?

   a. Your estimated time of arrival
   b. The patient's age and sex
   c. Complete and detailed past medical history
   d. Brief, pertinent past medical history

10. A good rule to follow when speaking into a radio microphone is to:

    a. Talk louder than normal while holding the microphone right next to your mouth
    b. Speak in a normal voice with the microphone a few inches away from your mouth
    c. Speak more slowly than normal and in a low voice
    d. Speak in a normal voice with the microphone touching your mouth

11. As a general rule, how many inches should the microphone be held away from your mouth while speaking?

    a. 2 to 3
    b. 5 to 6
    c. 8 to 10
    d. 10 to 12

12. As a rule, radio communication allows for:

    a. Both parties to speak at the same time
    b. One person to speak at a time
    c. Interruption for a more serious patient
    d. A dispatcher to connect both parties

13. Proper radio transmission consists of all the following *except*:

    a. Use of clear, concise words
    b. Use of the standard medical reporting format
    c. Use of the word "we" instead of the word "I"
    d. Giving the patient's name over the radio

14. Which of the following is not acceptable practice for radio communications?

    a. The use of profanity over the airwaves
    b. The use of words such as "we" instead of "I"
    c. The use of standard radio codes
    d. A radio transmission that takes longer than 30 seconds

15. The governmental agency responsible for regulating all aspects of radio communication in the United States is called the:

    a. Radio Communications Center (RCC)
    b. Dispatch Communications Center (DCC)
    c. Federal Communications Commission (FCC)
    d. Center for Federal Communications (CFC)

16. The governmental agency that regulates radio communication in the United States does so by providing all the following services *except*:

    a. Establishing technical standards for radio equipment
    b. Allocating radio frequencies
    c. Issuing licenses to agencies that sell radio equipment
    d. Issuing licenses to agencies that use and repair radio equipment

17. Focusing your attention on the patient, telling the truth, and using language the patient will understand are all components of:

    a. The standard medical presentation format
    b. The governmental agency that regulates radio communications in the United States
    c. The primary assessment
    d. Interpersonal communication skills

18. Speaking clearly, slowly, and distinctly and using the patient's proper name are examples of:

    a. Nonverbal communication skills
    b. Verbal communication skills
    c. Body communication skills
    d. Radio communication skills

19. All the following are effective components of general communication with patients, family members, and bystanders *except*:

    a. Allowing sufficient time for responses
    b. Avoiding medical terminology when possible
    c. Being personal by using terms such as "dear" or "honey"
    d. Incorporating effective body language in communicating

20. Which of the following may be appropriate when communicating with a patient who speaks another language?

    a. Shout in a very loud voice
    b. Do not attempt any further communication until you arrive at the hospital
    c. Use a translator if one is available and time permits
    d. Do not initiate transport until a translator arrives at the scene

21. It is appropriate to use medical terms when communicating with:

    a. The patient
    b. The patient's family
    c. Other EMTs
    d. Bystanders

List three special problems or techniques that the EMT may encounter or perform when dealing with elderly patients.

22. ______________________________

23. ______________________________

24. ______________________________

List four special problems or techniques that the EMT may encounter or perform when dealing with the sick or injured child.

25. ______________________________

26. ______________________________

27. ______________________________

28. ______________________________

List four special problems or techniques that the EMT may encounter or perform when dealing with a deaf patient.

29. ______________________________

30. ______________________________

31. ______________________________

32. ______________________________

List three special problems or techniques that the EMT may encounter or perform when dealing with a blind patient.

33. ______________________________

34. ______________________________

35. ______________________________

List five special problems or techniques that the EMT may encounter or perform when dealing with a confused patient.

36. ______________________________

37. ______________________________

38. ______________________________

39. ______________________________

40. ______________________________

List four special problems or techniques that the EMT may encounter or perform when dealing with patients who are mentally challenged.

41. ______________________________

42. ______________________________

43. ______________________________

44. ______________________________

Questions 45 to 47 refer to the following scenario.

> You are called to respond to the local community college, where you encounter a 19-year-old woman who was stung by a bee. The patient tells you that her sister is allergic to bees and she is afraid that she might be also. She has some slight swelling on her arm at the site of the sting but no other complaints.

45. You call medical control and speak with a physician to determine if you should administer an Epi-Pen to this patient. This type of communication is called:

    a. Online medical control
    b. Offline medical control
    c. Standing orders
    d. Protocols

46. In the past, your radio communication system from your ambulance to the base physician has not been reliable because of poor signal strength. The recent addition of a ____________ to your radio system boosts the signal strength and allows for more reliable communications.

47. While you are concluding your call with the base physician, a local taxicab company begins to break into your radio communication. You are concerned that this type of radio interference could jeopardize emergency communications and you report this incident to your supervisor. Your supervisor reports this incident to the governmental agency responsible for regulating radio communications in the United States. This agency is the:

    a. Center for Radio Control (CRC)
    b. Emergency Medical Services Dispatching Coordinator (EMSDC)
    c. Frequency Allocation Agency (FAA)
    d. Federal Communications Commission (FCC)

Across

1. Person who gets the calls for assistance
3. Radios that transmit with low power and limited range
7. Governmental agency responsible for regulating radio communications
8. Method by which biologic data are transferred from one location to another by radio
9. Receives requests for emergency assistance
12. Trained personnel who give medical instructions to the person who placed the call for help
14. To sort calls by priority
16. The person who communicates with field personnel
17. _____ is used to transmit a patient's electrocardiogram
19. History of the present illness
20. The hub for communications throughout the EMS network

Down

2. PTT feature on a radio
4. A parent should be allowed to _____ a child
5. Real-time medical direction is given by an _____ _____
6. Government agency that developed the EMS Dispatcher National Standard Curriculum
8. _____ patients have heightened senses
9. The central nervous system of EMS
10. Device that retransmits a radio signal at a higher power
11. A term used to describe a hazardous materials incident
13. Radios that are capable of transmitting and receiving information in the vehicles
15. _____ patients should be treated with respect
18. Electrocardiogram

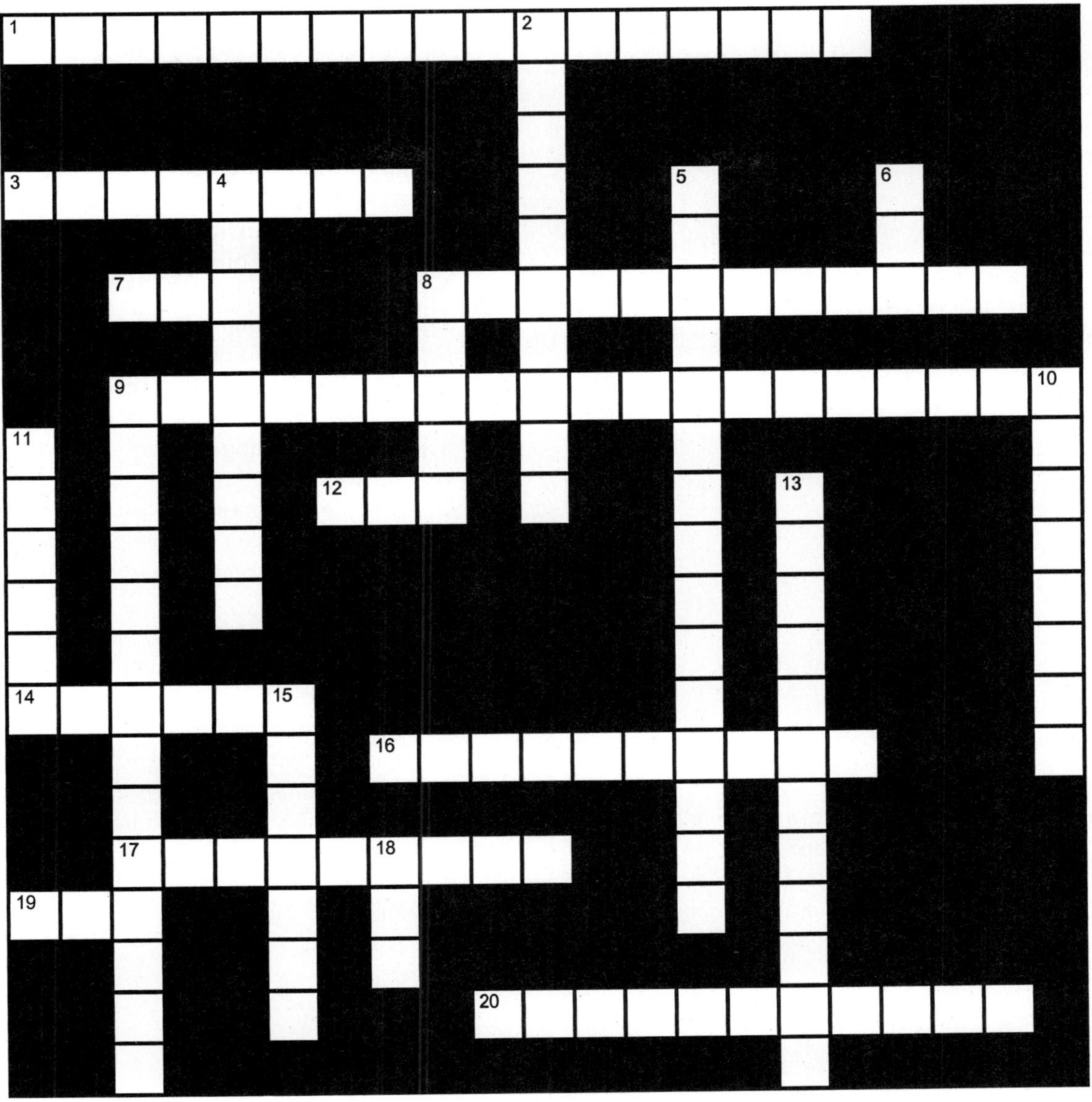
1
2
3
4
5
6
7
8
9
10
11
12
13
14
15
16
17
18
19
20

ANSWER KEY

1. d
2. a
3. b
4. d
5. b
6. b
7. a
8. c
9. c
10. b
11. a
12. b
13. d
14. a
15. c
16. c
17. d
18. b
19. c
20. c
21. c
22. Treat with special respect
23. Move the elderly with extra care
24. Be sensitive to the spouse's concerns
25. Allow the parent to accompany the child
26. Bring along objects that help make the child feel more secure
27. Interact with both the parent and the child
28. Be honest with the child
29. If the patient can read lips, look directly at his or her face and speak in a normal, slow voice
30. Uses short written questions as necessary
31. Be patient
32. Explain to the patient what you are doing
33. Maintain physical contact with the blind patient
34. Describe in detail what you are doing
35. If the patient has a support dog, bring the dog with the patient or arrange for care of the dog
36. Use simple terms
37. Give simple explanations
38. Reinforce orientation and simple explanations
39. Allow the patient ample time to respond to questions
40. Assume that the patient can understand what you are saying
41. Give simple explanations and reinforcement
42. Determine the capability of the patient to understand
43. Distinguish mental from physical disability
44. Assume that the patient can understand what you are saying
45. a
46. Repeater
47. d

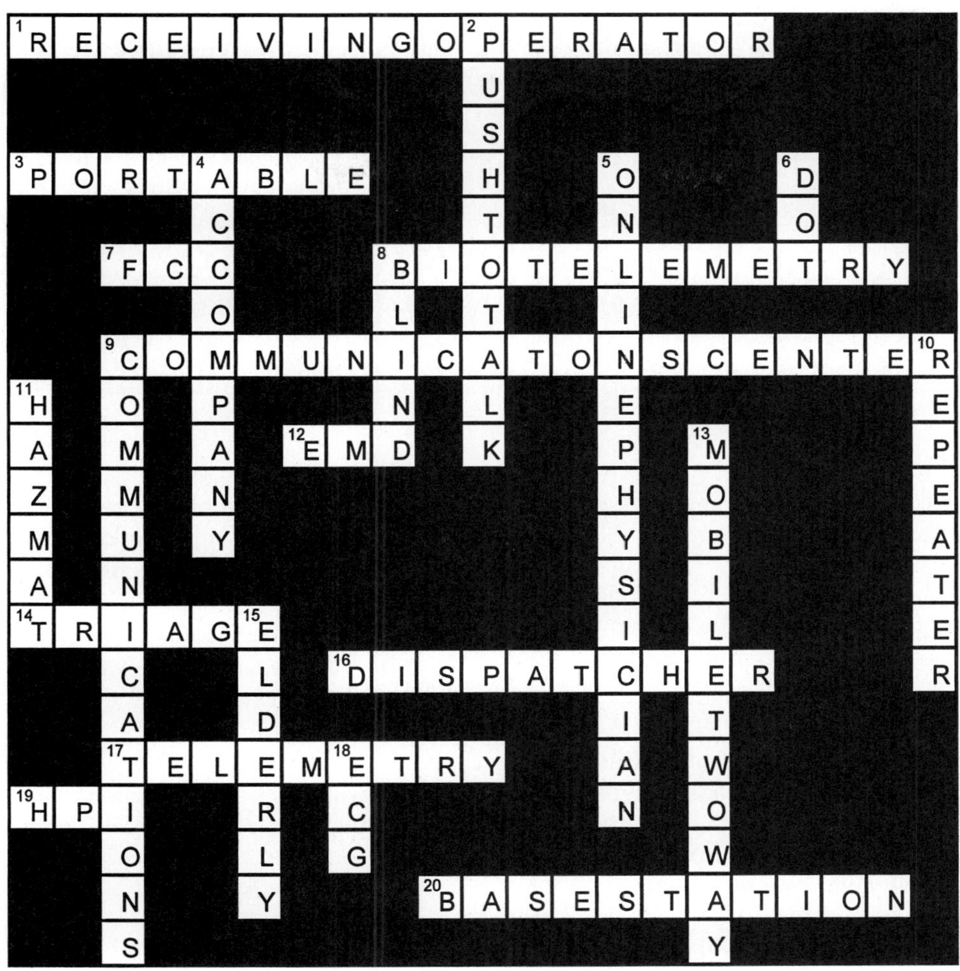
RECEIVINGOPERATOR
PUSHTOTALK
PORTABLE
ACCOCOMPANY
ONLINEPHYSICIAN
DO
FCC
BIOTELEMETRY
BLN
COMMUNICATIONSCENTER
REPEATER
HAZMAT
COMMUNICATIONS
EMD
MOBILETWOWAY
TRIAGE
ELDERLY
DISPATCHER
TELEMETRY
ECG
HPI
BASESTATION

Chapter 15 Documentation

1. Which of the following is not a component of the written prehospital care report?

   a. Patient data
   b. Administrative information
   c. Accurate accounting of time
   d. Mechanical condition of the ambulance

2. The written prehospital care report should include all the following essential information *except*:

   a. A statement that the patient is drunk
   b. The patient's skin color and temperature
   c. The patient's pulse rate
   d. The time the ambulance arrived on the scene

3. The narrative section of the written prehospital care report is used to:

   a. Relay the facts regarding how you found the patient
   b. Definitively conclude what happened to the patient
   c. Document the radio codes used on the call
   d. Record the patient's vital signs

4. Run data include all the following *except*:

   a. The date of the call
   b. The time the call was received
   c. The name of the patient
   d. The names of the crew members

5. Effective record keeping includes the systematic collection of data from the dispatch phase through the transfer of care to the emergency department staff. Which of the following information is least desirable?

   a. The location of the call
   b. The name of the person calling for assistance
   c. The patient assessment
   d. Changes in patient condition

6. In what section of the prehospital care report are the patient's chief complaint, level of consciousness, and blood pressure recorded?

   a. Assessment data
   b. Treatment data
   c. Patient disposition
   d. Run data

7. In what section of the prehospital care report is the application of a splint documented?

   a. Patient disposition
   b. Run data
   c. Patient data
   d. Treatment data

8. In what section of the prehospital care report are the receiving hospital and the emergency department staff member accepting the patient documented?

   a. Patient disposition
   b. Run data
   c. Patient data
   d. Treatment data

9. The information ascertained during the treatment of the patient, such as vital signs, is part of the:

   a. Dispatch data
   b. Patient data
   c. Assessment data
   d. Treatment data

10. Most emergency medical services systems use military times to document the respective phases of a call. In military time, 3:00 PM is expressed as:

    a. 1300 hours
    b. 1400 hours
    c. 1500 hours
    d. 1600 hours

11. Noon is expressed in military time as:

    a. 0000 hours
    b. 1200 hours
    c. 2400 hours
    d. 0100 hours

12. Which of the following represents the best or objective documentation of a suspected case of alcohol intoxication on an ambulance call report?

    a. The patient appeared intoxicated with an alcohol-like compound
    b. There was an alcohol-like smell on the patient's breath
    c. The patient was speaking as if he was intoxicated
    d. The patient was extremely intoxicated

13. Which of these statements is least effective when documenting biologic death in the patient data section of the written prehospital care report?

    a. The patient was dead for 30 minutes before our arrival
    b. The patient has extreme dependent lividity on the back and posterior legs
    c. The patient has evidence of rigor mortis in all extremities
    d. The patient has sustained severe destruction of the skull and brain from the fall

14. The effectiveness of a written prehospital care report depends on which of the following four major factors?

    a. Accuracy, clarity, chronology, completeness
    b. Legibility, clarity, judgment, accuracy
    c. Clarity, accuracy, completeness, judgment
    d. Legibility, honesty, accuracy, completeness

15. The refusal signature is of no value unless you:

    a. Inform the patient of the potential consequences of refusal
    b. Have at least two copies of the refusal
    c. Have a police officer witness the refusal
    d. Have rendered at least some first aid care

16. Which of the following people is least effective as a witness to refusal of care?

    a. The patient's family member
    b. A bystander
    c. Your partner
    d. A police officer

17. Information you receive concerning a patient's condition can:

    a. Be told to the general public
    b. Be told only to a friend
    c. Be told to reporters as requested
    d. Be documented and told to the emergency department staff

18. Which of the following patients has the right to refuse medical aid?

    a. An unconscious patient with a diabetic history
    b. A competent adult patient with a wrist injury
    c. A 6-year-old girl who was struck by a car
    d. A diabetic patient with an altered level of consciousness

19. Which of the following actions is not appropriate for the competent adult patient who refuses medical aid?

    a. Consultation with your local medical control physician
    b. Ensuring that the patient can make a rational, informed decision
    c. Attempting to persuade the patient to seek medical attention
    d. Applying restraints and transporting the patient to the nearest emergency department

20. If you are treating a minor or unconscious patient, it is best to:

    a. Render care to your level of training and transport the patient
    b. Withhold transport until a relative can be located
    c. Have a bystander accompany the patient to the hospital
    d. Transport the patient with a police officer

21. Reviewing written prehospital care reports to evaluate effectiveness of prehospital care is called:

    a. Legal protection
    b. Peer review
    c. Continuing education
    d. Continuous quality improvement

22. When an error of omission occurs, the EMT should:

    a. Falsify the information on the written prehospital care report
    b. Document what would have been done according to local protocol
    c. Rewrite the written prehospital care report to reflect what should have happened
    d. Document what actually did or did not happen and what steps, if any, were taken to correct the situation

23. To correct an error that occurs while writing the prehospital care report, you should:

    a. Obliterate the error and start over
    b. Draw a single horizontal line through the error, initial, and rewrite the correct information
    c. Draw two diagonal lines that form an **x** through the error, initial, and rewrite the correct information
    d. Destroy all copies and start over

24. The distribution and use of the written prehospital care report are determined by:

    a. The patient
    b. State and local protocol
    c. The chief of your ambulance agency
    d. Your EMT instructor

Write in the abbreviation or symbol for the each of the following:

25. Male ________________

26. Female ________________

27. Before ________________

28. Blood pressure ________________

29. Bag-valve-mask ________________

30. With ________________

31. Complaining of ________________

32. Cardiopulmonary resuscitation

    ____

33. Date of birth ________________

34. History ________________

35. Left lower quadrant ________________

36. Left upper quadrant ________________

37. Nitroglycerin ________________

38. Oxygen ________________

39. By mouth ________________

40. Patient ________________

41. Physical examination ________________

42. Right lower quadrant ________________

43. Right upper quadrant ________________

44. Sublingual ________________

45. Shortness of breath ________________

46. Treatment ________________

47. Years old ________________

Questions 48 to 50 refer to the following scenario.

> You are dispatched to a call at 2355 hours to care for a patient with injuries from a fall. On arrival you find a 15-year-old boy who injured his left thumb when he tripped into a wall. The patient is staying with a 16-year-old friend; there are no adults present. The patient tells you that the injury is very minor and that he will wait until his parents arrive in approximately 2 hours.

48. You arrive at the scene of this call at 10 minutes after midnight. The proper way to document this time is:

    a. 12:10 AM
    b. 0010 hours
    c. 2410 hours
    d. 0110 hours

49. The patient data that you document on the prehospital care report for this patient include all the following *except:*

    a. Patient's name
    b. Patient's age
    c. Time of arrival at the scene
    d. Patient's date of birth

50. This patient wants to refuse aid. You know that:

    a. The patient can refuse aid because he is an emancipated minor
    b. The patient must be treated under the concept of implied consent because of the injury and transported to the hospital
    c. The patient is a minor and cannot refuse medical aid
    d. The friend can sign the refusal for the patient

Across

2. The expression of the patient's main problem in his or her own words
5. History (abbreviation)
7. Bag-valve-mask (abbreviation)
8. By mouth (abbreviation)
10. Physical examination (abbreviation)
12. A medical record and legal document that is a complete record of a call
15. Treatment (abbreviation)
16. Information regarding the dispatch of a call
17. Nitroglycerin (abbreviation)
18. Muscle rigidity following death
21. _____ and honesty are vital in avoiding jeopardizing care of patients
23. Demographic information about the victim
24. No information should be given to anyone other than essential personnel regarding the patient's condition as it is _____
25. Sublingual (abbreviation)

Down

1. Time relationships
3. c/o
4. Mnemonic used to remember the assessment of a patient's mental status
6. Call review sessions are a primary means of _____ _____ for EMTs
7. Blood pressure (abbreviation)
9. Mottling of the dependent areas of the body
11. _____ _____ improvement reports are reviewed to evaluate the effectiveness of prehospital care
13. Patient (abbreviation)
14. y/o
19. During a disaster, _____ _____ are used for notation of a patient's status
20. Mnemonic to remember the key questions in a patient's history
22. PCRs should be written with _____ so that they are easily understood by the reader

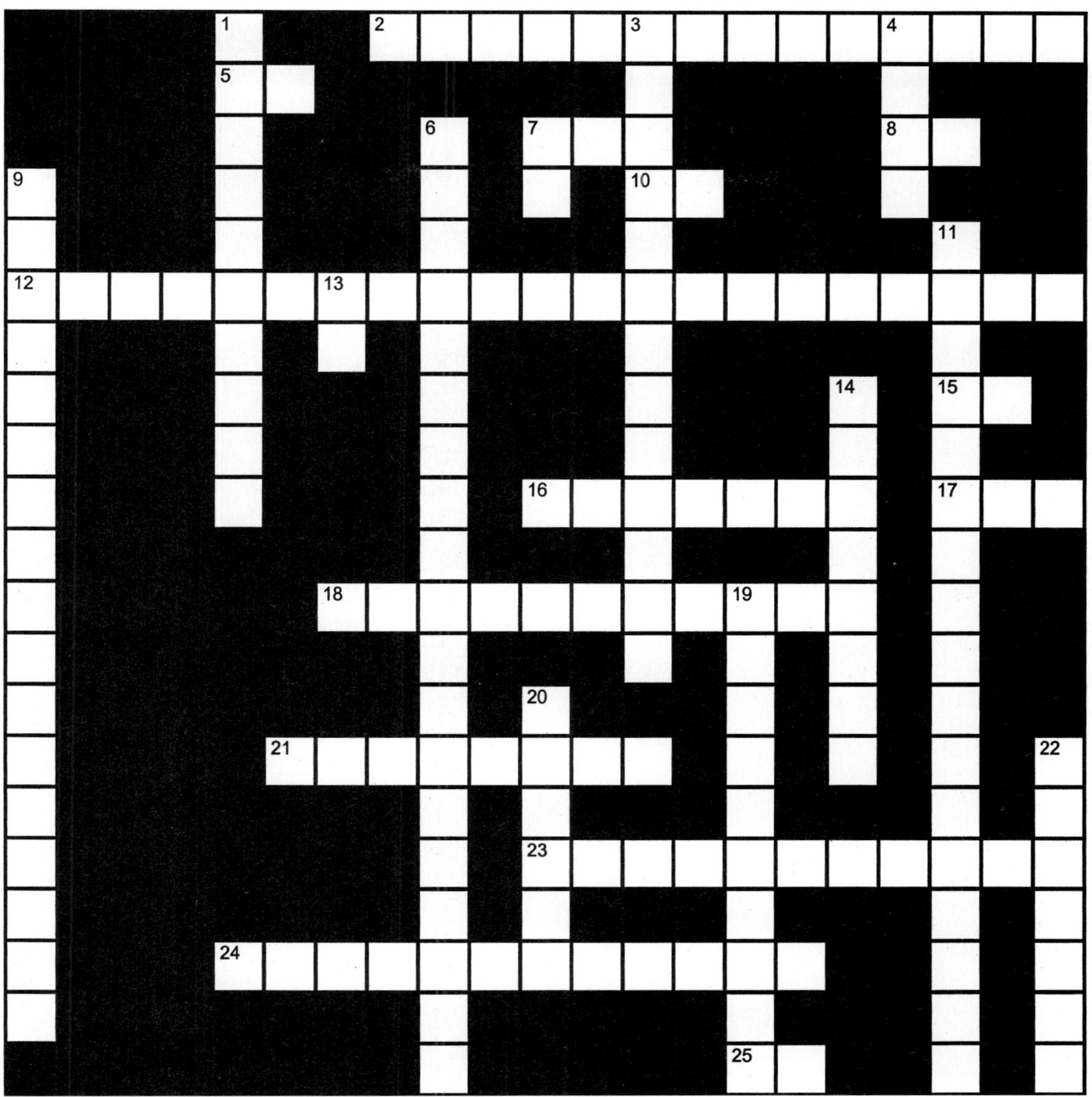

ANSWER KEY

1. d
2. a
3. a
4. c
5. b
6. a
7. d
8. a
9. c
10. c
11. b
12. b
13. a
14. a
15. a
16. c
17. d
18. b
19. d
20. a
21. d
22. d
23. b
24. b
25. ♂
26. ♀
27. $\bar{a}$
28. BP
29. BVM
30. $\bar{c}$
31. c/o
32. CPR
33. DOB
34. Hx
35. LLQ
36. LUQ
37. NTG
38. O_2
39. po
40. pt
41. Px
42. RLQ
43. RUQ
44. SL
45. SOB
46. Tx
47. y/o
48. b
49. c
50. c

<table>
<tr><td></td><td></td><td></td><td></td><td>1 C</td><td></td><td></td><td>2 C</td><td>H</td><td>I</td><td>E</td><td>F</td><td>3 C</td><td>O</td><td>M</td><td>P</td><td>L</td><td>4 A</td><td>I</td><td>N</td><td>T</td></tr>
<tr><td></td><td></td><td></td><td></td><td>5 H</td><td>X</td><td></td><td></td><td></td><td></td><td></td><td></td><td>O</td><td></td><td></td><td></td><td></td><td>V</td><td></td><td></td><td></td></tr>
<tr><td></td><td></td><td></td><td></td><td>R</td><td></td><td></td><td></td><td>6 C</td><td></td><td>7 B</td><td>V</td><td>M</td><td></td><td></td><td></td><td></td><td>8 P</td><td>O</td><td></td><td></td></tr>
<tr><td>9 D</td><td></td><td></td><td></td><td>O</td><td></td><td></td><td></td><td>O</td><td></td><td>P</td><td></td><td>10 P</td><td>X</td><td></td><td></td><td></td><td>U</td><td></td><td></td><td></td></tr>
<tr><td>E</td><td></td><td></td><td></td><td>N</td><td></td><td></td><td></td><td>N</td><td></td><td></td><td></td><td>L</td><td></td><td></td><td></td><td></td><td></td><td>11 C</td><td></td><td></td></tr>
<tr><td>12 P</td><td>R</td><td>E</td><td>H</td><td>O</td><td>S</td><td>13 P</td><td>I</td><td>T</td><td>A</td><td>L</td><td>C</td><td>A</td><td>R</td><td>E</td><td>R</td><td>E</td><td>P</td><td>O</td><td>R</td><td>T</td></tr>
<tr><td>E</td><td></td><td></td><td></td><td>L</td><td></td><td>T</td><td></td><td>I</td><td></td><td></td><td></td><td>I</td><td></td><td></td><td></td><td></td><td></td><td>N</td><td></td><td></td></tr>
<tr><td>N</td><td></td><td></td><td></td><td>O</td><td></td><td></td><td></td><td>N</td><td></td><td></td><td></td><td>N</td><td></td><td></td><td></td><td>14 Y</td><td></td><td>15 T</td><td>X</td><td></td></tr>
<tr><td>D</td><td></td><td></td><td></td><td>G</td><td></td><td></td><td></td><td>U</td><td></td><td></td><td></td><td>I</td><td></td><td></td><td></td><td>E</td><td></td><td>I</td><td></td><td></td></tr>
<tr><td>E</td><td></td><td></td><td></td><td>Y</td><td></td><td></td><td></td><td>I</td><td></td><td>16 R</td><td>U</td><td>N</td><td>D</td><td>A</td><td>T</td><td>A</td><td></td><td>17 N</td><td>T</td><td>G</td></tr>
<tr><td>N</td><td></td><td></td><td></td><td></td><td></td><td></td><td></td><td>N</td><td></td><td></td><td></td><td>G</td><td></td><td></td><td></td><td>R</td><td></td><td>U</td><td></td><td></td></tr>
<tr><td>T</td><td></td><td></td><td></td><td></td><td></td><td>18 R</td><td>I</td><td>G</td><td>O</td><td>R</td><td>M</td><td>O</td><td>R</td><td>19 T</td><td>I</td><td>S</td><td></td><td>O</td><td></td><td></td></tr>
<tr><td>L</td><td></td><td></td><td></td><td></td><td></td><td></td><td></td><td>E</td><td></td><td></td><td></td><td>F</td><td></td><td>R</td><td></td><td>O</td><td></td><td>U</td><td></td><td></td></tr>
<tr><td>I</td><td></td><td></td><td></td><td></td><td></td><td></td><td></td><td>D</td><td></td><td>20 S</td><td></td><td></td><td></td><td>I</td><td></td><td>L</td><td></td><td>S</td><td></td><td></td></tr>
<tr><td>V</td><td></td><td></td><td></td><td></td><td>21 A</td><td>C</td><td>C</td><td>U</td><td>R</td><td>A</td><td>C</td><td>Y</td><td></td><td>A</td><td></td><td>D</td><td></td><td>Q</td><td></td><td>22 C</td></tr>
<tr><td>I</td><td></td><td></td><td></td><td></td><td></td><td></td><td></td><td>C</td><td></td><td>M</td><td></td><td></td><td></td><td>G</td><td></td><td></td><td></td><td>U</td><td></td><td>L</td></tr>
<tr><td>D</td><td></td><td></td><td></td><td></td><td></td><td></td><td></td><td>A</td><td></td><td>23 P</td><td>A</td><td>T</td><td>I</td><td>E</td><td>N</td><td>T</td><td>D</td><td>A</td><td>T</td><td>A</td></tr>
<tr><td>I</td><td></td><td></td><td></td><td></td><td></td><td></td><td></td><td>T</td><td></td><td>L</td><td></td><td></td><td></td><td>T</td><td></td><td></td><td></td><td>L</td><td></td><td>R</td></tr>
<tr><td>T</td><td></td><td></td><td></td><td>24 C</td><td>O</td><td>N</td><td>F</td><td>I</td><td>D</td><td>E</td><td>N</td><td>T</td><td>I</td><td>A</td><td>L</td><td></td><td></td><td>I</td><td></td><td>I</td></tr>
<tr><td>Y</td><td></td><td></td><td></td><td></td><td></td><td></td><td></td><td>O</td><td></td><td></td><td></td><td></td><td></td><td>G</td><td></td><td></td><td></td><td>T</td><td></td><td>T</td></tr>
<tr><td></td><td></td><td></td><td></td><td></td><td></td><td></td><td></td><td>N</td><td></td><td></td><td></td><td></td><td></td><td>25 S</td><td>L</td><td></td><td></td><td>Y</td><td></td><td>Y</td></tr>
</table>

Chapter 16 General Pharmacology

1. All the following medications are likely to be carried on the EMT ambulance *except:*

   a. Nitroglycerin
   b. Glucose gel
   c. Oxygen
   d. Activated charcoal

2. Which of the following prescribed medications may an EMT assist with administration when a patient has the medication available?

   a. Epinephrine
   b. Atropine
   c. Digoxin
   d. Lidocaine

3. A simple form of the chemical name of a medication is called the:

   a. Trade name
   b. Biochemical name
   c. Basic name
   d. Generic name

4. Situations in which a drug should not be used because it may cause harm to the patient or have no effect is called a:

   a. Side effect
   b. Complication
   c. Contraindication
   d. Adverse reaction

Match the name of a drug in column B to the correct form of the drug in column A.

Column A	Column B
5. _____ Tablet	a. Activated charcoal
6. _____ Suspension	b. Epinephrine
7. _____ Gel	c. Oxygen
8. _____ Liquid for injection	d. Nitroglycerin
9. _____ Gas	e. Oral glucose

10. What is a common route of administration for nitroglycerin?

    a. Intramuscular
    b. Sublingual
    c. Intravenous
    d. Inhaler

11. Which of the following doses is equivalent to 1 g?

    a. 10 mg
    b. 100 mg
    c. 1000 mg
    d. 1000 μg

12. What is a key consideration when administering activated charcoal?

    a. Drinking it very slowly to ensure absorption
    b. Mixing it with milk to create the appropriate mixture
    c. Drinking 2 teaspoons at a time
    d. Shaking it before administration

13. The effects of a drug on organs other than the desired action are called:

    a. Adverse reactions
    b. Side effects
    c. Contraindications
    d. Complications

14. Which of the following patients is most likely to be a candidate for glucose administration?

    a. A patient who is dehydrated
    b. A patient who is vomiting
    c. A patient with an altered mental state
    d. A patient with chest pain

Match the drug names in column A with their type in column B.

Column A	Column B
15. ____ Glucose	a. Generic
16. ____ Epi-Pen	b. Trade
17. ____ Actidose	
18. ____ Alupent	
19. ____ Nitrostat	
20. ____ Epinephrine	
21. ____ Albuterol	

22. The science that deals with the origin, nature, chemistry, effects, and uses of drugs is called

    ___________.

23. A ___________ is any chemical compound that may be administered to someone as an aid in the treatment or improvement of an abnormal condition.

List the four rights of medication administration:

24. ___________________________________

25. ___________________________________

26. ___________________________________

27. ___________________________________

28. A child weighs 22 lbs. How many kilograms does this child weigh? ___________

29. The medication that is carried on the ambulance, which is often packaged as a suspension and may be used to treat certain suspected toxic ingestions at the direction of medical control, is called

    ___________.

30. 1 L of fluid contains ___________ mL.

Questions 31 to 33 refer to the following scenario.

> You are called to the scene of an attempted suicide. The scene is secured and the police are present. Your patient is a 16-year-old girl who tells you that she wanted to kill herself and that she took 20 tablets of acetaminophen, each containing 500 mg. The patient weighs 110 pounds. At the present time the patient is stable with a pulse rate of 80, blood pressure of 116/72 mm Hg, and a respiratory rate of 16 breaths/min.

31. As per your protocol, you call the regional poison control center to determine if any interventions should be initiated on the scene. The nurse specialist on the phone asks you to calculate the patient's weight in kilograms so that they can determine if the quantity of medication taken is at the toxic level. This patient weighs:

    a. 40 kg
    b. 50 kg
    c. 60 kg
    d. 70 kg

32. You would anticipate that the poison control center would advise you to:

    a. Administer an Epi-Pen
    b. Administer an Epi-Pen Jr.
    c. Provide emotional and medical support for the patient and transport her to the hospital
    d. Induce vomiting by placing your gloved finger in the back of the patient's mouth

33. Albuterol is a:

    a. Trade name
    b. Biochemical name
    c. Basic name
    d. Generic name

Questions 34 to 36 refer to the following scenario.

> You respond to a call in an apartment complex and find a 53-year-old man complaining of left-sided chest pressure that radiates down his left arm. The patient appears pale and sweaty. The patient has a cardiac history and has a bottle of nitroglycerin with him. He has not taken the nitroglycerin and you notice that the medication is prescribed to him and it is not out of date. The patient has a blood pressure of 156/88 mm Hg, heart rate is 88 beats/min and regular, and the respiratory rate is 14 breaths/min. The patient tells you that he is not allergic to anything, his only past medical history is a heart attack 2 years ago, and he took Viagra about 1 hour ago.

34. In this scenario you would not assist this patient in taking a nitroglycerin tablet because you know that Viagra may interact with the nitroglycerin and produce unwanted and possibly harmful effects. This is called:

    a. A contraindication
    b. A complication
    c. A side effect
    d. An adverse reaction

35. After the call is over, you critique the call with your partner and review the reasons for not assisting the patient in taking nitroglycerin. Your partner, who is studying to be an EMT, tells you that on a previous call a patient took a nitroglycerin tablet but then complained of a headache. You tell him that that was:

    a. A contraindication in taking the drug
    b. A complication in taking the drug
    c. A side effect of taking the drug
    d. An adverse reaction that is life threatening

36. You remember that if you were to assist a patient in taking a nitroglycerin tablet that this medication is administered:

    a. By a nebulizer connected to an oxygen source
    b. Rectally
    c. With an auto injector
    d. Sublingually

Across

2. Common means of administering drugs through the skin such as a nitroglycerin patch
5. A condition or disease for which a drug is expected to have a beneficial effect
9. Premeasured amounts of drug to be administered
10. The generic name for an Epi-Pen
12. The trade name for Ventolin
14. Solid particles mixed in a liquid
17. A way of administering medications through the bone
19. Medication carried by the EMT-Basic that is a gas
20. Method of administration of a medication by swallowing
21. Medication in spray form

Down

1. Chemical compound administered to someone for treatment of disease or relief from pain
3. After administration of a drug a patient must be _______ for the effects and side effects the drug may have had
4. Layer of fat and connective tissue beneath the skin where epinephrine is injected
6. The amount of drug necessary to provide the desired effect, yet low enough to minimize side effects
7. This name of a medication is a simple form of its chemical name
8. The generic name for SuperChar
11. Quantity of a drug to be administered at one time
13. Metric term for the weight of drugs
14. Under the tongue
15. The trade name for nitroglycerin
16. The desired effect a drug has on the body or target organ
18. This name of a medication is given to it by the pharmaceutical company that makes it

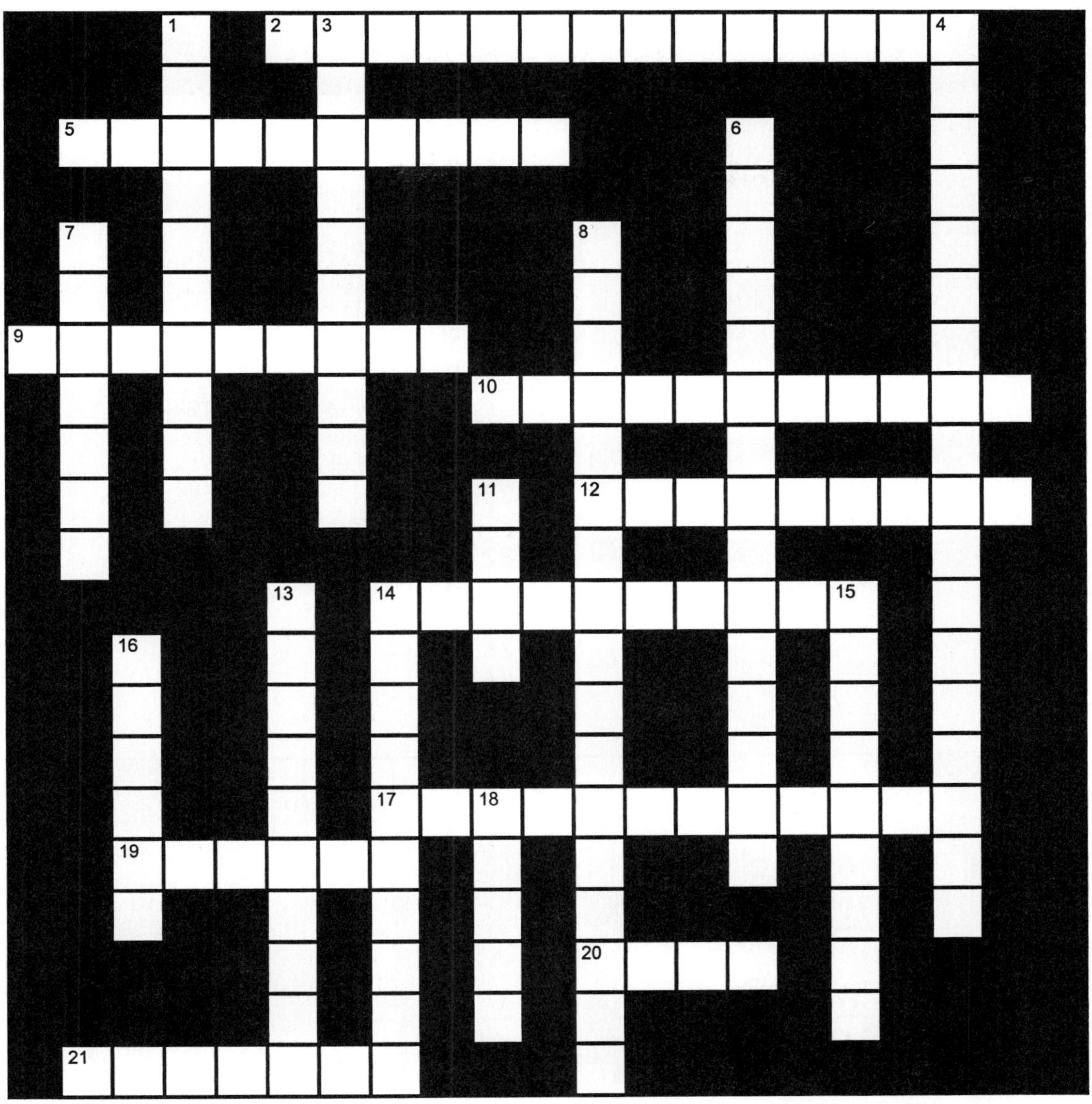
1
2
3
4
5
6
7
8
9
10
11
12
13
14
15
16
17
18
19
20
21

ANSWER KEY

1. a
2. a
3. d
4. c
5. d
6. a
7. e
8. b
9. c
10. b
11. c
12. d
13. b
14. c
15. a
16. b
17. b
18. b
19. b
20. a
21. a
22. Pharmacology
23. Medication (drug)
24. Right patient
25. Right drug
26. Right dose
27. Right route of administration
28. 10 kg
29. Activated charcoal
30. 1000
31. b
32. c
33. d
34. a
35. c
36. d

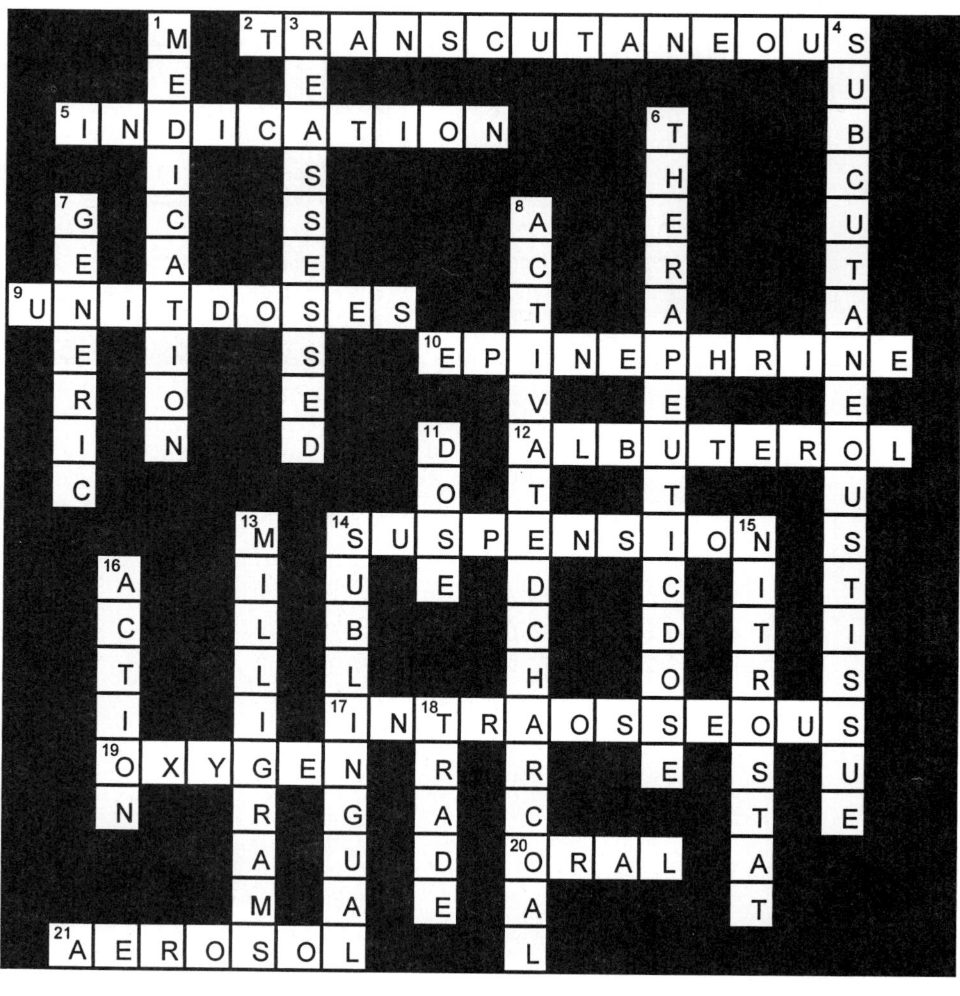

Chapter 17 Respiratory Emergencies

1. The structure that covers the trachea during swallowing to prevent aspiration is called the:

   a. Pharynx
   b. Epiglottis
   c. Thyroid cartilage
   d. Cricoid cartilage

2. The respiratory structure that is palpable just above the sternum is the:

   a. Bronchus
   b. Trachea
   c. Carina
   d. Bronchiole

3. The muscle that separates the chest and abdomen is called the:

   a. Diaphragm
   b. Intercostals
   c. Abdominis recti
   d. None of the above

4. The normal resting tidal volume for an adult is approximately:

   a. 500 mL
   b. 800 mL
   c. 1000 mL
   d. 2000 mL

5. The process by which gases move from an area of higher concentration to an area of lower concentration is called:

   a. Ventilation
   b. Respiration
   c. Diffusion
   d. Transportation

6. The portion of the lung where diffusion takes place is called the:

   a. Bronchi
   b. Pleura
   c. Bronchiole
   d. Alveoli

7. The amount of air inhaled and exhaled during a given breath is called the:

   a. Residual volume
   b. Expiratory reserve
   c. Total volume
   d. Tidal volume

8. Normal atmospheric air contains approximately what percentage of oxygen?

   a. 15%
   b. 21%
   c. 28%
   d. 50%

9. A term commonly used to describe a feeling of difficulty breathing is:

   a. Hemoptysis
   b. Tachypnea
   c. Dyspnea
   d. Ischemia

10. A bluish discoloration of the skin caused by oxygen-poor hemoglobin is called:

    a. Mottling
    b. Ecchymosis
    c. Cyanosis
    d. Anoxic erythema

11. The accessory muscles of inspiration are noted primarily by observing the:

    a. Chest wall
    b. Neck
    c. Abdominal wall
    d. Back

12. A high-pitched sound that is emitted from the lower airway that usually occurs on expiration and may be caused by asthma or chronic obstructive pulmonary disease is called:

    a. Wheeze
    b. Stridor
    c. Rhonchi
    d. Crackles

13. During positive-pressure ventilation, effective tidal volume is evaluated primarily on the basis of:

    a. Chest rise
    b. Skin color
    c. Pupil response
    d. None of the above

14. The most common complication of excessive or forceful ventilation is:

    a. Pneumothorax
    b. Gastric distention
    c. Oxygen toxicity
    d. Air embolism

15. A patient who is exhibiting wheezing, stridor, accessory muscle use, and a weak, ineffective cough probably has a:

    a. Complete airway obstruction
    b. Partial airway obstruction with good air exchange
    c. Partial airway obstruction with poor air exchange
    d. None of the above

16. All the following signs are associated with complete upper airway obstruction *except*:

    a. Hand on the throat
    b. Inability to speak
    c. Absent breath sounds on one side
    d. Inability to cough

17. The most definitive sign of a complete airway obstruction in a conscious patient is:

    a. Cyanosis of the skin
    b. Wheezing on inspiration
    c. Snoring on expiration
    d. Inability to speak

18. In a pregnant woman, the correct location for a chest thrust to relieve a foreign body obstruction is:

    a. The upper portion of the sternum
    b. The sternum on the nipple line
    c. The lower half of the sternum
    d. Directly over the xiphoid process

19. If the initial attempt at ventilation is unsuccessful in an unconscious patient, you should next:

    a. Deliver four back blows
    b. Deliver four abdominal thrusts
    c. Reopen the airway and attempt ventilation
    d. Perform a finger sweep

20. When attempting to clear a complete airway obstruction in the unconscious patient, how many abdominal thrusts should you administer?

    a. Up to 2
    b. Up to 5
    c. Up to 8
    d. Up to 10

21. In a child or infant with a complete airway obstruction, you should perform a finger sweep only if:

    a. The patient is conscious
    b. The epiglottis is visible
    c. Three attempts at ventilation are unsuccessful
    d. You can visualize the object

22. In which of the following patients can back blows be used in the treatment of a complete airway obstruction?

    a. Less than 1 year old
    b. 1 to 8 years old
    c. 8 to 10 years old
    d. More than 10 years old

23. A patient who is breathing rapidly and shallowly at a rate of 36 breaths/min and who is unresponsive should receive:

    a. Oxygen by nonrebreather mask
    b. Positive-pressure ventilation
    c. Oxygen by nasal cannula
    d. Oxygen by Venturi mask

24. A possible complication of high-concentration oxygen administration for a chronic obstructive pulmonary disease patient is:

    a. Pneumothorax
    b. Pulmonary embolism
    c. Pneumonia
    d. Respiratory arrest

25. An inflammation of the alveolar spaces caused by various types of infectious organisms or by aspiration of fluid into the tracheobronchial tree is called:

    a. Pneumonia
    b. Pleurisy
    c. Pneumothorax
    d. Pulmonary embolism

26. A condition that results from air entering the pleural space and causes total or partial collapse of the lungs is called:

    a. Hemothorax
    b. Pneumothorax
    c. Pleurisy
    d. Pulmonary embolism

27. The most common breath sound associated with a pneumothorax is:

    a. Diminished or absent
    b. Wheezes
    c. Rhonchi
    d. Friction rub

Match the inhaler medications in column A with their drug types in column B.

Column A	Column B
28. _____ Albuterol	a. Generic
29. _____ Atrovent	b. Trade
30. _____ Ventolin	
31. _____ Alupent	
32. _____ Proventil	
33. _____ Metaproterenol	

34. All the following are steps of administration of an inhaler *except*:

    a. Check expiration date on the inhaler
    b. Shake the inhaler vigorously several times
    c. Have patient inhale deeply before administration
    d. Check to see if the patient has taken previous doses

35. Immediately after inhaling the medication, the patient should:

    a. Hyperventilate several times
    b. Cough vigorously to clear airways
    c. Hold his or her breath for as long as comfortable
    d. Lay supine to facilitate absorption

36. A child with epiglottitis may be found sitting upright and leaning forward with his or her weight distributed on the hands, which is known as the

    ____________ position.

37. The number of breaths per minute multiplied by the quantity of air exchanged with each breath is

    called ____________.

38. What is the colorful term used to describe patients

    with emphysema? ____________

39. Inflammation of alveolar spaces caused by

    infection or aspiration is called ____________.

40. A common respiratory problem characterized by a voluntary increase in the rate and volume of breathing often accompanied by anxiety is termed

    ____________.

41. The mnemonic used to assess the mental status of

    a patient is ____________.

42. The rate of artificial ventilation for a nonbreathing

    adult is ____________.

43. The rate of artificial ventilation for a nonbreathing child (ages 1-8 years) is ___________.

44. The rate of artificial ventilation for a nonbreathing infant (<1 year of age) is ___________.

List the six key questions to ask the patient with a respiratory emergency.

45. ____________________________________

46. ____________________________________

47. ____________________________________

48. ____________________________________

49. ____________________________________

50. ____________________________________

Questions 51 to 55 refer to the following scenario.

> You are called to respond to the local elementary school where you find a 7-year-old girl in the nurse's office. The school nurse tells you that the girl has a history of asthma and came into the office complaining of difficulty breathing while participating in her gym class. Your evaluation reveals a patient in severe respiratory distress, with a respiratory rate of 36 breaths/min and labored, heart rate of 132 beats/min, and blood pressure of 84/60 mm Hg.

51. As part of your assessment to help determine the severity of the respiratory distress in this child, you would examine the child for signs of severe respiratory distress, which may include all the following *except:*

    a. Nasal flaring
    b. Accessory muscle use in the neck
    c. Pink skin color
    d. Inability to speak in full sentences

52. Your evaluation of this patient's blood pressure reveals a reading that:

    a. Is very low for this patient
    b. Is very high for this patient
    c. Should decrease significantly once the patient's respiratory distress is relieved
    d. Is in the normal range for this patient

53. If this patient is having an asthma attack you would generally expect that auscultation of the lungs will reveal:

    a. Absent breath sounds on one side
    b. Full and clear bilateral breath sounds
    c. Wheezes
    d. Crackles (rales)

54. During transport to the hospital you administer oxygen to your patient by a nonrebreather mask. The patient's respiratory rate decreases from 36 breaths/min to 10 breaths/min. The patient still appears to be in severe respiratory distress. This decrease in respiratory rate is:

    a. An ominous sign that respiratory failure/arrest may be imminent
    b. A sign of oxygen toxicity
    c. An indication that the patient's airway has become obstructed
    d. A good sign that the patient is improving

55. You are approximately 3 minutes from the hospital when the patient stops breathing but still has a pulse at a rate of 124 beats/min. You should:

    a. Begin positive-pressure ventilation at a rate of 12 times per minute until the pop-off valve on your bag-valve-mask is triggered
    b. Begin positive-pressure ventilation at a rate of 20 times per minute until the pop-off valve on your bag-valve-mask is triggered
    c. Begin positive-pressure ventilation at a rate of 12 times per minute until you see chest rise
    d. Begin positive-pressure ventilation at a rate of 20 times per minute until you see chest rise

Questions 56 to 58 refer to the following scenario.

> You respond to a call and find a 63-year-old man in the kitchen in severe respiratory distress. The patient is breathing through pursed lips and his skin appears pink. The patient tells you that he has a history of emphysema and that his breathing difficulty has been worsening for the past 6 hours. The patient's pulse is 104 beats/min, blood pressure is 142/86 mm Hg, and respiratory rate is 24 breaths/min. The patient tells you that he normally smokes three packs of cigarettes a day but today he has only smoked two packs because of his trouble breathing.

56. The type of disease that this patient has is considered:

    a. A type of chronic obstructive pulmonary disease
    b. A severe form of pneumonia
    c. Caused by coronary artery disease
    d. One that can be cured with proper medical care

57. As part of your treatment of this patient you:

    a. Withhold any supplemental oxygen because of the patient's medical history
    b. Administer oxygen by a nasal cannula at 2 L/min
    c. Administer oxygen by a nonrebreather mask
    d. Administer oxygen by a bag-valve-mask device

58. As you further examine the patient you observe that he can be described as having a barrel chest appearance. This is caused by:

    a. Continuous use of supplemental oxygen in the home
    b. Excessive smoking
    c. Excessive alcohol consumption
    d. Air trapping in the lungs

Questions 59 to 60 refer to the following scenario.

> You are called to the scene of the local community college and encounter a 20-year-old woman who is breathing very rapidly. The patient's friends tell you that the patient has anxiety attacks and became very nervous after the final examination scores were posted in her class. The patient is alert and complains only of difficulty breathing associated with tingling about the mouth and fingers. Vital signs are a pulse of 104 beats/min and regular, blood pressure of 116/72 mm Hg, and respiratory rate of 28 breaths/min; the patient has full clear bilateral breath sounds. The patient tells you that she does not take any medications, is not allergic to anything, and only has a history of anxiety attacks.

59. Your treatment for this patient includes:

    a. Having the patient breathe in and out with a paper bag over her mouth and nose
    b. Having the patient hold her breath in an attempt to "break" the attack
    c. Administering oxygen by a nonrebreather oxygen mask
    d. Performing positive-pressure ventilations

60. You have been treating the patient for the past 10 minutes while you transport her to the hospital. Your estimated arrival time at the hospital is 5 minutes. You reevaluate your patient and now her vital signs are pulse of 92 beats/min and regular, blood pressure 112/68 mm Hg, and respiratory rate of 16 breaths/min; the patient has full clear bilateral breath sounds. The change in this patient's respiratory rate is:

    a. An ominous sign of impending respiratory failure/arrest
    b. A good indication that the patient is responding appropriately to treatment
    c. An indication of oxygen toxicity
    d. An indication that that the patient's underlying medical problem may be a pneumothorax

Across

1. Flap of cartilage that covers the larynx during swallowing
4. Term used to describe patients with chronic bronchitis
5. Physical finding that may be found in the neck indicating air leakage under the skin
6. The normal regulation for breathing is the amount of _____ _____ in our blood
11. Place the head of an infant in the _____ position to avoid bending and kinking the soft trachea
12. Medication delivery device commonly used by an asthmatic patient
14. Breathing is controlled by the _____
19. Voluntary increase in the rate and volume of breathing, often accompanied by anxiety
20. In infants and children the internal diameter of the airway is _____ than in adults
25. Whistling noise associated with narrowed bronchioles that may be heard without a stethoscope
27. A way to administer inhalation therapy as a mist
28. Colorful term used to describe patients with emphysema
29. Wet sounds generated by air moving through fluid in the airway

Down

2. Low-pitched sounds associated with partial obstruction of the airway by the tongue
3. Air sacs in the lungs where gas exchange takes place
5. The narrowest part of the pediatric airway
7. Mnemonic used to obtain specific facts regarding a patient's chest pain
8. Diaphragm contracts and pulls downward during _____
9. Bacterial infection causing swelling of the epiglottis
10. Difficult and labored breathing
13. The _____ is large in relation to the airway in a child
14. Bluish discoloration of the mucous membranes or skin
15. A likely side effect of prescribed inhaler administration
16. The high-pitched breath sound heard with narrowing of the upper respiratory tract
17. Acute obstructive respiratory disease with narrowing of the airways
18. Amount of air inspired and expired during one respiratory cycle
21. After the trachea the airway splits into the two main _____
22. Crackles or _____ is a sound similar to rubbing hair together caused by fluid in the airway
23. Position characterized by posture that is upright and leaning forward
24. Chronic obstructive pulmonary disease
26. Respirator mask used to protect against tuberculosis

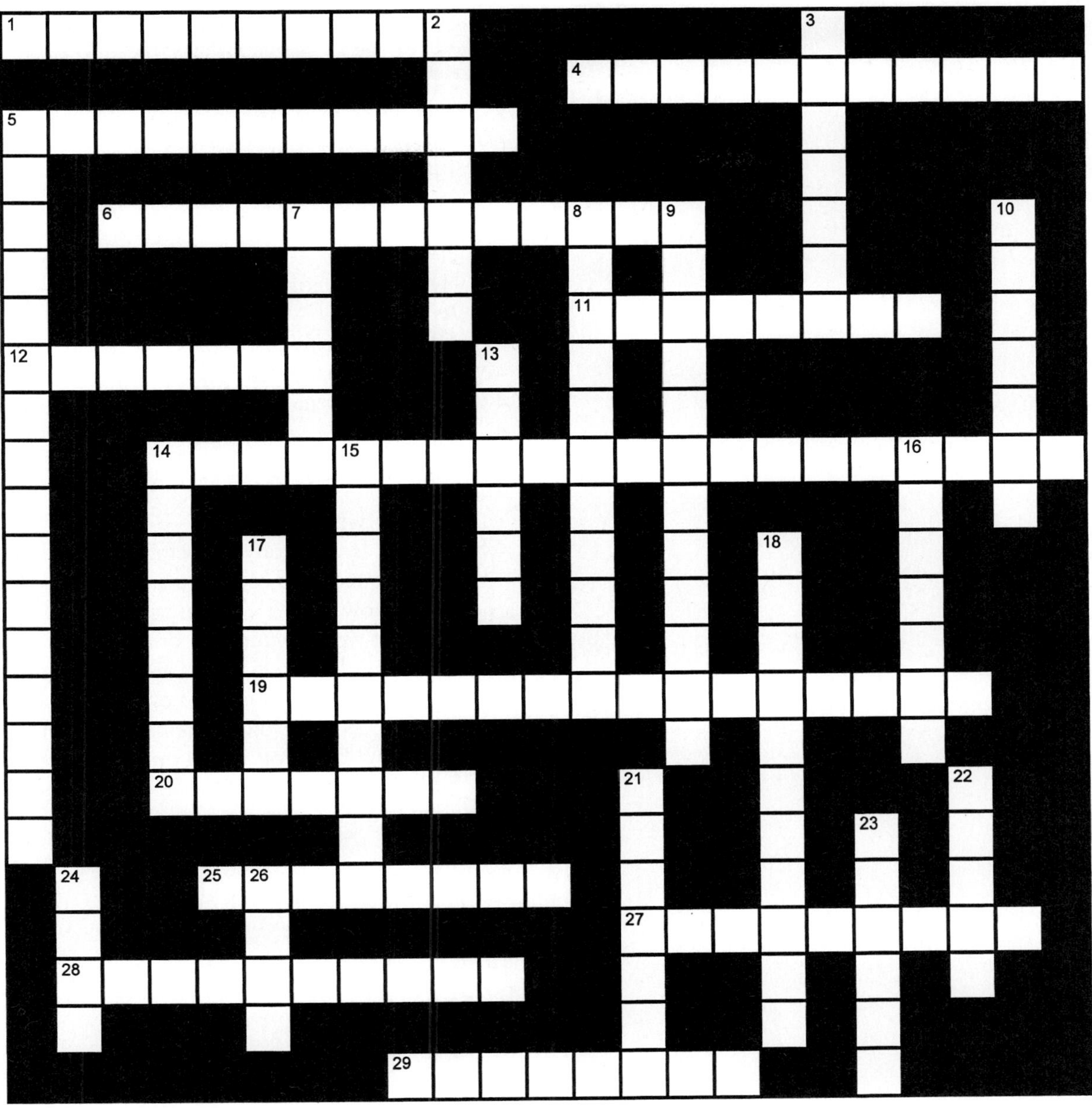
1
2
3
4
5
6
7
8
9
10
11
12
13
14
15
16
17
18
19
20
21
22
23
24
25
26
27
28
29

ANSWER KEY

1. b
2. b
3. a
4. a
5. c
6. d
7. d
8. b
9. c
10. c
11. b
12. a
13. a
14. b
15. c
16. c
17. d
18. c
19. c
20. b
21. d
22. a
23. b
24. d
25. a
26. b
27. a
28. a
29. b
30. b
31. b
32. b
33. a
34. c
35. c
36. Tripod
37. Minute volume
38. Pink puffer
39. Pneumonia
40. Hyperventilation syndrome
41. AVPU
42. 12 times per minute
43. 20 times per minute
44. 20 times per minute
45. Onset: What were you doing when the symptoms began?
46. Provocation: Does anything make your breathing problem worse?
47. Quality: Is there any associated pain? If there is, where is the pain, can you point to it with one finger, how would you describe it, and does the pain get worse when you breathe?
48. Radiation: If you do have pain, does the pain go anywhere, such as to your arm, neck or jaw?
49. Severity: How severe is the shortness of breath (or the pain)? Can you rate it on a scale of 1 to 10?
50. Time: How long have you had the respiratory distress and/or the pain?
51. c
52. d
53. c
54. a
55. d
56. a
57. c
58. d
59. c
60. b

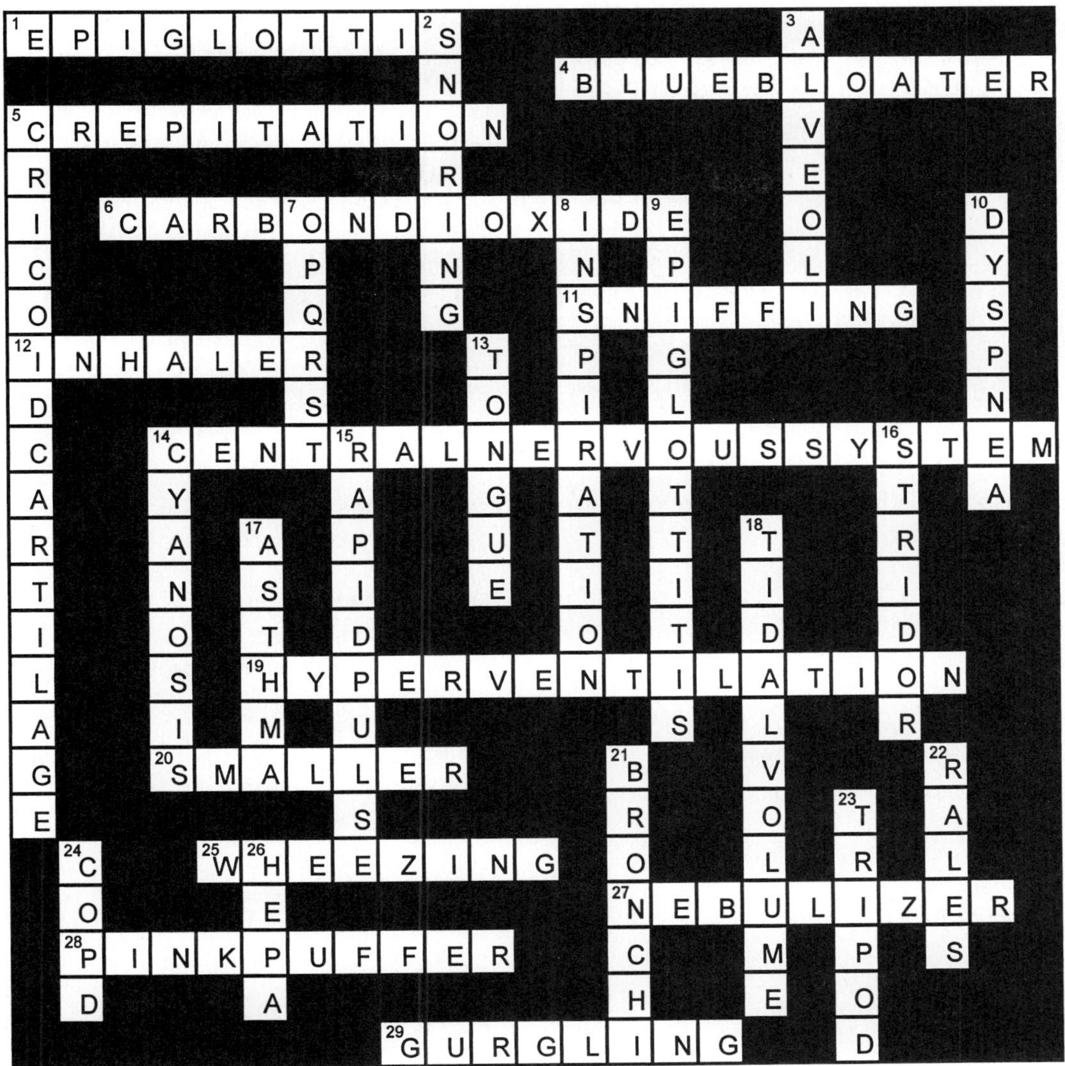

Chapter 18 Cardiovascular Emergencies

1. The protein responsible for the transport of oxygen and carbon dioxide is called:

   a. Protoplasm
   b. Platelets
   c. Plasma
   d. Hemoglobin

2. The cellular portions of the blood that are responsible for combating infection are the:

   a. Platelets
   b. Red blood cells
   c. White blood cells
   d. Hemoglobin

3. The portion of blood responsible for clotting:

   a. Platelets
   b. Red blood cells
   c. White blood cells
   d. Plasma

4. The portion of the heart that pumps blood to the body (systemic circulation) is called the:

   a. Left atrium
   b. Right atrium
   c. Left ventricle
   d. Right ventricle

5. The valve that directs blood into the pulmonary artery during systole and prevents backflow into the right ventricle during diastole is called the:

   a. Aortic valve
   b. Pulmonary semilunar valve
   c. Tricuspid valve
   d. Mitral valve

6. The portion of the conduction system that is the primary pacemaker of the heart is called the:

   a. Sinoatrial node
   b. Purkinje fiber
   c. Atrioventricular node
   d. Bundle of His

7. The amount of blood ejected from the heart with each contraction is called the:

   a. Cardiac output
   b. Tidal volume
   c. Cardiac reserve
   d. Stroke volume

8. Which of the following vessels are most muscular?

   a. Arteries
   b. Veins
   c. Capillaries
   d. Venules

9. The femoral, popliteal, and dorsalis pedis arteries are all located in the:

   a. Head
   b. Lower extremities
   c. Upper extremities
   d. Trunk

10. Which phase of the cardiac cycle does the diastolic pressure best reflect?

    a. Contraction
    b. Relaxation
    c. Intermediate
    d. Rapid firing

Match the layer of the heart in column A with the description in column B.

Column A	**Column B**
11. _____ Myocardium	a. Smooth inner lining
12. _____ Epicardium	b. Outermost layer
13. _____ Endocardium	Thick muscular layer

14. The upper receiving chambers of the heart are called the:

    a. Ventricles
    b. Septum
    c. Atria
    d. Pleura

15. The circulation originating from the left side of the heart is the:

    a. Pulmonary circulation
    b. Systemic circulation
    c. Arterial circulation
    d. Venous circulation

16. The circulation originating from the right side of the heart is the:

    a. Pulmonary circulation
    b. Systemic circulation
    c. Arterial circulation
    d. Venous circulation

17. The valves that control flow from the atria to the

    ventricles are the ___________ valves.

    a. Semilunar
    b. Atrioventricular
    c. Atrial
    d. Ventricular

18. Gas exchange occurs in which of the following vessels?

    a. Arteries
    b. Veins
    c. Capillaries
    d. Venules

19. Shock that occurs from a myocardial infarction (heart attack) is called:

    a. Cardiogenic shock
    b. Distributive shock
    c. Obstructive shock
    d. Hypovolemic shock

20. The progressive narrowing of vessels because of plaque formation on the innermost lining best describes:

    a. Angioedema
    b. Atherosclerosis
    c. Angina pectoris
    d. Ischemia

21. A patient who is demonstrating generalized signs of hypoxia (i.e., cyanosis or altered mental state) and severe chest pain should receive oxygen by a:

    a. Nasal cannula
    b. Nonrebreather mask
    c. Simple face mask
    d. Venturi mask

22. Which is routinely used to self-administer nitroglycerin?

    a. Subcutaneous injection
    b. Intramuscular injection
    c. Ingest solution
    d. Spray or tablet placed under tongue

23. An insufficient supply of blood through a vessel that results in oxygen deprivation to tissue best describes:

    a. Ischemia
    b. Hypoxia
    c. Anoxia
    d. Anemia

24. Blockage of a coronary artery resulting in death of heart tissue defines:

    a. Coronary insufficiency
    b. Myocardial infarction
    c. Angina pectoris
    d. Cardiac arrest

25. Nausea, vomiting, weakness, shortness of breath, palpitations, light-headedness, sweating, dizziness, and loss of consciousness are all possible associated signs of:

    a. Cardiac arrest
    b. Angina pectoris
    c. Myocardial infarction
    d. Oxygen toxicity

26. Chest pain brought on by emotional or physical exertion and relieved by rest best describes:

 a. Pleuritic chest pain
 b. Angina pectoris
 c. Myocardial infarction
 d. Cardiogenic shock

27. The patient should be questioned about high blood pressure, heart disease, chronic obstructive pulmonary disease, and diabetes during the:

 a. Chief complaint
 b. History of present illness
 c. Medications and allergies
 d. Past medical history

28. Nitroglycerin acts to relieve chest pain by which of the following mechanisms?

 a. Increases heart rate
 b. Increases the force of contraction
 c. Causes vasodilation
 d. Increases blood pressure

29. Which of the following terms best describes the classic pain of cardiovascular disease, such as angina or myocardial infarction?

 a. Sharp
 b. Squeezing
 c. Pleuritic
 d. Stabbing

30. The pulse of a patient having a myocardial infarction is usually:

 a. Rapid
 b. Almost any variation
 c. Slow
 d. Irregular

31. A common reaction to serious illness, including myocardial infarction, that often causes the patient to not seek help is referred to as:

 a. Rationalization
 b. Denial
 c. Confabulation
 d. Anxiety syndrome

32. Myocardial infarction patients who have shortness of breath usually prefer to be placed in what position?

 a. Sitting
 b. Supine
 c. Prone
 d. Lateral recumbent

33. Patients who take nitroglycerin may commonly have which of the following side effects?

 a. Hives
 b. Arrhythmias
 c. Headache
 d. Edema

34. The two most important factors in the treatment of prehospital cardiac arrest are CPR and:

 a. Defibrillation
 b. Drug therapy
 c. Intubation
 d. Catheterization

Match the type of heart failure in column B with the signs and symptoms in column A.

Column A	Column B
35. _____ Rales	a. Right-sided heart failure b. Left-sided heart faliure
36. _____ Ankle edema	
37. _____ Frothy sputum	
38. _____ Distended neck veins	
39. _____ Ascites	

40. A 55-year-old man has had severe pressurelike chest pain for the last 3 minutes after walking up two flights of stairs. He is alert and his skin is pale, cool, and sweaty. His vital signs are pulse 100 beats/min and regular, respirations 20 breaths/min and normal, and blood pressure 160/90 mm Hg. What position should this patient be placed in?

 a. Supine
 b. Lateral recumbent
 c. Prone
 d. A position of comfort

41. What is the first and most important treatment provided by the EMT for the patient with chest pain?

    a. Administering oxygen
    b. Rapidly transporting to the hospital
    c. Attaching the automated external defibrillator (AED)
    d. Assisting the patient in the administration of nitroglycerin

42. The patient tells you that he has angina pectoris and is prescribed nitroglycerin but has not taken any today. How should you assist this patient in the administration of a nitroglycerin tablet?

    a. Have him swallow one tablet and drink 10 mL of water
    b. Do not administer the tablet; 3 minutes after the start of the pain is too late to take the tablet
    c. Place one tablet under the tongue and do not drink water
    d. Have him swallow 3 tablets and drink 10 mL of water

43. What is the maximum number of nitroglycerin tablets that a patient can take?

    a. One
    b. Two
    c. Three
    d. Four

44. A patient usually takes one nitroglycerin tablet and achieves relief of chest pain. After taking three tablets today the patient's chest pain decreases slightly. The patient does not want to go to the hospital. The reason that this patient must be urged to go to the hospital is:

    a. Malignant hypertension
    b. Poor brain perfusion
    c. Sweaty skin
    d. Changing pattern of disease

45. If an angina patient's chest pain continues for 20 minutes, which of the following conditions should you suspect?

    a. Angina pectoris
    b. Myocardial infarction
    c. Cardiogenic shock
    d. Heart failure

46. You respond to a call and find a 62-year-old woman complaining of crushing chest pain for 1 hour with pale, sweaty skin. She states that the pain radiates to her left arm and she also feels nausea and dizziness. On physical examination, you note vital signs of a pulse of 110 beats/min and very irregular, blood pressure of 160/100 mm Hg, and respirations of 28 breaths/min and slightly labored. You suspect:

    a. Angina pectoris
    b. Congestive heart failure
    c. Cardiogenic shock
    d. Myocardial infarction

47. What is the most common cause of death from myocardial infarction?

    a. Shock
    b. Ventricular fibrillation
    c. Pulmonary edema
    d. Respiratory failure

48. What is the most common cause of myocardial infarction?

    a. Poor circulation caused by arrhythmias
    b. Blockage of a coronary artery
    c. Overstretching of the ventricle
    d. Bleeding into the arterial wall

49. Besides the prompt application of CPR, which variable will most affect the survival of a cardiac arrest patient?

    a. The size of the heart attack
    b. Time to defibrillation
    c. The ventilation device used during CPR
    d. The compression rate

50. The chaotic electrical rhythm that causes sudden clinical death in most cardiac arrest patients is called:

    a. Ventricular asystole
    b. Ventricular fibrillation
    c. Ventricular tachycardia
    d. Ventricular standstill

51. The origin of prehospital defibrillation dates back to the:

    a. 1940s
    b. 1950s
    c. 1960s
    d. 1970s

52. Defibrillation pads are positioned just below the right clavicle on the right sternal border and:

    a. Just below the left clavicle
    b. Directly over the mid-sternum
    c. Just left of the left nipple, mid-axillary line
    d. Just above the left nipple, mid-clavicular line

53. When treating a patient in cardiac arrest the AED is applied and shocks the patient three times in a row. After the third shock, the appropriate action would be to:

    a. Perform CPR and transport immediately
    b. Perform a precordial thump to stimulate the heart
    c. Press analyze and shock as indicated
    d. Check for signs of circulation; if there are no signs of circulation, perform CPR for 1 minute and reanalyze

54. While en route to the hospital, the patient becomes unconscious and pulseless. While your partner prepares the AED, what immediate action should you take?

    a. Administer oxygen by nonrebreather mask
    b. Perform cardiopulmonary resuscitation
    c. Give nitroglycerin
    d. Monitor the pulse and breathing

55. You defibrillate the patient and the machine advises you to defibrillate again. How many defibrillations should you provide before reevaluating the pulse?

    a. One
    b. Two
    c. Three
    d. Four

56. To apply an AED, a patient must be:

    a. Having a confirmed heart attack
    b. Unconscious and pulseless
    c. At least 20 years old
    d. In the prone position

57. AEDs are useful to treat:

    a. Asystole and bradyarrhythmias
    b. Pulseless electrical activity
    c. Ventricular fibrillation and ventricular tachycardia
    d. Atrial fibrillation and atrial tachycardia

58. Which of the following patients should have an AED attached?

    a. A 6-year-old boy having a seizure
    b. A 46-year-old man complaining of chest pain
    c. A pulseless 25-year-old woman
    d. A 58-year-old man complaining of fluttering in his chest

59. The EMT is responsible for all the following in an emergency cardiac care system *except*:

    a. Early defibrillation
    b. Early CPR
    c. Prescribing nitroglycerin
    d. Collecting a history

60. If you apply the AED and it has advised "no shock," you should:

    a. Check for signs of circulation; if there are no signs of circulation, perform CPR for 1 minute and reanalyze
    b. Continue analyzing for 1 hour until it advises you to shock
    c. Always pronounce the patient dead in the field
    d. Check the machine for the correct operation

61. Applying an AED, analyzing, and defibrillating in a moving ambulance:

    a. Is not appropriate because it may shock a normal rhythm
    b. Is important to reduce time to defibrillation
    c. Should be done if the patient is pulseless
    d. Helps facilitate rapid analysis of the rhythm

62. All the following are types of AEDs *except*:

    a. Fully automated
    b. Semiautomated
    c. Fully manual with paddles
    d. Semiautomated with an electrocardiogram (ECG) screen

63. The major advantage of an AED over a manual defibrillator is the ability to:

    a. Provide defibrillation with little or no operator knowledge of an ECG
    b. Deliver higher energy with the use of pads
    c. Provide voice prompts that calm the operator during the emergency
    d. Shock asystole, which an AED will not shock

64. When using an AED you should check a pulse in all the following circumstances *except:*

    a. After each set of three stacked shocks
    b. When the machine advises no shock indicated
    c. Before using the AED
    d. After every shock that is delivered

65. Some AEDs allow for conversion of the defibrillator to manual mode:

    a. For rhythm monitoring and advanced cardiac life support procedures
    b. To avoid spontaneous shocks
    c. For stopping a defibrillation in progress
    d. For shocking asystole

66. When a patient remains in ventricular fibrillation after two sets of stacked shocks in an EMS system where there is no advanced life support care, the EMT should:

    a. Transport or follow local protocols
    b. Perform CPR for 3 minutes and analyze
    c. Shock continuously without CPR
    d. Pronounce the patient dead

67. After shocking a patient back to a normal rhythm, the patient becomes pulseless during transport to the hospital. You should:

    a. Stop the vehicle, analyze, and shock if advised
    b. Continue CPR until you arrive at the hospital
    c. Continue driving and analyze and shock while en route
    d. Administer a precordial thump and start CPR

68. When a patient remains in a shockable rhythm, the primary reason for not checking pulses between the three shocks with an AED is:

    a. The machine may shock during the analyze mode
    b. It would delay the three sequential shocks
    c. Pulses are irrelevant with AEDs
    d. To avoid interruption of carotid blood flow

69. The national organization that designs training programs and establishes guidelines for defibrillator use is the:

    a. American Board of EMTs
    b. American College of Cardiology
    c. American Heart Association
    d. American Association of Emergency Physicians

70. The best method for ensuring competency with AEDs is:

    a. Frequent hands-on practice
    b. Written reviews
    c. Device maintenance
    d. Mental drills

71. The review of scene events after a cardiac arrest patient encounter with an AED is usually performed by:

    a. The EMT who managed the case
    b. Another EMT
    c. The medical director or designee
    d. The EMS administrator

72. Which statement best describes the relation between cardiovascular compromise and cardiac arrest?

    a. All patients who have cardiovascular compromise will sustain a cardiac arrest
    b. Cardiovascular compromise will rarely evolve into a cardiac arrest situation
    c. Patients who sustain cardiovascular compromise are at high risk of sudden cardiac arrest
    d. Cardiac arrest usually occurs after several hours of cardiovascular compromise

73. Patients with chest pain should be routinely attached to an AED.

    a. True
    b. False

74. If you are alone with a pulseless patient and you have an AED, what action should you take first after determining breathlessness and pulselessness?

    a. Perform CPR for 1 minute
    b. Attach the AED and begin operation
    c. Perform CPR until helps arrives
    d. Perform one shock and start CPR

List the six key questions that you should ask the patient with a cardiac emergency.

75. ______________________________

76. ______________________________

77. ______________________________

78. ______________________________

79. ______________________________

80. ______________________________

List the four links in the chain of survival.

81. ______________________________

82. ______________________________

83. ______________________________

84. ______________________________

List nine common associated complaints that may be present in the patient with chest pain.

85. ______________________________

86. ______________________________

87. ______________________________

88. ______________________________

89. ______________________________

90. ______________________________

91. ______________________________

92. ______________________________

93. ______________________________

Questions 94 to 97 refer to the following scenario.

> You respond to a call at the local gym and encounter an approximately 50-year-old man on the floor next to an exercise bicycle. Bystanders tell you that the patient got off the exercise equipment, sat on the floor, and then collapsed. Your patient has a blood pressure of 72/40 mm Hg, the heart rate is 30 beats/min, and his respiratory rate is 4 breaths/min.

94. Your initial management for this patient includes:

    a. Connecting the AED to the patient and analyzing the patient's heart rhythm
    b. Positioning the patient supine with his head elevated and providing positive-pressure ventilations
    c. Positioning the patient supine with his legs elevated and providing positive-pressure ventilations
    d. Positioning the patient supine with his legs elevated and delivering supplemental oxygen with a nonrebreather mask

95. You are en route to the hospital when you no longer feel the patient's pulse and respirations cease. Your estimated drive time to the hospital is 20 minutes. You should:

    a. Have your partner continue driving to the hospital while you connect the AED and analyze the patient's heart rhythm
    b. Have your partner pull over to the side of the road and then connect the AED and analyze the patient's heart rhythm
    c. Begin CPR and continue CPR until you reach the hospital
    d. Perform CPR for 5 minutes and if the patient is still in cardiac arrest connect the AED and analyze the patient's heart rhythm

96. Approximately 5 minutes before arriving at the hospital the patient has a return of spontaneous circulation. You reevaluate the patient and the heart rate is 72 beats/min, blood pressure is 142/76 mm Hg, and the respiratory rate is 14 breaths/min. Respirations are now adequate. You should:

    a. Continue positive-pressure ventilations
    b. Administer oxygen at 2 to 3 L/min with a nasal cannula
    c. Open the airway with the head tilt/chin lift method; no supplemental oxygen is required
    d. Administer oxygen with a nonrebreather mask

97. You are now 2 minutes from the hospital when the patient begins to vomit. The best position to place this patient in is:

    a. Supine
    b. Prone
    c. Left lateral recumbent
    d. Supine with the patient's legs elevated

Questions 98 to 101 refer to the following scenario.

Your EMS unit is on standby at the high school football game. You are summoned to the sidelines to treat a 42-year-old man who was coaching the game when he became very dizzy. The patient informs you that he has a cardiac history and sometimes takes nitroglycerin. He has the nitroglycerin pills with him that are prescribed for him and have not expired. Vital signs are pulse of 86 beats/min regular and weak, blood pressure of 120/60 mm Hg, and respiratory rate 20 breaths/min and normal. Your drive time to the hospital is approximately 12 minutes.

98. You continue to evaluate your patient and begin to ask questions specific to the patient's chief complaint. You would ask the patient:

    a. Do you have any chest pain or chest discomfort?
    b. Do you have any sharp chest pain?
    c. Do you have any pressure in your chest?
    d. Do you have a squeezing sensation in your chest?

99. Your treatment for this patient includes:

    a. Oxygen by nonrebreather mask and assisting the patient in taking one nitroglycerin tablet
    b. Oxygen by nonrebreather mask and connecting the AED to the patient
    c. Oxygen by nonrebreather mask and rapid transport
    d. Assisting the patient in taking one nitroglycerin tablet

100. While placing the patient on your ambulance stretcher, he patient appears to have seizurelike activity that last for approximately 30 seconds. You reevaluate your patient and determine that he is now in cardiac arrest. You should:

    a. Begin CPR and transport the patient to the hospital
    b. Withhold CPR because CPR is not indicated in a patient who has had a seizure
    c. Withhold CPR until an AED is available
    d. Begin CPR and connect the AED to the patient as soon as possible

101. If you use the AED, you know that if the patient is in a shockable rhythm, and the AED delivers three shocks, you should now:

    a. Press the analyze button again
    b. Begin CPR; a pulse check is not indicated
    c. Check for a pulse; if no pulse is present begin CPR
    d. Begin rapid transport and press the analyze button again en route to the hospital

Across

1. Major artery of the arm
3. Early defibrillation is accomplished through the use of _____ _____ defibrillation
8. The smaller, upper chambers of the heart that contract first
11. Patients with left-sided heart failure are at risk for respiratory compromise related to the decrease of oxygen exchange in the _____ in the lungs
12. Fluid accumulation in the lower back and abdomen
16. Ischemic chest pain is usually located in the _____ _____
17. Computerized device that allows EMTs and lay rescuers to deliver electrical energy to the heart
19. Activity with an organized heart rhythm but no effective pumping
20. Mechanical device used to deliver electrical shock to the victim
21. The force exerted by the blood volume on the walls of the vessels
22. The ability for cells in the heart to generate an electrical impulse and discharge on their own
25. In _____ circulation the right ventricle pumps blood through the lungs to pick up oxygen
26. State of poor circulation in which the vital tissues are poorly perfused
28. Unit of energy used by the AED
30. Pressure in the vessels when the heart relaxes
31. _____ waveform AEDs deliver current in one direction
33. The SA node is located in the _______
34. Vessels that direct blood flow returning to the heart
35. A common human response of a patient who is having a heart attack
36. _____ neck veins indicate the signs of right and left heart failure

Down

1. _____ waveform AEDs deliver current in two directions
2. Organ responsible for generating blood flow to all parts of the body
4. Early 911 access, early CPR, early defibrillation, and early advanced care
5. _____ disease is the leading cause of death in the United States
6. Mnemonic to remember the key questions in a patient history
7. The SA node is the _____ of the heart
9. Flatline ECG
10. Vessels that direct blood flow away from the heart
13. Decreased blood flow through an organ
14. In _____ circulation, the left ventricle pumps oxygen-rich blood to the body
15. AEDs are attached to the patient by cables connected to monitoring-defibrillation _____ _____
18. Lightheadedness is a common side effect of nitroglycerin because it causes _____ of the veins
20. The definitive treatment for ventricular fibrillation
23. The larger, lower chambers of the heart
24. Major artery of the leg
27. Major artery of the neck
29. Mnemonic used to obtain specific facts regarding a patient's chest pain
32. Method used to sustain life by circulating oxygenated blood to the brain

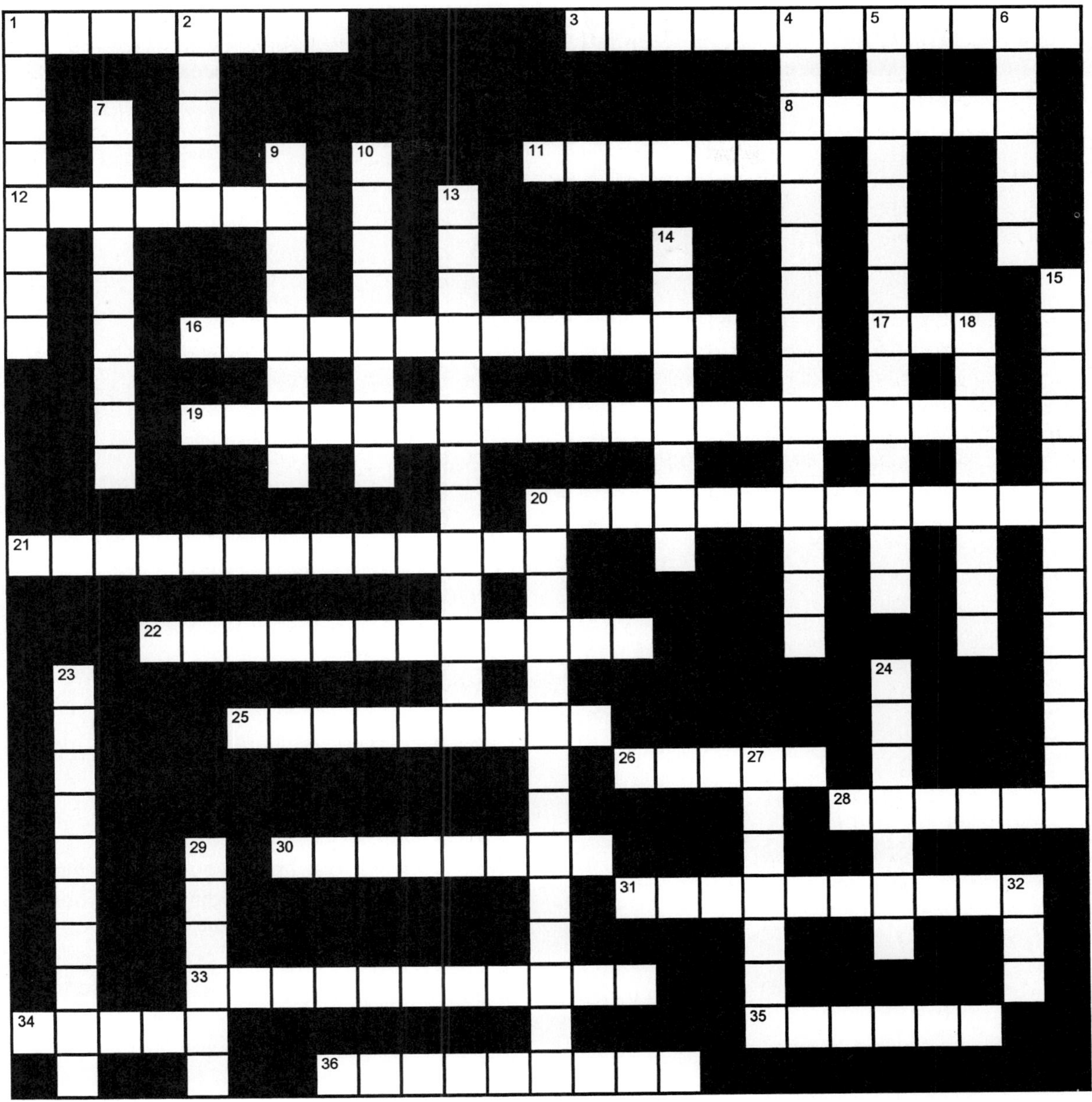

ANSWER KEY

1. d
2. c
3. a
4. c
5. b
6. a
7. d
8. a
9. b
10. b
11. c
12. b
13. a
14. c
15. b
16. a
17. b
18. c
19. a
20. b
21. b
22. d
23. a
24. b
25. c
26. b
27. d
28. c
29. b
30. b
31. b
32. a
33. c
34. a
35. b
36. a
37. b
38. a
39. a
40. d
41. a
42. c
43. c
44. d
45. b
46. d
47. b
48. b
49. b
50. b
51. c
52. c
53. d
54. b
55. c
56. b
57. c
58. c
59. c
60. a
61. a
62. c
63. a
64. d
65. a
66. a
67. a
68. b
69. c
70. a
71. c
72. c
73. b
74. b
75. Onset: What were you doing when the symptoms began?
76. Provocation: Does anything make the pain better or worse?
77. Quality: How would you describe the pain?
78. Radiation: Does the pain go anywhere, such as to your arm, neck, or jaw?
79. Severity: Describe the pain on a scale of 1 to 10 and compare it with previous episodes, if appropriate.
80. Time: How long have you had the pain?
81. Early access to 911
82. Early CPR
83. Early defibrillation
84. Early advanced care
85. Nausea
86. Vomiting
87. Weakness
88. Shortness of breath
89. Palpitations
90. Lightheadedness
91. Sweating
92. Dizziness
93. Loss of consciousness
94. c
95. b
96. d
97. c
98. a
99. a
100. d
101. c

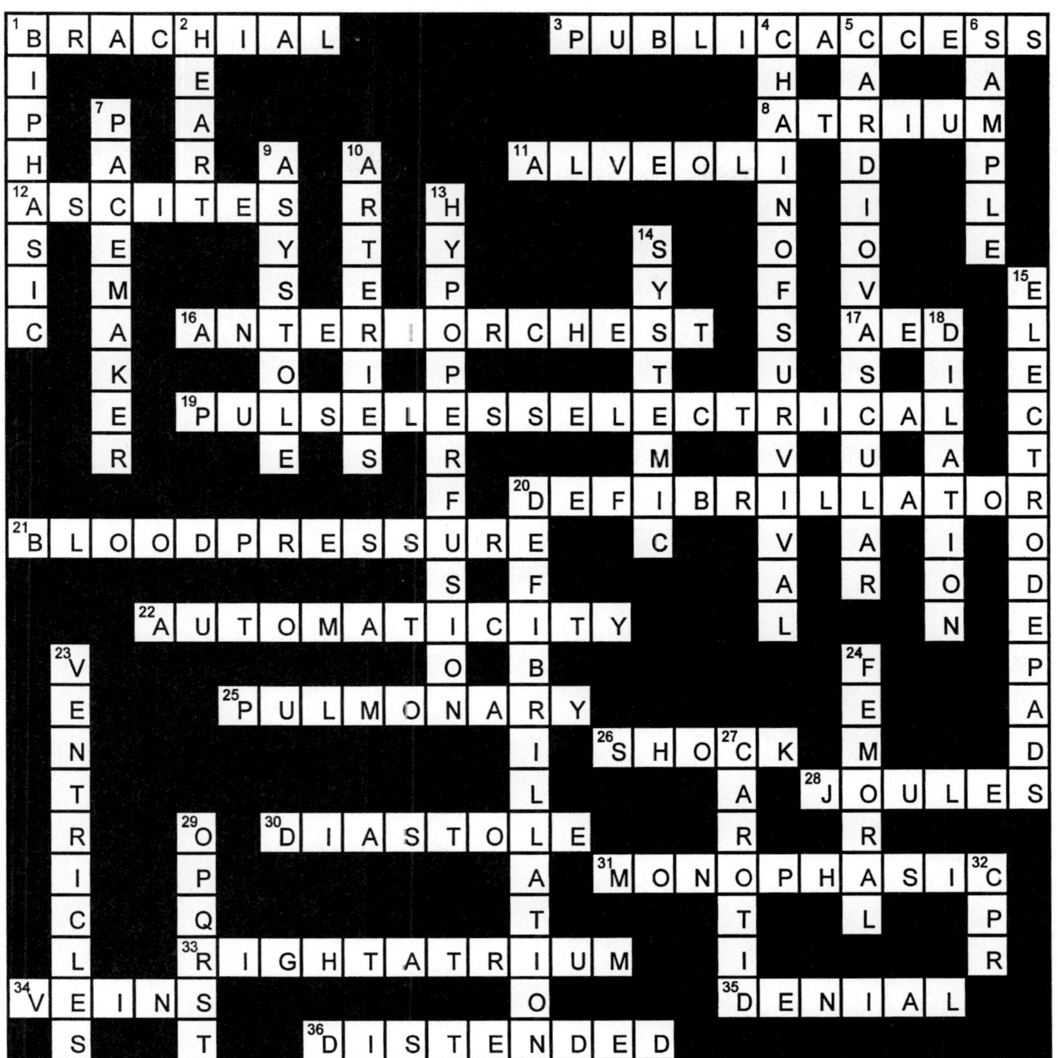
1 BRACHIAL
2 HEART
3 PUBLICACCESS
4 CHAINOFSURVIVAL
5 CARDIOVASCULAR
6 SAMPLE
7 PACEMAKER
8 ATRIUM
9 ASYSTOLE
10 ARTERIES
11 ALVEOLI
12 ASCITES
13 HYPOPERFUSION
14 SYSTEMIC
15 ELECTRODEPADS
16 ANTERIORCHEST
17 AED
18 DILATION
19 PULSELESSELECTRICAL
20 DEFIBRILLATOR
20 DEFIBRILLATION
21 BLOODPRESSURE
22 AUTOMATICITY
23 VENTRICLES
24 FEMORAL
25 PULMONARY
26 SHOCK
27 CAROTID
28 JOULES
29 OPQRST
30 DIASTOLE
31 MONOPHASIC
32 CPR
33 RIGHTATRIUM
34 VEINS
35 DENIAL
36 DISTENDED

Chapter 19 Altered Mental Status

1. Stored forms of glucose can be released between meals. This process is initiated by the hormone:

   a. LDH
   b. Progesterone
   c. Glycogen
   d. Glucagon

2. Patients who have a severe or absolute lack of insulin are called:

   a. Non-insulin-dependent diabetics
   b. Insulin-dependent diabetics
   c. Glucose-dependent diabetics
   d. Glycogen-dependent diabetics

3. Non-insulin-dependent diabetics usually take medication that stimulates the pancreas to produce:

   a. Glucose
   b. Fructose
   c. Glycogen
   d. Insulin

4. Diabetes is a disease that results from an inadequate secretion of the hormone:

   a. Insulin
   b. Epinephrine
   c. Glucagon
   d. Progesterone

5. Insulin helps regulate the use and storage of:

   a. Ketones
   b. Isotones
   c. Glucose
   d. Epinephrine

6. What does the brain primarily rely on for nourishment?

   a. Insulin
   b. Glycogen
   c. Glucose
   d. Glucagon

7. Insulin is produced within specialized cells in the:

   a. Liver
   b. Spleen
   c. Pancreas
   d. Adrenal gland

8. Some glucose is stored in the liver and muscle as a larger molecule called:

   a. Glucagon
   b. Glycogen
   c. Fructose
   d. Insulin

9. A diabetic emergency that develops from a lack of insulin and elevated blood glucose causing dehydration and acidosis is:

   a. Diabetic encephalopathy
   b. Diabetic ketoacidosis
   c. Diabetic syndrome
   d. Insulin shock

Match the signs and symptoms in column A with the diabetic emergency in column B.

Column A	Column B
10. ____ Increased thirst	a. Hypoglycemia b. Diabetic ketoacidosis
11. ____ Sweaty skin	
12. ____ Pale skin	

13. _____ Increased urination

14. _____ Salivation

15. _____ Combative behavior

16. _____ Acetone and deep respiration

17. _____ Fruity breath odor

---

18. The most common and treatable diabetic problem encountered in prehospital care that results from a lack of available sugar in the blood is:

    a. Diabetic coma
    b. Hypoglycemia
    c. Hyperosmolar coma
    d. Diabetic encephalopathy

19. Signs of hypoglycemia may include hunger, nausea, weakness, and:

    a. Dry mouth
    b. Bizarre behavior
    c. Slow pulse
    d. Hypotension

20. A drug that is given intramuscularly for hypoglycemia and that may be carried at times by the patient is:

    a. Glucose
    b. Glucagon
    c. Glycogen
    d. Insulin

21. Before giving a conscious diabetic an oral glucose gel, you should:

    a. Check for a gag reflex
    b. Take two sets of vital signs
    c. Lay the patient supine
    d. Give the patient two glasses of water

22. Which of the following is a trade name for oral glucose:

    a. Glucometer
    b. Glucagon
    c. Glutose
    d. Glugel

23. All the following are steps of administration of oral glucose gel *except:*

    a. Obtain an online or offline order from medical direction
    b. Check for altered mental status
    c. Check for history of diabetes
    d. Take blood pressure in both sitting and lying positions

24. If a situation is unclear regarding the history and physical assessment of a suspected diabetic patient, you should:

    a. Disregard the history and proceed with the treatment
    b. Discuss the situation with your partner and proceed with the treatment
    c. Consult with medical direction before treatment
    d. Not be concerned, as the history and physical assessment are not important for these patients

25. A reversible episode of focal neurologic dysfunction that typically lasts a few minutes to a few hours and resolves within 24 hours is called a(n) ___________.

26. ___________ is the most common cause of intracerebral hemorrhage.

27. A stroke is also referred to as a(n) ___________.

28. A blood clot that moves in the blood stream and migrates to the brain causing a stroke is referred to as a(n) ___________.

29. A clot that develops within a brain artery itself is referred to as a(n) ___________.

TRUE OR FALSE

30. _____ Hemorrhagic strokes are the most common type.

31. _____ Hypotension is commonly caused by a stroke.

32. _____ The use of a prehospital stroke scale is useful to predict the patient's neurologic outcome.

33. _____ The presence of an acute stroke is an indication for rapid transport.

34. _____ Patients with a hemorrhagic stroke can often be treated with "clot busting" medications if they arrive at the hospital within a few hours of symptom onset.

35. _____ A history of transient ischemic attacks is a significant indicator of stroke risk.

36. _____ Stroke is the leading cause of death in the United States in adults.

Questions 37 to 40 are based on the following scenario.

> You respond to a local nursing home and encounter an 82-year-old woman who is found in her bed and is unresponsive to verbal or painful stimuli. The nurse's aide informs you that the patient is in the nursing home for rehabilitation after surgery to replace her left hip. Normally the patient is alert and oriented and can ambulate with a walker. It is now 1400 hours. The patient has a history of "irregular" heartbeats but is not taking any medications. The patient was last seen awake and alert at approximately 1000 hours. The patient's vital signs are pulse of 88 beats/min and irregular, blood pressure of 156/92 mm Hg, and respiratory rate of 16 breaths/min and adequate.

37. The best term to describe this patient's altered mental state is:

    a. Lethargy
    b. Stupor
    c. Semicoma
    d. Coma

38. Based on the patient's clinical presentation you suspect that the patient is experiencing:

    a. An acute cardiac condition
    b. A drug overdose
    c. Hypoglycemia
    d. A stroke

39. As you further evaluate your patient you determine that the patient does not open her eyes, does not make any verbal sounds, and does not move despite painful stimuli. What would this patient's score be on the Glasgow Coma Scale?

    a. 0
    b. 3
    c. 10
    d. 15

40. Prehospital management of this patient includes:

    a. Administration of oral glucose and transport to the closest hospital
    b. Airway management and rapid transport to the appropriate hospital
    c. Contact with poison control for permission to administer a cathartic
    d. Connecting the patient to the AED to be prepared if she goes into cardiac arrest

List 10 possible causes of a seizure:

41. ______________________________

42. ______________________________

43. ______________________________

44. ______________________________

45. ______________________________

46. ______________________________

47. ______________________________

48. ______________________________

49. ______________________________

50. ______________________________

Questions 51 to 53 refer to the following scenario.

> You respond to a business office and find a 37-year-old woman who is lying on the floor and has a depressed level of consciousness and is confused. Coworkers tell you that the patient appeared to have a seizure. You ask the coworkers exactly what the patient was exhibiting during the seizure and they describe intermittent contractions and relaxations of the muscles, which they also tell you "looked like jerking movements."

51. The activity that is described to you by the coworkers is termed the:

    a. Tonic phase of a seizure
    b. Clonic phase of a seizure
    c. Postictal period
    d. Aura

52. While you continue to examine your patient she slowly begins to awake but still appears to be confused. This stage of a seizure is called the:

    a. Tonic phase of a seizure
    b. Clonic phase of a seizure
    c. Postictal period
    d. Aura

53. While you begin transport of the patient to the ambulance she begins to exhibit signs of a grand mal seizure. The seizure continues as you prepare the patient for transport. If the seizure continues for more than 5 minutes this would be termed:

    a. A petit mal seizure
    b. Irreversible brain damage
    c. Status epilepticus
    d. Convulsions

Across

1. Disease caused by an inadequate secretion of insulin
9. Bluish discoloration of mucous membranes or skin
10. The area that is the center for receiving and processing visual stimuli
11. Medication that converts glycogen back to glucose
14. "Stroke"
17. Seizure phase characterized by intermittent contractions and relaxations of the skeletal muscles resulting in rapid, jerky movements
18. High body temperature
20. Glucose deprivation
22. On finding a patient with an alteration in mental status, the EMT must first assess the adequacy of _____
26. Bluish skin color is a sign of _____
31. A patient who is easily aroused but drifts into a sleepy state without continued stimulation
33. Low body temperature
35. Damage to one side of the brain shows examination findings that are one-sided or _____
37. Scale used to measure a patient's mental status
38. Hormone that regulates the utilization and storage of glucose

Down

2. A condition of a lack of awareness of one's own environment from which the patient may be aroused
3. _____ odor on the breath may be a sign of diabetic ketoacidosis
4. The cerebrum is divided down the middle into right and left halves called _____
5. The largest and most superior portion of the brain
6. Lower part of the brain
7. Final phase of a seizure with depressed level of consciousness and confusion
8. Symptoms for which no cause can be found
12 Stroke that occurs as the result of an occluded blood vessel supplying the brain
13. Toxemia of pregnancy—a potential for seizures
15. If the brain is deprived of oxygen, _____ _____ can occur in 4-6 minutes
16. A patient who can be aroused but does not reach a normal level of consciousness and function
19. Phase of seizure with sustained contraction of all voluntary muscles
20. Warm, hot, dry skin suggests _____
21. Third leading cause of death in the United States
23. Temporary alteration in behavior caused by abnormal electrical activity in the brain
24. Seizure in a child precipitated by a high fever and infection
25. A generalized seizure affecting the entire body
27. Seizures that may affect only a portion of the body or manifest as an alteration in consciousness
28. The area of the brain that receives smell and hearing signals
29. Artery that joins the carotids in the center of the brain
30. A patient in a _____ has no responsiveness to external stimuli
32. A carbohydrate used by the cells for energy
34. Sensations or motor events that may warn the patient of an oncoming seizure
36. The patient's ability to respond to stimuli is measured using this mnemonic

1 2 3 4 5 6 7 8 9 10 11 12 13 14 15 16 17 18 19 20 21 22 23 24 25 26 27 28 29 30 31 32 33 34 35 36 37 38

ANSWER KEY

1. d
2. b
3. d
4. a
5. c
6. c
7. c
8. b
9. b
10. b
11. a
12. a
13. b
14. a
15. a
16. b
17. b
18. b
19. b
20. b
21. a
22. c
23. d
24. c
25. Transient ischemic attack
26. Hypertension
27. Cerebrovascular accident
28. Embolism
29. Thrombus
30. False
31. False
32. True
33. True
34. False
35. True
36. False
37. d
38. d
39. b
40. b
41. Alcohol withdrawal
42. Drug withdrawal
43. Eclampsia (toxemia of pregnancy)
44. Epilepsy
45. Fever
46. Hypoglycemia
47. Hypoxia
48. Infections
49. Poisonings
50. Trauma
51. b
52. c
53. c

1 DIABETES
2 SEMICOMA
3 FRUITY
4 HEMISPHERES
5 CEREBRUM
6 BRAINSTEM
7 POSTICTAL
8 IDIOPATHIC
9 CYANOSIS
10 OCCIPITAL
11 GLUCAGON
12 ISCHEMIC
13 ECLAMPSIA
14 CEREBROVASCULARACCIDENT
15 BIOLOGICALDEATH
16 STUPOROUS
17 CLONIC
18 HYPERTHERMIA
19 TONIC
20 HYPOGLYCEMIA / HEATSTROKE
21 STROKE
22 VENTILATIONS
23 SEIZURE
24 FEBRILE
25 GRANDMAL
26 HYPOXIA
27 FOCAL
28 TEMPORAL
29 BASILAR
30 COMA
31 LETHARGIC
32 GLUCOSE
33 HYPOTHERMIA
34 AURA
35 UNILATERAL
36 AVP
37 GLASGOWCOMA
38 INSULIN

Chapter 20 Allergies

1. Anaphylaxis is a serious allergic reaction after patients come into contact with substances called

   ___________ to which they have been previously sensitized.

   a. Antigens
   b. Antibodies
   c. Histamines
   d. Antihistamines

2. A substance that is released from cells during an anaphylactic reaction that can trigger blood vessels to dilate and capillaries to leak is called:

   a. An antigen
   b. An endorphin
   c. Histamine
   d. Adrenaline

3. Which of the following is a common agent for producing an anaphylactic reaction?

   a. Vegetables
   b. Shellfish
   c. Milk
   d. Fruit

Match the physiologic effects in column A to the signs and symptoms of anaphylaxis in column B.

Column A	Column B
4. _____ Constriction of bronchial smooth muscle	a. Hypotension
5. _____ Increased permeability of capillaries and fluid leakage	b. Swelling of the skin and stridor caused by obstruction
6. _____ Dilation of the arteries	c. Sneezing and nasal congestion
7. _____ Increased mucus secretions in the respiratory tree	d. Wheezing breath sounds

8. Some anaphylactic patients may carry a kit that contains antihistamine agents and:

   a. Morphine
   b. Dilantin
   c. Epinephrine
   d. Phenobarbital

9. Anaphylactic reactions may present with raised, red patches of skin called:

   a. Erythema
   b. Purpura
   c. Urticaria (hives)
   d. Papules

10. The major lethal complications of anaphylaxis are circulatory collapse and:

    a. Arrhythmias
    b. Airway obstruction
    c. Heart failure
    d. Fluid overload

11. Epinephrine is usually administered to an adult through an autoinjector at a dose of:

    a. 0.3 mg
    b. 0.1 mg
    c. 0.2 mg
    d. 0.5 mg

12. Epinephrine is usually administered to a child through an autoinjector at a dose of:

    a. 0.15 mg
    b. 0.2 mg
    c. 0.25 mg
    d. 0.3 mg

13. The trade name for epinephrine is:

    a. Norepinephrine
    b. Acetylcholine
    c. Adrenalin
    d. Isoproterenol

14. What is the location for administration of an epinephrine autoinjector?

    a. Mid-lateral shoulder region
    b. Lower and outer quadrant of the buttocks
    c. Mid-lateral thigh region
    d. Mid-biceps muscle

15. Patients in anaphylaxis who are exhibiting signs of shock should be transported in what position?

    a. Left lateral recumbent
    b. Supine
    c. Supine position with the legs elevated
    d. Supine with the head elevated

16. A patient with severe difficulty breathing; hives; and swelling of the mouth, neck, and tongue is likely to be experiencing:

    a. A minor allergic reaction
    b. Anaphylaxis
    c. Asthma or chronic obstructive pulmonary disease
    d. Epiglottitis

17. Complete airway obstruction from anaphylaxis can be treated by the emergency medical technician with:

    a. Abdominal thrusts
    b. Extreme hyperextension
    c. Patient positioning
    d. Continued attempts at positive-pressure ventilation

18. The definitive treatment of complete airway obstruction in the hospital might include all the following *except:*

    a. Cricothyroidotomy
    b. Intubation
    c. Placement of a chest tube
    d. Tracheostomy

19. A patient with anaphylaxis shows some improvement after epinephrine administration but deteriorates during transport. You should

    ____________.

List 10 of the 20 symptoms (patient complaints) that may be present in the anaphylactic patient.

20. ________________________________

21. ________________________________

22. ________________________________

23. ________________________________

24. ________________________________

25. ________________________________

26. ________________________________

27. ________________________________

28. ________________________________

29. ________________________________

List 10 of the 16 signs of anaphylaxis.

30. ________________________________

31. ________________________________

32. ________________________________

33. ________________________________

34. ________________________________

35. ________________________________

36. ________________________________

37. ________________________________

38. ________________________________

39. ________________________________

List the six key questions to ask the patient with an allergic reaction.

40. ______________________________

41. ______________________________

42. ______________________________

43. ______________________________

44. ______________________________

45. ______________________________

List the eight possible side effects that a patient may exhibit after the administration of epinephrine.

46. ______________________________

47. ______________________________

48. ______________________________

49. ______________________________

50. ______________________________

51. ______________________________

52. ______________________________

53. ______________________________

Questions 54 to 57 refer to the following scenario.

> You respond to a ball field and encounter a 23-year-old man who is in severe respiratory distress. His friends tell you that the patient was stung by a bee on his arm. Approximately 5 minutes after he was stung he began to have difficulty breathing and a bystander called 911. Your evaluation reveals a patient with hives on his arm, torso, and chest. His lips appear to be slightly swollen. The patient's blood pressure is 72/40 mm Hg, heart rate is 110 beats/min, and the respiratory rate is 28 breaths/min. Your partner suggests that you administer epinephrine to this patient.

54. Based on the physical examination of this patient you:

    a. Withhold any epinephrine because of the patient's low blood pressure
    b. Withhold any epinephrine because of the patient's age
    c. Administer an Epi-Pen Jr. containing 0.15 mg of epinephrine
    d. Administer an Epi-Pen containing 0.30 mg of epinephrine

55. Your continued treatment of this patient includes:

    a. Remaining at the scene for 3 to 5 minutes to see if your initial treatment has any effect
    b. Initiating humidified oxygen administration by a nasal cannula at 2 to 4 L/min
    c. Initiating high-concentration oxygen administration by a nonrebreather mask and rapid transport
    d. Administering a Mark I Kit

56. If you administer epinephrine to this patient you would expect that:

    a. The patient's heart rate will quickly decrease
    b. The patient's heart rate will remain unchanged
    c. The patient's heart rate will quickly increase
    d. Any change in the patient's heart rate would depend on the specific cause of the allergic reaction

57. During transport to the hospital the patient's airway becomes totally obstructed by swelling in the neck and tongue. You should:

    a. Immediately perform abdominal thrusts
    b. Immediately perform chest thrusts
    c. Perform a jaw thrust and maintain oxygen delivery with a nonrebreather mask
    d. Attempt to deliver positive-pressure ventilations

Questions 58 and 59 refer to the following scenario.

> You respond to a patient's home where you encounter a 33-year-old woman who tells you that she is having a severe allergic reaction to antibiotics that she just began to take that morning. The patient has a history of asthma but no other medical history or known allergies. The patient is alert, has a respiratory rate of 14 breaths/min, full clear bilateral breath sounds, a pulse of 92 beats/min and regular, and blood pressure is 124/72 mm Hg. The patient does not have any difficulty speaking or swallowing. You notice a few hives on the patient's upper torso.

58. Your immediate treatment for this patient includes:

    a. Administering an Epi-Pen Jr. containing 0.15 mg of epinephrine
    b. Administering an Epi-Pen containing 0.30 mg of epinephrine
    c. Administering oxygen and transporting the patient to the hospital
    d. Advising the patient that hospital evaluation is not needed and to call back if the symptoms progress

59. Based on your evaluation of the patient you suspect the patient may be having:

    a. A minor allergic reaction
    b. An anaphylactic reaction
    c. An acute asthma attack
    d. Chronic obstructive pulmonary disease

Across

1. Location for Epi-Pen injection
6. Skin color that results from vasoconstriction
7. An antihistamine, also known as Benadryl
10. Trade name for epinephrine
11. A substance recognized as foreign to the body
13. A protein helpful in fighting infections and neutralizing toxins
14. Substance within the body that is released during anaphylaxis, causing vessel dilation and hypotension, which may lead to shock

Down

2. Preloaded syringe for self-administration of epinephrine
3. A life-threatening allergic reaction
4. Cardiac system's common response to the administration of epinephrine
5. Rash
8. Shock
9. Potent drug that can block the effects of histamine and slow the anaphylactic process
11. Condition resulting from vasodilation, causing hives and swelling of the face, lips, tongue, and airway
12. High-pitched noise heard at inspiration caused by obstruction of the upper airway

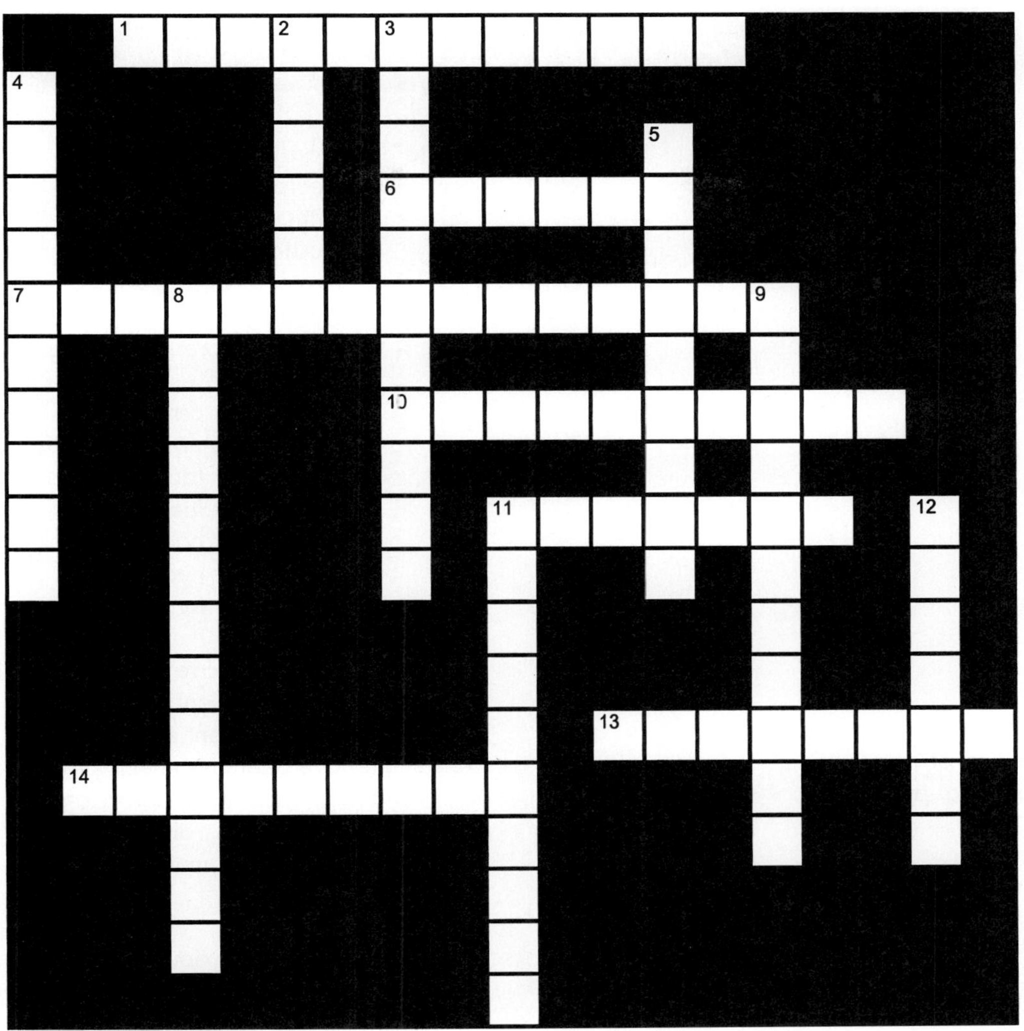
1
2
3
4
5
6
7
8
9
10
11
12
13
14

ANSWER KEY

1. a
2. c
3. b
4. d
5. b
6. a
7. c
8. c
9. c
10. b
11. a
12. a
13. c
14. c
15. c
16. b
17. d
18. c
19. Consult medical direction for the possibility of a second injection of epinephrine

20. to 29. Abdominal pain
Anxiety
Coughing
Cramping
Diarrhea
Facial edema
Fainting
Hoarseness
Itching
Itchy and watery eyes
Laryngeal edema
Loss of voice
Pharyngeal edema
Runny nose
Sense of impending doom
Sneezing
Tightness in throat
Tingling feeling
Vomiting
Wheezing

30. to 39. Cardiac arrest
Decreased mental state
Difficulty breathing
Flushing of skin
Hives
Hypotension
Rapid, labored breathing
Rapid pulse
Respiratory arrest
Stridor and noisy breathing
Swelling of face
Swelling of feet
Swelling of hands
Swelling of neck
Swelling of tongue
Wheezing

40. Does the patient have a history of allergies?
41. What was the patient exposed to?
42. How was the patient exposed?
43. What have been the effects of the exposure?
44. What has been the progression (speed of onset, specific complaints) of the exposure?
45. What, if any, interventions have already occurred?
46. Chest pain
47. Dizziness
48. Excitability and anxiousness
49. Headache
50. Increased heart rate
51. Nausea
52. Pallor
53. Vomiting
54. d
55. c
56. c
57. d
58. c
59. a

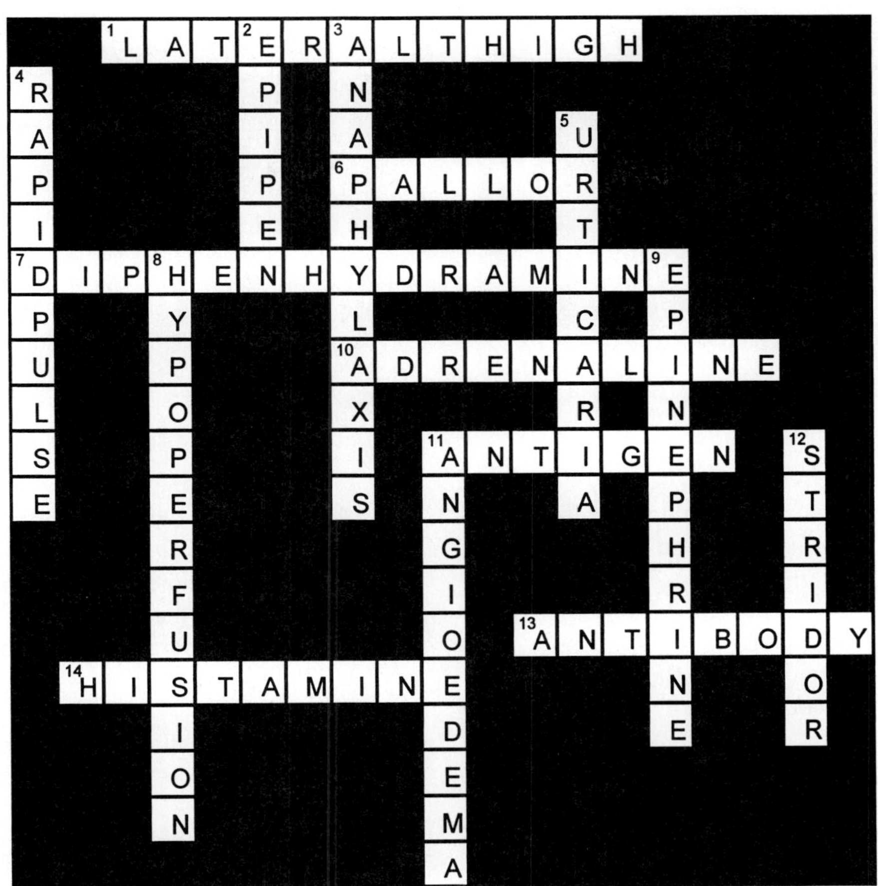
1 LATERALTHIGH
2 EPIPEPE
3 ANAPHYLAXIS
4 RAPIDPULSE
5 URTICARIA
6 PALLOR
7 DIPHENHYDRAMINE
8 HYPOPERFUSION
9 EPINEPHRINE
10 ADRENALINE
11 ANTIGEN
11 ANGIOEDEMA
12 STRIDOR
13 ANTIBODY
14 HISTAMINE

Chapter 21 Poisoning and Overdoses

1. A regional agency available for phone consultation in the event of a poisoning is called a(n):

   a. Toxicology center
   b. Abused substance center
   c. Poison control center
   d. Toxic ingestion center

Match the type of poisoning in column A with the substance in column B.

Column A	Column B
2. _____ Ingestion	a. Carbon monoxide
3. _____ Inhalation	b. Organophosphates (insecticide) on skin
4. _____ Injection	c. Methanol
5. _____ Absorption	d. Scorpion sting

6. The first priority in managing an unconscious suspected poison patient is to:

   a. Induce vomiting
   b. Provide cardiorespiratory support
   c. Hasten elimination of the poison
   d. Keep the patient awake

7. Three important questions regarding a poisoning incident are what was taken, how much was taken, and:

   a. Why it was taken
   b. The age of the patient
   c. Whether it was a suicide attempt
   d. When it was taken

8. Administering activated charcoal is designed to:

   a. Hasten elimination
   b. Neutralize the poison
   c. Prevent absorption by the body
   d. Provide an antidote

9. The primary antidote for a carbon monoxide poisoning is:

   a. Carbon dioxide
   b. Naloxone
   c. Oxygen
   d. Epi-Pen

10. The most common pupillary finding in opioid (narcotic) overdoses (e.g., heroin) is:

    a. Dilated
    b. Midpositional
    c. Unequal
    d. Pinpoint

11. The major complication of a narcotic overdose is:

    a. Arrhythmia
    b. Cardiac arrest
    c. Respiratory arrest
    d. Bleeding

12. Fast heart rates, hypertension, chest pain, anxious behavior, delirium, and paranoia best describe an overdose of:

    a. Depressants
    b. Narcotics
    c. Sedative-hypnotics
    d. Stimulants

13. Alcohol is a central nervous system:

    a. Depressant
    b. Stimulant
    c. Hypnotic
    d. Hallucinogenic

14. A drug that may exhibit few or no symptoms immediately after taken in overdose but that may lead to severe liver failure days later is:

    a. Aspirin
    b. Valium
    c. Amphetamine
    d. Acetaminophen

15. The first and most important step in the management of an inhalation poisoning is:

    a. Removal from the toxic environment
    b. Administration of oxygen
    c. Positive-pressure ventilation
    d. Cardiopulmonary resuscitation

16. Eyes that have been exposed to corrosive chemicals should be irrigated for a minimum of:

    a. 5 minutes
    b. 10 minutes
    c. 15 minutes
    d. 20 minutes

17. All the following are commonly injected drugs *except:*

    a. Amphetamine
    b. Acetaminophen
    c. Cocaine
    d. Heroin

Questions 18 to 20 refer to the following scenario.

> You respond to a call and find a 5-year-old girl who is suspected of a having ingested 100 acetaminophen (Tylenol) tablets 10 minutes earlier. The mother shows you an empty bottle, but the child appears perfectly normal and has normal vital signs. The child is alert and oriented.

18. Normal vital signs in this type of overdose are:

    a. Possible but not likely
    b. Likely in the first 24 hours
    c. Possible only in the first few minutes
    d. Highly unlikely after 5 minutes

19. You contact medical direction for advice in treating this child. What first step would they likely advise under these circumstances?

    a. Give 15 mL of ipecac
    b. Give several glasses of water
    c. Give activated charcoal
    d. Rapid transport only

20. What would the likely treatment be for an ingestion of an alkali poison?

    a. Give 15 mL (1 tablespoon) of ipecac
    b. Give one or two glasses of water or milk
    c. Give activated charcoal
    d. Rapid transport only

Questions 21 to 23 refer to the following scenario.

> You respond to a call and find 50-year-old man locked in his garage with his car motor running. He is unresponsive and his skin is pink.

21. Your immediate action should be to:

    a. Open the garage door, turn off the car engine, and give high-concentration oxygen
    b. Remove the patient from the garage and give high-concentration oxygen
    c. Immediately transport the patient to the hospital to be intubated
    d. Give humidified oxygen by nasal cannula and transport

22. The pink skin color associated with carbon monoxide poisoning is from:

    a. Unsaturated hemoglobin
    b. Hemoglobin saturated with carbon dioxide
    c. Hemoglobin saturated with carbon monoxide
    d. Hemoglobin saturated with cyanide

23. Which of the following definitive treatments would be most helpful for treating a patient with carbon monoxide poisoning?

    a. Hyperbaric oxygen
    b. Intubation and ventilation
    c. Heart-lung machine
    d. Dialysis

Questions 24 to 26 refer to the following scenario.

> You respond to an overdose and find a 22-year-old man with track marks on his arm who is unresponsive to painful stimuli. Physical examination reveals pinpoint pupils, and snoring is heard with each breath. His vital signs are respirations 10 breaths/min and shallow, pulse 62 beats/min and thready, and blood pressure 90/60 mm Hg.

24. Your immediate action is to:

    a. Open the airway and begin positive-pressure ventilation
    b. Suction and administer oxygen by nasal cannula
    c. Apply the pneumatic anti-shock garment
    d. Induce vomiting

25. Based on the signs and symptoms of the patient, you suspect:

    a. Amphetamine overdose
    b. Barbiturate overdose
    c. Opiate overdose
    d. Sedative-hypnotic overdose

26. You are en route to the hospital when the patient begins to vomit. Your immediate action is to:

    a. Perform the Heimlich maneuver
    b. Place the patient prone and continue transport
    c. Change your oxygen delivery mask to a nonrebreather oxygen mask
    d. Use suction to clear the airway

27. A patient has ingested a substance that might contraindicate the use of activated charcoal. What actions should you take?

    a. Contact medical direction for clarification
    b. Proceed with administration of activated charcoal
    c. Provide a lower dose of the activated charcoal
    d. Do not administer the activated charcoal

28. ___________ is the toxic substance contained in antifreeze.

29. ___________ is the toxic substance found in automobile windshield washing fluid.

30. The national toll-free number that should be accessed to contact the regional poison control center is ___________.

List the seven key questions to ask the patient with a poisoning/overdose.

31. ______________________________

32. ______________________________

33. ______________________________

34. ______________________________

35. ______________________________

36. ______________________________

37. ______________________________

Match the diagnostic odor in column A with the possible substance in column B

Column A	Column B
38. ____ Acetone (sweet, fruity)	a. Organophosphate
39. ____ Disinfectants	b. Methyl salicylate
40. ____ Eggs (rotten)	c. Ethanol, isopropyl alcohol, diabetic ketoacidosis
41. ____ Garlic	d. Hydrogen sulfide
42. ____ Wintergreen	e. Phenol, creosote

Questions 43 to 45 refer to the following scenario.

> You respond to a suburban home where you find a neighbor frantically yelling that she can see her neighbors lying on the floor in their living room not moving. The neighbor tells you that she has been banging on the door but no one is answering. The neighbor saw a fuel oil service truck leave the home about 3 hours ago.

43. Your first consideration in gaining access to these patients is to:

    a. Immediately break a window and enter the home to access the patients
    b. Call for the specialized self-contained breathing apparatus team to access the house
    c. Summon personnel to the scene with appropriate self-contained breathing devices
    d. Enter the house while wearing an oxygen mask

44. Once the patients are removed from the house you begin your evaluation and determine that there are a total of three patients. All are responsive only to painful stimuli. One patient has a "pink" appearance; the other two patients appear pale. Based on the scene and your patient evaluations you determine that the patients may have:

    a. Food poisoning
    b. Carbon monoxide poisoning
    c. An unknown drug overdose
    d. Smoke inhalation

45. The best treatment for these patients includes:

    a. Low-flow oxygen and transport to the local hospital 5 minutes away
    b. High-flow oxygen and transport to the local hospital 5 minutes away
    c. Low-flow oxygen and transport to the hyperbaric center 12 minutes away
    d. High-flow oxygen and transport to the hyperbaric center 12 minutes away

Questions 46 to 49 refer to the following scenario.

> You respond to the local bus station and encounter an approximately 33-year-old man lying on the ground. The patient does not have any visible trauma. Vital signs are pulse 92 beats/min and regular, respiratory rate is 2 breaths/min, blood pressure is 142/76 mm Hg, and the patient's pupils are very constricted. The patient's lips appear to be bluish in color.

46. Your immediate treatment for this patient is:

    a. Rapid transport
    b. Administration of oxygen by a nonrebreather mask
    c. Initiation of positive-pressure ventilations
    d. Administration of a cathartic

47. Based on your evaluation you suspect:

    a. Carbon monoxide poisoning
    b. A narcotic overdose
    c. An acetaminophen overdose
    d. Anaphylactic shock

48. The bluish coloration in the patient's lips is caused by:

    a. Hemoglobin saturated with carbon monoxide
    b. Oxygen toxicity
    c. The patient's hyperventilating
    d. Unsaturated hemoglobin

49. While you are en route to the hospital with this patient, you determine that the patient has gone into cardiac arrest (no pulse and no respirations). Your estimated time of arrival at the hospital is 7 minutes. The use of the automated external defibrillator for this patient is:

    a. Contraindicated because of the cause of the cardiac arrest
    b. Indicated and should be performed as soon as possible
    c. Contraindicated because of the patient's age
    d. Indicated only after there is no response to 5 minutes of cardiopulmonary resuscitation

Across

1. Adsorbent material that binds most toxins
8. Antifreeze
9. Medication that may be necessary to treat victims of organophosphate poisoning
10. Medication used to induce vomiting
12. The study of poisons
13. Drug that induces sleep
16. A remedy to counteract a poison
19. Substance that through its chemical action usually kills, injures, or impairs an organism
20. A spider is a type of _____ that may sting or bite, possibly causing an allergic reaction
23. Poisoning occurring from insect or snake bite
26. Taken into the body through the airway
27. Taken into the body through the skin
28. Most commonly abused drug in the United States
29. Drug that minimizes activity and excitement

Down

2. Hospital facility used to treat a victim of carbon monoxide poisoning
3. Organophosphate antidote
4. Opiate-type drugs
5. Gas that smells like rotten eggs, used in petroleum and rubber processing
6. Agent found in electroplating, photography, and metal cleaning that can be poisonous
7. The most severe type of food poisoning
11. Antidote for cyanide poisoning
14. Wood alcohol
15. Tearing
17. Taken into the body through the gastrointestinal tract
18. Pain relievers
21. Poisonous
22. Self-administration of drugs, taken in excess or in combination with other agents, to the point of poisoning
24. Antidote to an opioid overdose; also known as Narcan
25. Organophosphate used in war gases

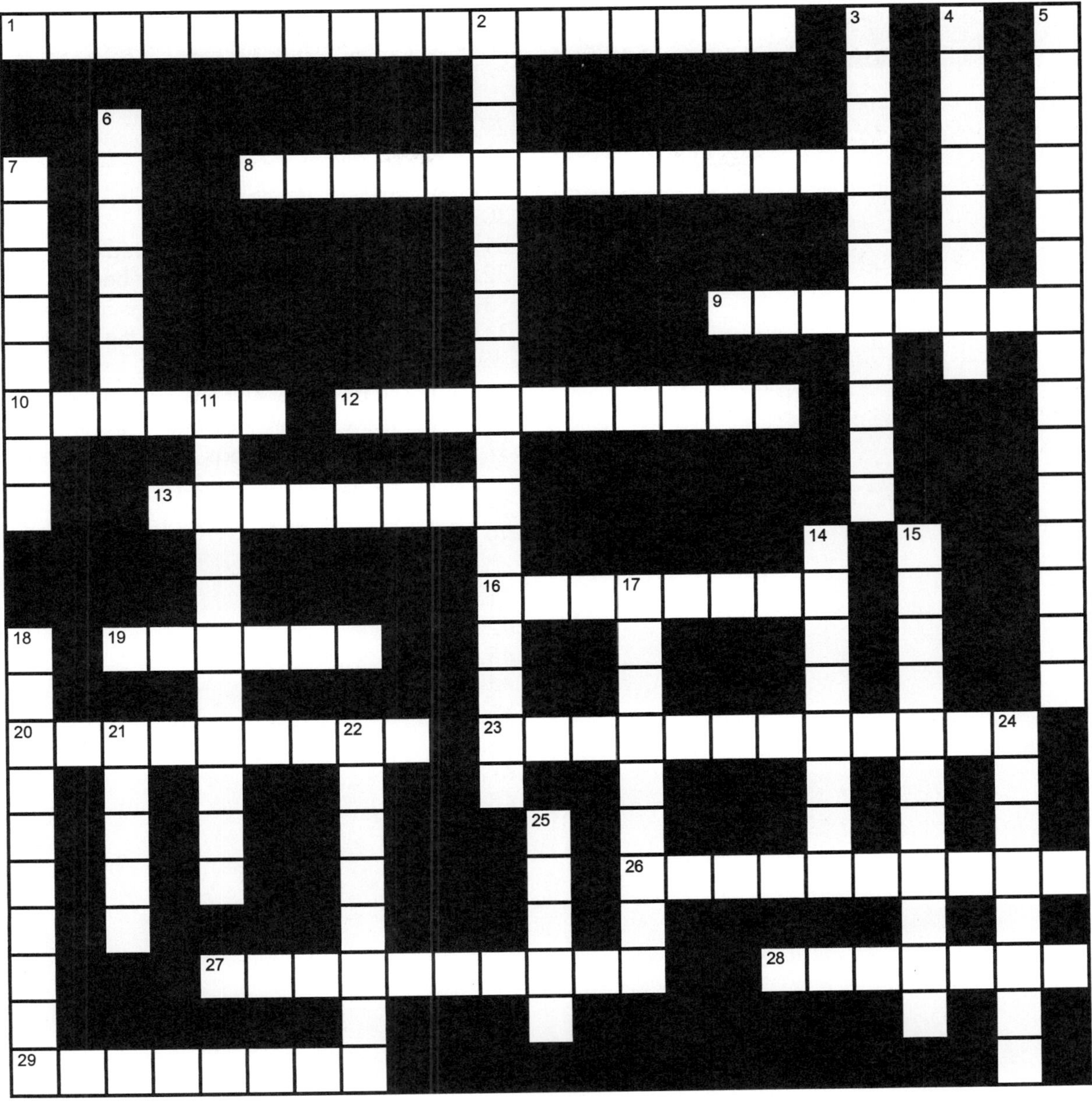

ANSWER KEY

1. c
2. c
3. a
4. d
5. b
6. b
7. d
8. c
9. c
10. d
11. c
12. d
13. a
14. d
15. a
16. d
17. b
18. b
19. c
20. b
21. b
22. c
23. a
24. a
25. c
26. d
27. a
28. Ethylene glycol
29. Methanol
30. 800-222-1222
31. What was the substance involved?
32. When did the patient ingest or become exposed?
33. How much of the substance was ingested?
34. Over what period of time was the substance ingested?
35. What, if any, interventions have already occurred?
36. What is the patient's estimated weight?
37. What effects, if any, has the patient experienced since the ingestion/exposure?
38. c
39. e
40. d
41. a
42. b
43. c
44. b
45. d
46. c
47. b
48. d
49. b

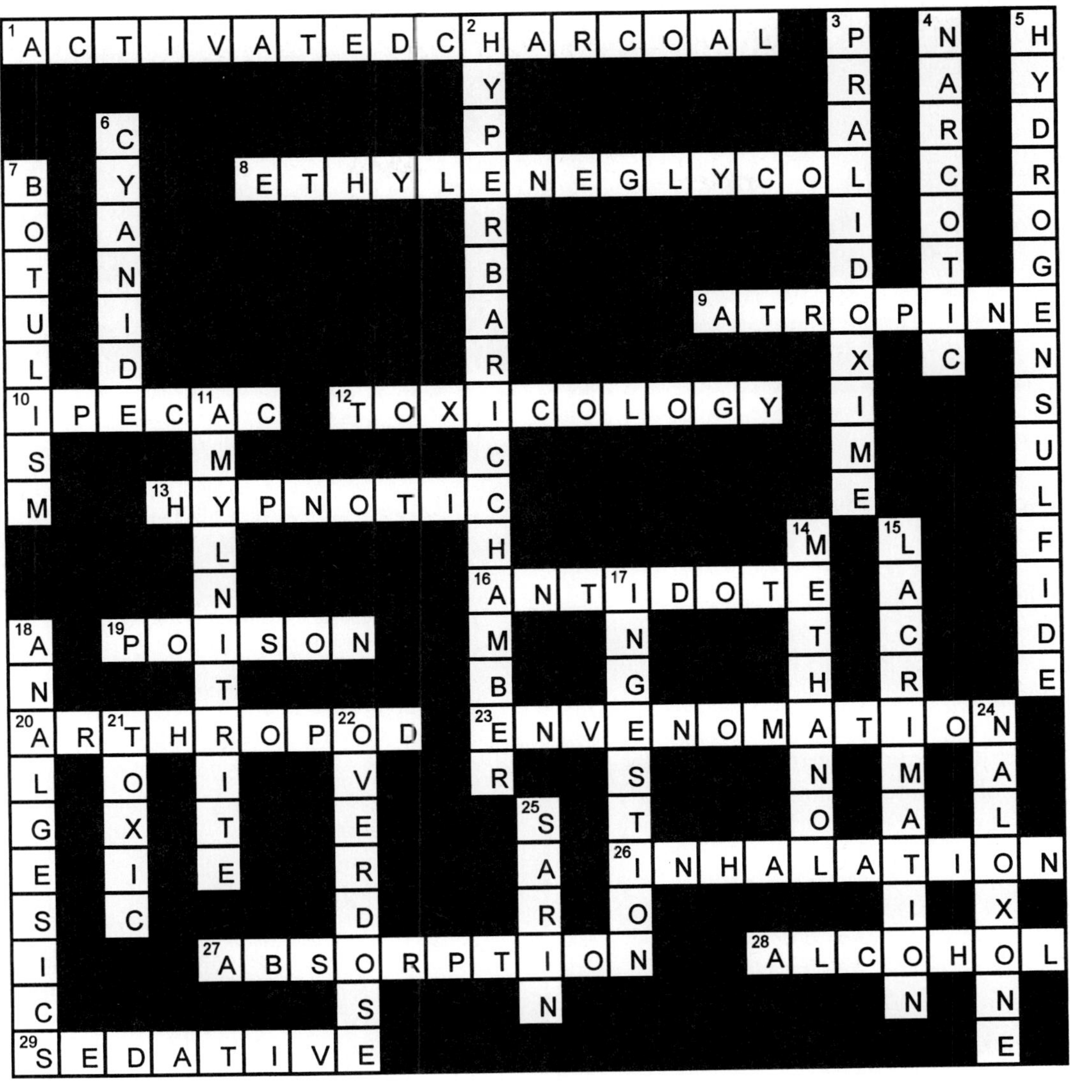
ACTIVATEDCHARCOAL
HYPERBARICCHAMBER
PRALIDOXIME
NARCOTIC
HYDROGENSULFIDE
CYANIDE
ETHYLENEGLYCOL
BOTULISM
ATROPINE
IPECAC
AMYLNITRITE
TOXICOLOGY
HYPNOTIC
METHANOL
LACRIMATION
ANTIDOTE
INGESTION
ANALGESIC
POISON
ARTHROPOD
TOXIC
OVERDOSE
ENVENOMATION
NALOXONE
SARIN
INHALATION
ABSORPTION
ALCOHOL
SEDATIVE

Chapter 22 Environmental Emergencies

1. Heat production in the body is primarily a function of:

   a. Metabolism
   b. The skin
   c. The gastrointestinal tract
   d. The kidneys

2. The transfer of heat from a warmer to a cooler environment not in direct contact with the body is called:

   a. Evaporation
   b. Conduction
   c. Convection
   d. Radiation

3. The transfer of heat to objects in direct contact with the body is called:

   a. Evaporation
   b. Conduction
   c. Convection
   d. Radiation

4. The transfer of heat to circulating air currents is called:

   a. Evaporation
   b. Conduction
   c. Convection
   d. Radiation

5. The loss of heat when moisture vaporizes on the body surface is called:

   a. Evaporation
   b. Conduction
   c. Convection
   d. Radiation

6. Under normal conditions, most heat loss occurs by:

   a. Evaporation
   b. Conduction
   c. Convection
   d. Radiation

7. Loss of heat by respiration is:

   a. Large
   b. Moderate
   c. Minimal
   d. Not possible

8. The body's "thermostat" that regulates temperature by influencing heat production, heat distribution, and heat loss is located in the:

   a. Cerebellum
   b. Brainstem
   c. Hypothalamus
   d. Pituitary

9. Heat distribution and heat loss are a primary responsibility of the:

   a. Cardiovascular system
   b. Respiratory system
   c. Digestive system
   d. Urinary system

10. When heat loss is needed, the body responds by initiating:

    a. Vasoconstriction
    b. Vasodilation
    c. Shivering
    d. Piloerection

11. High humidity in the environment will decrease the rate of:

a. Convection
b. Conduction
c. Respiration
d. Evaporation

12. Excessive losses of salt during exercise can cause heat:

a. Exhaustion
b. Cramps
c. Prostration
d. Stroke

13. Which of the following drinks will help ensure a balanced intake of water and electrolytes?

a. Sugar water
b. Gatorade
c. Orange juice
d. Seltzer

14. Which of the following age groups is most susceptible to heat emergencies?

a. Teenagers
b. Elderly
c. Middle-aged
d. None of the above

Match the predisposing factors of heat-related emergencies in column A with the explanations in column B.

Column A	Column B
15. _____ Heart disease	a. Compromised cardiovascular response
16. _____ Obesity	b. Increased insulation results in less heat loss
17. _____ Parkinson's disease	c. Inability to care for themselves
18. _____ Mental retardation	d. Muscle tremors produce heat

19. Alcohol can cause a gain in heat when the environmental temperature is above the body temperature because of:

a. Vasoconstriction
b. Vasodilation
c. Increased pulse
d. High blood pressure

20. Muscle cramping in heavily used muscles either during or immediately after exertion best describes:

a. Heat exhaustion
b. Heat stroke
c. Heat prostration
d. Heat cramps

21. The problem in the previous question should be treated by all the following *except*:

a. Rapid cooling with ice water
b. Placing the patient in a cool location
c. Providing an electrolyte drink
d. Stretching crampy muscles

22. The heat disorder that results from widespread vasodilation and fluid loss from sweating is called:

a. Heat exhaustion
b. Heat stroke
c. Heat prostration
d. Heat cramps

23. The treatment of the above condition includes all the following *except*:

a. Rapid cooling with ice water
b. Removal to cool environment
c. Removal excessive clothing
d. Replacement of electrolyte fluids

Match the heat-related condition in column A to the signs and symptoms in column B.

Column A	Column B
24. _____ Heat exhaustion	a. Very high temperature, dry skin, and altered mental state
25. _____ Heat cramps	b. Muscular cramps after exercise
26. _____ Heat stroke	c. Weakness, cool sweaty skin, rapid pulse, and elevated core temperature

27. The treatment of heat stroke involves all the following *except:*

a. Rapid cooling with ice at arterial points
b. Fanning with wet sheets on body
c. Rapid transport and oxygen
d. Cooling with alcohol sponge bath

28. On a hot, dry, and windless day (99°F), the body relies primarily on which of the following mechanisms to lose heat?

    a. Convection
    b. Evaporation
    c. Radiation
    d. Respiration

29. A core body temperature of less than 35°C best defines:

    a. Frostbite
    b. Hyperthermia
    c. Hypothermia
    d. Frostnip

30. A normal body response to cold emergencies involves:

    a. Increased metabolism and vasoconstriction at skin
    b. Increased metabolism and vasodilation at skin
    c. Slowed metabolism and vasoconstriction at skin
    d. Slowed metabolism and vasodilation at skin

31. Acute immersion hypothermia is a very severe form of cold injury because:

    a. Water is a very good conductor of heat
    b. Water vapors freeze your nasal mucosa
    c. Inhalation of water causes bronchoconstriction
    d. Cold water causes vasodilation and shock

32. A person who is drug intoxicated, ill, and lying on the floor of his apartment (70°F) for 2 days becomes hypothermic. This is an example of:

    a. Subacute hypothermia
    b. Acute hypothermia
    c. Chronic hypothermia
    d. Frostnip

Categorize the items in column A as either mild, moderate, or severe signs or symptoms of hypothermia in column B.

Column A	**Column B**
33. ____ Significant hypotension	a. Mild (35°-33°C)
34. ____ Unresponsive to pain.	b. Moderate (32°-27°C)
35. ____ Difficulty in speech	c. Severe (26°-22°C)
36. ____ Muscular rigidity	
37. ____ Slowing of pulse and respirations	
38. ____ Ventricular fibrillation	
39. ____ Shivering	

40. Which of the following statements regarding active external rewarming (i.e., placing the patient in a tub with 105°F water) is most correct?

    a. It is essential for all patients to avoid brain damage
    b. It should only be used for severe hypothermia
    c. It should only be used when transport is significantly delayed
    d. It should never be used

41. Which of the following statements regarding stimulation of hypothermic patients is most correct?

    a. They should receive vigorous tactile stimulation so that they do not lapse into a coma
    b. They should be handled very gently to avoid abnormal heart rhythms
    c. They should receive strong verbal stimulation to increase circulation to the brain
    d. They should receive only vigorous stimulation when they are in a coma

42. With severe hypothermia patients, hyperventilation should be:

    a. Avoided
    b. Performed at 24 breaths/min
    c. Performed at 32 breaths/min
    d. Performed at 40 breaths/min

43. Which of the active rewarming techniques is recommended for field use?

    a. Gastric lavage with warm fluids through a nasogastric tube
    b. Warm IV fluids and peritoneal lavage
    c. Warmed humidified oxygen and warm packs at arterial points (e.g., armpits)
    d. Applying battery-operated heated electric blankets

44. Cardiopulmonary resuscitation should be started on hypothermic patients when:

    a. The pulse drops below 50 beats/min
    b. The pulse drops below 40 beats/min
    c. The pulse drops below 30 beats/min
    d. Pulselessness is absolutely certain

45. A major complication of active external rewarming is:

    a. Burns to the skin
    b. Respiratory arrest caused by brainstem stimulation
    c. Rewarming shock caused by vasodilation of peripheral vessels
    d. Damage to the respiratory mucosa

46. Which of the following areas of the body is most subject to localized cold injury?

    a. Nose
    b. Genitalia
    c. Legs
    d. Arms

47. Ironically, which of the following mechanisms that protect against hypothermia is the major contributor to localized cold injury?

    a. Increased heart rate
    b. Peripheral vasoconstriction
    c. Shivering
    d. Peripheral vasodilation

48. A completely reversible cold injury characterized by blanching of the skin and loss of sensation in the affected area is called:

    a. Frostbite
    b. Deep frostbite
    c. Frostnip
    d. Superficial frostbite

49. A localized cold injury that is characterized by white and waxy skin that is firm to the touch but in which the tissue beneath the skin is soft and resilient is called:

    a. Deep frostbite
    b. Focal hypothermia
    c. Frostnip
    d. Superficial frostbite

50. The most severe form of localized cold injury that appears white and feels deeply frozen and resists depression to the touch is called:

    a. Deep frostbite
    b. Focal hypothermia
    c. Frostnip
    d. Superficial frostbite

51. Active rewarming of a frostbitten extremity is not recommended in the field because:

    a. Of the time needed to effectively rewarm the part
    b. Arrhythmias may develop
    c. It can lead to rewarming shock
    d. It is performed with electrical equipment

52. If a frostbitten foot should thaw before arrival at the hospital, you should:

    a. Break blisters to relieve pressure
    b. Cover with sterile dressings
    c. Encourage the person to walk to improve circulation
    d. Do nothing to the affected part

Questions 53 to 56 refer to the following scenario.

> You are on an ice fishing trip with two friends when you find a hiker who was lost in the woods. The hiker has been walking in deep snowdrifts for the past 3 hours. You bring the camper into your cabin and examine his feet, which appear white and deeply frozen. It is not possible to evacuate the patient to a hospital for at least 8 more hours.

53. You should

    a. Keep the extremities frozen until the patient can be transported to the hospital
    b. Give the patient alcoholic beverages to hasten rewarming
    c. Begin rewarming of the extremities because of the long transport time
    d. Rub the extremities vigorously in the snow

54. Rewarming of a localized cold injury should be performed at a water temperature of:

    a. 100°F
    b. 102°F
    c. 105°F
    d. 110°F

55. During the active rewarming process, water should:

    a. Remain perfectly still in the container to avoid irritation to the affected part
    b. Be continuously circulated to maintain an even temperature
    c. Be allowed to cool to body temperature during the rewarming process
    d. Be continuously heated slowly up to the patient's tolerance (not to exceed 120°F)

56. Following the rewarming of a deeply frostbitten extremity, pain is:

    a. Common
    b. Very rare
    c. Occasional
    d. Highly unlikely

57. Prolonged exposure (10-12 hours) to above-freezing temperatures and dampness (generally below 10°C, 50°F) can result in cold injury to wet extremities, which is called:

    a. Deep frostbite
    b. Immersion foot
    c. Frost foot
    d. Cold foot

58. You are called to the scene and find a 35-year-old man who is unconscious and unresponsive lying on the sidewalk. The temperature is 20°F and you suspect the patient may be experiencing hypothermia. Before beginning cardiac compressions, you should assess for a pulse for:

    a. 5 to 10 seconds
    b. 10 to 20 seconds
    c. 20 to 30 seconds
    d. 30 to 45 seconds

Questions 59 and 60 refer to the following scenario.

> A 78-year-old man is found on a park bench on a hot and humid summer day. He is unresponsive to painful stimulus. The physical exam reveals hot, flushed, dry skin and a strong bounding pulse. His vital signs are respirations 28 beats/min and shallow, pulse 120 beats/min and regular, and blood pressure 190/110 mm Hg.

59. This patient probably has:

    a. A severe infection
    b. Heat stroke
    c. Heat exhaustion
    d. Heat cramps

60. The initial treatment for this patient consists of:

    a. Rapid cooling with alcohol soaks
    b. Rapid cooling with water and convection
    c. Gradual cooling in shade and with salt water drinks
    d. Rapid transport only

Questions 61 and 62 refer to the following scenario.

> You respond to a marathon race and find a 23-year-old man who collapsed in the twenty-first mile of the race on a very hot (98°F) and dry day. Physical examination reveals the patient is lethargic and has pale and sweaty skin that is cool to the touch, weakness, dizziness, and a headache. His vital signs are pulse 90 beats/min and regular, respirations 20 breaths/min and shallow, and blood pressure 120/80 mm Hg. However, the blood pressure drops to 90/70 mm Hg when the patient sits up.

61. This patient probably has:

    a. Cardiac syncope
    b. A heat stroke
    c. Heat exhaustion
    d. Heat cramps

62. The initial treatment for this patient consists of:

    a. Rapid cooling with alcohol soaks
    b. Rapid cooling with water and convection
    c. Gradual cooling in the shade and replacement of fluids
    d. Rapid transport only

Questions 63 to 65 refer to the following scenario.

> You respond to a schoolyard on a very hot and humid day and find a 16-year-old girl complaining of severe leg cramps and sweating profusely. Otherwise, her physical examination and vital signs are normal. The coach advises you that she was running just before the episode.

63. This patient is probably having:

    a. Cardiac syncope
    b. Simple muscle cramps
    c. Heat exhaustion
    d. Heat cramps

64. The primary reason for the cramping is:

    a. Excessive loss of body salt
    b. Widespread vasodilation
    c. Muscle injury
    d. Muscle weakness

65. The initial treatment for this patient consists of:

    a. Rapid cooling with alcohol soaks
    b. Rapid cooling with water and convection
    c. Gradual cooling in shade and fluids
    d. Rapid transport only

Questions 66 and 67 refer to the following scenario.

You respond to an apartment and find a 78-year-old man who fell approximately 2 days ago and was found by his son 30 minutes before your arrival. The room is about 65°F. Physical examination reveals the patient is responsive to painful but not verbal stimuli, his skin is cool and dry to the touch, and he is shivering very slightly. His vital signs are pulse 80 beats/min and irregular, respirations 10 breaths/min and shallow, and blood pressure 90/60 mm Hg.

66. The primary problem with this patient is:

    a. Cardiogenic shock
    b. Shock because of pain in the leg
    c. Cardiac arrhythmia
    d. Moderate hypothermia

67. The initial treatment for this patient consists of:

    a. Warming with blankets
    b. Hot drinks en route to the hospital
    c. Rapid warming with electric blankets
    d. Rapid transport only

Questions 68 to 70 refer to the following scenario.

You respond to a call for a swimming pool injury. At the scene, you find a 7-year-old boy floating supine and slightly submerged in an indoor pool. The patient is unconscious and appears to be cyanotic from the shoulders up. His grandmother (who cannot swim) states that he dove into a shallow part of the pool and did not come up for 2 to 3 minutes.

68. What major consideration should you exercise during removal from the water?

    a. A quick abdominal thrust as soon as possible
    b. Spinal immobilization precautions
    c. Beginning compressions in the water
    d. Suctioning before ventilation

69. On removal, what manual airway maneuver would you use to evaluate breathing?

    a. Head tilt/chin lift
    b. Chin pull maneuver
    c. Head tilt/neck lift
    d. Jaw thrust without head tilt

70. On removal you note vital signs are pulse 80 beats/min, blood pressure 80/60 mm Hg, and respirations 2 breaths/min. The patient is unresponsive and cyanotic. Your next treatment will be to:

    a. Provide positive-pressure ventilation at a rate of 12 times per minute
    b. Provide positive-pressure ventilation at a rate of 20 times per minute
    c. Place the patient on a nonrebreather oxygen mask
    d. Provide humidified oxygen with a nasal cannula

Match the distinguishing features in column A with the type of snake in column B.

Column A	**Column B**
71. ____ Elliptical eyes	a. Nonpoisonous
72. ____ Round eyes	b. Pit vipers
73. ____ Pit between eyes and nostrils	
74. ____ Fangs	
75. ____ Triangular head	

76. In the treatment of poisonous snake bites, attempts to suck out the venom:

    a. Are required in every case
    b. Remove 90% of the venom
    c. Are highly controversial
    d. Should be done after swelling occurs

77. Which of the following is a useful technique to minimize distribution of the poison of a coral snake bite?

    a. Immobilizing the affected part with an elastic bandage
    b. Applying an arterial tourniquet
    c. 6 ounces of alcohol
    d. Placing the part on ice

Questions 78 and 79 refer to the following scenario.

> While on stand-by at an EMS picnic, you are called for a snake bite case. A 24-year-old man was bitten in the ankle by a snake, and his friend killed the snake just before your arrival. You examine the snake and note elliptical eyes, a pit between the eyes and nose, and a triangular head.

78. You conclude that the snake is:

    a. Poisonous
    b. Not poisonous
    c. Poisonous only if it is brightly colored
    d. Poisonous only if it has a rattle tail

79. Your response time to a hospital will be approximately 1 hour. Which of the following actions is appropriate under these conditions?

    a. Apply ice to the ankle
    b. Apply an arterial tourniquet
    c. Apply an elastic bandage and immobilize the limb
    d. Cut an "X" at the site of the bite and suck out the venom

List the five key questions to ask the patient or things that you as the EMT want to look for, in a patient with an environmental emergency.

80. ______________________________

81. ______________________________

82. ______________________________

83. ______________________________

84. ______________________________

TRUE OR FALSE

85. _____ A patient with a heat-related emergency is found with moist skin at the time of collapse. Because of this physical finding, it is impossible for the patient to be having heat stroke.

86. _____ The highest priority in treating a patient with heat stroke is rapid transport to the hospital.

87. _____ The term "near drowning" means a patient survived at least 24 hours after a submersion episode.

88. _____ Abdominal thrusts should not be routinely used in an attempt to clear the lungs of water in a submersion episode.

89. _____ Approximately 10% to 20% of drownings are considered to be a "dry drowning."

90. _____ The mammalian diving reflex increases metabolism, thereby increasing the patient's chance for survival.

Match the insect or spider in column A with the identifying characteristics in column B.

Column A	Column B
91. _____ Brown recluse spiders	a. Encountered in loose mounds of dirt and each sting can give rise to a small, circumscribed, elevated lesion
92. _____ Black widow spiders	b. Causes a painful red spot, sometimes with a central blist
93. _____ Fire ants	c. Severe cases cause problems with vision, swallowing, and slurred speech
94. _____ Scorpions and tarantulas	d. Causes abdominal pain and lower extremity weakness

Across

4. Involuntary contraction of small groups of muscles, generating heat
8. Self-administration of drugs, taken in excess or in combination with other agents, to the point of poisoning
11. Life-threatening emergency caused by the victim's inability to sweat
12. Painful muscular contractions of heavily exercised muscles
16. The cardiovascular system's inability to respond to the demands for increased blood flow to the skin while still maintaining flow to the muscles and other organs
17. The organ whose primary role is heat regulation
18. The _____ _____ spider has a red hourglass shape on the abdomen
19. A reversible cold injury secondary to intense vasoconstriction to cold exposure
20. Suffocation in water or other liquid resulting in death within 24 hours
21. The transfer of heat from a warmer environment to a cooler environment that is not in direct contact with the body

Down

1. Venomous snake with elliptical pupils
2. Venomous snake with red, yellow, and black bands
3. The _____ _____ spider has a dark-colored band on its back resembling a violin
5. Deep _____ is characterized by freezing extending throughout the dermis and deeper structures, possibly to bone
6. A core body temperature lower than 35° F
7. Describes the effects of extremity and shell rewarming before the core temperature can be raised
9. The portion of the brain that sets the body's thermostat and regulates temperature
10. _____ diving reflex
13. The loss of heat that occurs when moisture vaporizes on the body's surface
14. _____ _____ is caused by prolonged exposure to above-freezing temperatures and dampness
15. The transfer of heat to objects in direct contact with the body

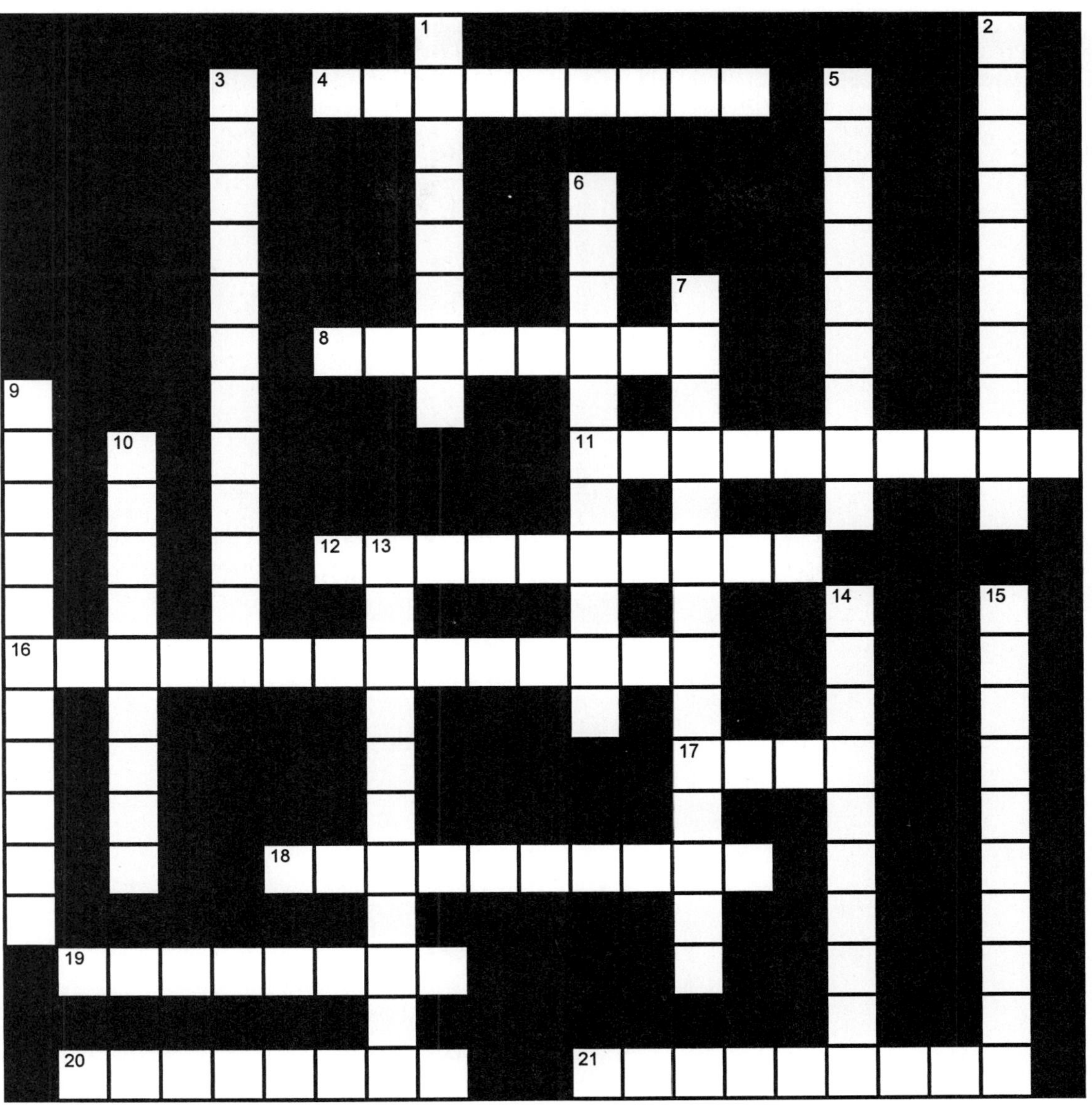
1
2
3
4
5
6
7
8
9
10
11
12
13
14
15
16
17
18
19
20
21

ANSWER KEY

1. a
2. d
3. b
4. c
5. a
6. d
7. c
8. c
9. a
10. b
11. d
12. b
13. b
14. b
15. a
16. b
17. d
18. c
19. b
20. d
21. a
22. a
23. a
24. c
25. b
26. a
27. d
28. b
29. c
30. a
31. a
32. c
33. c
34. c
35. a
36. b
37. b
38. c
39. a
40. c
41. b
42. a
43. c
44. d
45. c
46. a
47. b
48. c
49. d
50. a
51. a
52. b
53. c
54. c
55. b
56. a
57. b
58. d
59. b
60. b
61. c
62. c
63. d
64. a
65. c
66. d
67. a
68. b
69. d
70. b
71. b
72. a
73. b
74. b
75. b
76. c
77. a
78. a
79. d
80. What was the source of the environmental emergency?
81. What was the environment that the exposure occurred in?
82. What was the duration of the exposure?
83. Did the patient lose consciousness?
84. What effects, general or local, has the patient experienced?
85. False
86. False
87. True
88. True
89. True
90. False
91. b
92. d
93. a
94. c

1 PITVIPER
2 CORALSNAKE
3 BROWNRECLUSE
4 SHIVERING
5 FROSTBITE
6 HYPOTHERMIA
7 REWARMINGSHOCK
8 OVERDOSE
9 HYPOTHALMUS
10 MAMMALIAN
11 HEATSTROKE
12 HEATCRAMPS
13 EVAPORATION
14 TRENCHFOOT
15 CONDUCTION
16 HEATEXHAUSTION
17 SKIN
18 BLACKWIDOW
19 FROSTNIP
20 DROWNING
21 RADIATION

Chapter 23 Behavioral Emergencies

1. Which of the following age groups is most likely to commit suicide?

   a. Small children
   b. Persons in their 20s
   c. Middle-aged persons
   d. Elderly persons

2. You have a confused and agitated patient in your ambulance who thinks that he is in church and that you are his son. Your best approach would be to:

   a. Quietly go along with what he is saying or he will become more agitated
   b. Tell him that you are an EMT and that he is in an ambulance on the way to a hospital
   c. Let him think you are his son, but tell him where he is
   d. Restrain the patient and do not try to talk to him

3. An emotional response to sudden illness, a death in the family, or some other difficult personal experience that may be exhibited by anxiety, fear, paranoia, anger, hysteria, denial, or withdrawal is called a:

   a. Situational reaction
   b. Nervous breakdown
   c. Hysterical reaction
   d. Temporary breach

4. Nervousness, tension, pacing, hand wringing, and trembling are all symptoms of:

   a. Anxiety
   b. Paranoia
   c. Hysteria
   d. Suicidal tendencies

5. A patient who is afraid that you are trying to kill him with poison gas when you place an oxygen mask over his face may be experiencing:

   a. Anxiety
   b. Confusion
   c. Paranoia
   d. Hysteria

6. The patient who is having a heart attack and does not want to go in the ambulance because he "just has a little chest pain" is experiencing:

   a. Denial
   b. Hysteria
   c. Anxiety
   d. Confusion

7. A patient who has difficulty sleeping, loss of appetite, loss of sex drive, inability to feel pleasure, and feelings of hopelessness likely has:

   a. Denial
   b. Depression
   c. Hysteria
   d. Psychosis

8. A person who is about to commit suicide:

   a. Always exhibits signs of depression
   b. Never calls for help
   c. May appear very content and even happy
   d. Is never a danger to others

9. Distorted perceptions of reality, with hallucinations and inappropriate responses to the environment, best describes a:

   a. Phobia
   b. Situational reaction
   c. Psychosis
   d. Hysterical reaction

10. All the following are common signs of impending violent behavior *except*:

    a. Pacing
    b. Angry voice
    c. Pressured speech
    d. Crying

11. The first priority when faced with an emotionally disturbed patient is to:

    a. Restrain him or her immediately
    b. Consider possible medical causes
    c. Give sedation and then restrain
    d. Get permission from the family to restrain

12. The first priority with a potentially dangerous patient is:

    a. Self-protection
    b. The patient's protection
    c. The legal implications
    d. Restraining him or her

13. A suicidal patient who is explaining her reasons for wanting to commit suicide should be managed by:

    a. Comparing her problems to others and therefore minimizing their severity
    b. Acknowledging her perspective and offering her help at the hospital
    c. Being firm and taking a "parental role" in your relationship with her
    d. Waiting for an opportunity and quickly restraining her with the assistance of the police

14. In general, the best posture to assume when dealing with a violent patient is:

    a. Firm and authoritative
    b. Aggressive and self-assured
    c. Calm and reassuring
    d. Light-hearted and carefree

15. Responses such as guilt, grief, anger, hysteria, denial, withdrawal, or physical reactions are common reactions to:

    a. Phobias
    b. Pain
    c. Organic illness
    d. Death

Questions 16 and 17 refer to the following scenario.

> You have a female patient who appears to have been badly beaten and possibly raped. She refuses to answer questions about where she is hurt or what happened to her. She simply stares into space and refuses to look at you.

16. This patient's common reaction to a terrifying situation is known as:

    a. Denial
    b. Withdrawal
    c. Confusion
    d. Hysteria

17. Your first action in caring for this should be to:

    a. Examine her to see if she was raped
    b. Identify yourself in a gentle and reassuring manner
    c. Focus on injuries not emotional issues
    d. Have her describe the incident to experience an emotional catharsis

Questions 18 and 19 refer to the following scenario.

> You respond to a home and find a patient who is combative and angry. His family states that he never behaves in this manner and suddenly exhibited aggressive and dangerous behavior. The past medical history indicates no psychiatric disorders, but the patient has a history of heart disease, diabetes, and chronic obstructive lung disease.

18. This patient's condition is most likely related to:

    a. Psychosis
    b. Depression
    c. Hypoglycemia
    d. A drug reaction

19. Your action in caring for this patient should include:

    a. Administering glucose
    b. Administering epinephrine
    c. Restraining the patient with police and family
    d. Inducing vomiting

Questions 20 and 21 refer to the following scenario.

> You are dispatched to a call for a patient with terminal cancer. At the scene, you encounter a 34-year-old patient dying from leukemia. The patient is conscious and aware of his condition. He responds angrily to almost every request or comment made to him.

20. This patient's reaction:

    a. Is very common with dying patients
    b. Suggests insensitivity on your part
    c. Must be dealt with firmly
    d. Should be actively converted by cheerfulness

21. The most effective method for dealing with this patient is:

    a. Empathetic listening
    b. Firm interaction and directions
    c. A detached clinical approach
    d. Distract him from his problems

22. You are dispatched to a call for an emotionally disturbed patient. At the scene, you encounter a 78-year-old man who is disoriented and experiencing hallucinations. He states that he sees ants crawling on his chest and abdomen and that they are eating him alive. All the following are possible explanations for this patient's behaviors *except:*

    a. Alcohol withdrawal
    b. Organic brain syndrome
    c. LSD ingestion
    d. Depression

23. A situation in which a patient exhibits abnormal behavior within a given situation that is unacceptable or intolerable to the patient, family, or community best describes an:

    a. Anxiety reaction
    b. Behavioral emergency
    c. Psychosis
    d. Schizophrenic reaction

24. You encounter a 48-year-old patient who is exhibiting violent behavior. The patient attempted to cut his wrists. He now refuses to go to the hospital. After multiple attempts to convince him with a calm reassuring approach, you should:

    a. Work with police to restrain and remove the patient
    b. Allow the patient to refuse care because he is an adult
    c. Leave him alone with family members to convince him
    d. Use a contrived story to convince him to go

List the seven key questions to ask the patient with a behavioral emergency.

25. ______________________________

26. ______________________________

27. ______________________________

28. ______________________________

29. ______________________________

30. ______________________________

31. ______________________________

List the eight common medical and environmental causes of behavior alteration.

32. ______________________________

33. ______________________________

34. ______________________________

35. ______________________________

36. ______________________________

37. ______________________________

38. ______________________________

39. ______________________________

TRUE OR FALSE

40. _____ Suicide is the tenth leading cause of death in the United States.

41. _____ Paranoia is the most common mental disorder in elderly patients.

42. _____ A person about to commit suicide always shows signs of depression.

43. _____ The most important aspect of the *initial assessment* of the patient with a suspected behavioral emergency is to look for the possibility of an underlying medical cause.

44. _____ Visual, tactile (touch), or olfactory (smell) hallucinations almost always have an organic cause.

Questions 45 to 47 refer to the following scenario.

> You respond to the scene of an apartment house fire and encounter a 33-year-old man who is being restrained by the police. He tells you that his wife and two children are still trapped in the building. You continue to stay with this person until the fire is under control.

45. Your patient appears very tense and can't stay still. He continues to pace back and forth as he watches the efforts of the fire department to find his family. This patient is exhibiting signs of:

    a. Anxiety
    b. Paranoia
    c. Agitation
    d. Denial

46. Approximately 30 minutes elapse and the fire chief comes over and tells your patient that the bodies of his wife and two children have been found. Your patient begins to cry uncontrollably and starts beating his fists against a car. This patient is now exhibiting signs of:

    a. Anxiety
    b. Paranoia
    c. Agitation
    d. Denial

47. You continue to comfort your patient and offer to call a friend or relative to be with him. Initially the patient won't focus on what you are saying but after a while the patient sits on the ground and holds his head in his hands. You continue to reassure the patient but he is refusing to talk or interact with you. This patient is now exhibiting signs of:

    a. Anxiety
    b. Paranoia
    c. Agitation
    d. Withdrawal

Across

5. Senile _____ is an organic brain syndrome caused by degeneration of the brain
7. Appears as nervousness, tension, pacing, hand wringing, and trembling
8. Behavioral disorder present in at least 5% of the population
12. You may have a need to _____ a patient who is combative
14. The _____ patient displays confusion and agitation
17. The patient with _____ may be crying uncontrollably or beating fists against a wall
18. _____ hallucinations involve touch
19. _____ hallucinations involve smell

Down

1. A medical disorder causing a behavioral symptom
2. The _____ patient may hear voices or have bizarre thoughts
3. The tenth leading cause of death in the United States
4. The manner in which a person acts or performs
6. Medical information tag worn by many people
9. _____ disorders are character traits that interfere with a person's ability to function successfully in society
10. Patients with _____ hallucinations hear voices
11. Reasonable _____ is determined by what is necessary to prevent the patient from injuring himself or others
13. The patient with _____ feels threatened by people and his or her environment
15. Hallucinations may be due to an _____ cause rather than a behavioral disorder
16. An unconscious inability to accept or believe a situation

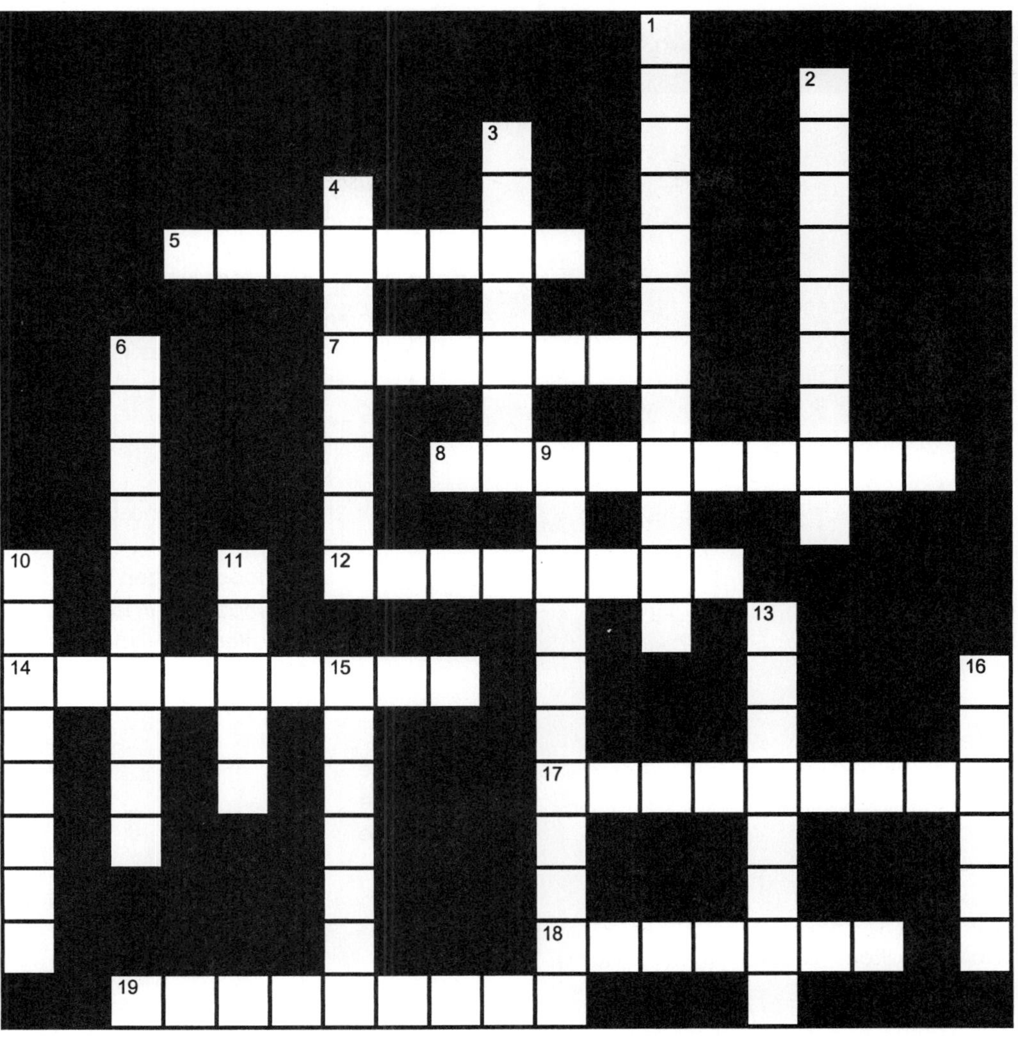
1
2
3
4
5
6
7
8
9
10
11
12
13
14
15
16
17
18
19

ANSWER KEY

1. d
2. b
3. a
4. a
5. c
6. a
7. b
8. c
9. c
10. d
11. b
12. a
13. b
14. c
15. d
16. b
17. b
18. c
19. a
20. a
21. a
22. d
23. b
24. a
25. How do you feel?
26. Ask appropriate questions to determine suicidal tendencies
27. Is the patient a threat to self or others?
28. Is there a medical problem along with the behavioral emergency?
29. What is the patient's past medical history?
30. Has the patient/family undertaken any interventions?
31. What medications does the patient take and does he or she take them as prescribed?

32. to 39. Excessive cold
Excessive heat
Head trauma
Inadequate blood flow to the brain (shock, stroke)
Low blood oxygen level
Low blood sugar level
Mind-altering substances
Psychogenic, resulting in psychotic thinking, depression, or panic

40. True
41. False
42. False
43. False
44. True
45. a
46. c
47. d

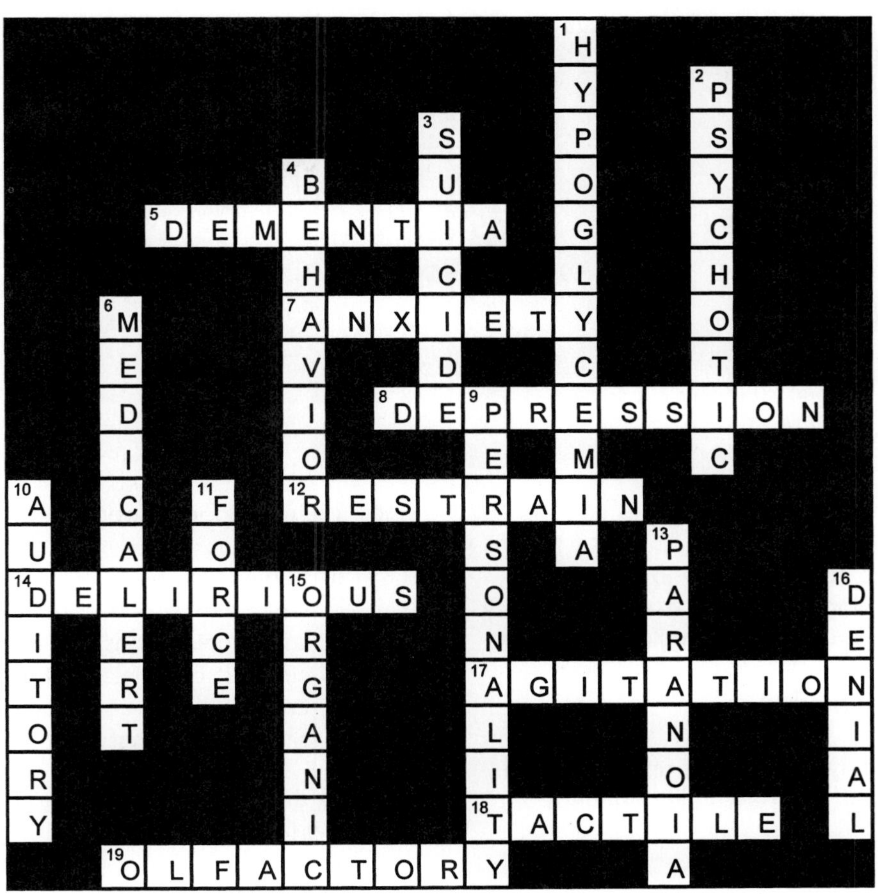

Chapter 24 Obstetrics and Gynecology

1. A major function of the fallopian tubes is:

   a. Carrying eggs from the ovary to the uterus
   b. The site of implantation of a normal pregnancy
   c. The connecting point between the cervix and the vagina
   d. The site of egg production

2. The part of the body where eggs are stored and become mature and where female hormones are produced is the:

   a. Fallopian tube
   b. Uterus
   c. Ovary
   d. Cervix

3. The section of the uterus that dilates during labor is the:

   a. Body
   b. Cervix
   c. Fundus
   d. Myometrium

4. The organ through which nutrients and waste products are exchanged between the baby and the mother is the:

   a. Uterus
   b. Placenta
   c. Liver
   d. Cervix

5. The umbilical cord contains:

   a. One vein and one artery
   b. One vein and two arteries
   c. Two veins and one artery
   d. Two veins and two arteries

6. The first stage of labor:

   a. Begins with full dilation of the cervix and ends when the baby is born
   b. Lasts from the onset of contractions until the cervix is completely dilated
   c. Ends at the onset of transition
   d. Should never last more than 1 hour

7. All the following are parts of the mechanism of childbirth *except*:

   a. Flexion
   b. Composition
   c. Internal rotation
   d. Expulsion

8. During the second stage of labor:

   a. The mother often has an urge to move her bowels
   b. Postpartum hemorrhage may occur
   c. You can expect to deliver the placenta
   d. Labor contractions stop

9. Your first action after the baby's head is born is to:

   a. Clamp the cord
   b. Suction the baby's mouth and nose with a bulb syringe
   c. Dry the baby thoroughly
   d. Deliver the placenta

10. During a normal vertex delivery, as soon as the baby's head is born, your second action is to:

    a. Immediately tell the mother to push before the cervix closes
    b. Ask the mother to pant while you check to see if there is a cord wrapped around the baby's neck
    c. Examine the baby's mouth to see if he or she has a cleft lip
    d. Tell the mother to push

11. If a baby's head is born and you find that the umbilical cord is wrapped tightly around the baby's neck, you should:

    a. Give the mother oxygen and transport rapidly
    b. Stretch the cord over the baby's head to unwind it
    c. Clamp the cord close together in two places and cut between the clamps
    d. Try to push the head back inside a little bit to ease tension around the baby's neck

12. In a vertex delivery with meconium-stained fluid, the mouth should be suctioned:

    a. Only after the nose is suctioned
    b. Before stimulating the baby to breathe
    c. Only after you check the heart rate
    d. The mouth should not be suctioned because you will contaminate the mouth with bacteria

13. When you find that the baby's leg is projecting out of the vagina in a laboring patient, you should:

    a. Grasp the leg firmly and pull until you can reach the other leg
    b. Transport rapidly while giving oxygen to the mother
    c. Try to push the leg back inside the vagina
    d. Press on the mother's fundus and ask her to push

14. After a baby is born and the cord is cut, you notice a sudden gush of blood from the mother's vagina and lengthening of the umbilical cord. This would indicate:

    a. Laceration of the vagina
    b. The onset of a postpartum hemorrhage
    c. The placenta is about to deliver
    d. Uterine rupture

15. Allowing the mother to nurse a healthy, full-term newborn after birth:

    a. Should never be done in the ambulance
    b. Can help to contract the uterus
    c. Can relieve cyanosis in a newborn
    d. Supplies the baby with the calories it needs

16. If the placenta does not spontaneously deliver within 15 to 20 minutes after the baby is born, you should:

    a. Ask the mother to push while you pull on the cord
    b. Proceed to the hospital
    c. Ask the mother to stand; gravity may deliver the placenta
    d. Perform McRobert's maneuver

17. When resuscitating a newborn, the heart rate is counted:

    a. For a full minute
    b. For 6 seconds
    c. Only after the Apgar score is done
    d. For 30 seconds

18. All the following are symptoms of respiratory distress in the newborn *except*:

    a. Grunting
    b. Nasal flaring
    c. Cyanosis of the hands and feet
    d. Sternal retractions

19. All the following are improper actions when resuscitating a newborn *except*:

    a. Hyperextending the neck before ventilating
    b. Quickly drying the baby immediately after birth
    c. Giving chest compressions with the heel of one hand
    d. Ventilating the baby at a rate of 80 breaths/min

20. Positive-pressure ventilation for a newborn should be done at a rate of:

    a. 20 to 30 breaths/min
    b. 40 to 60 breaths/min
    c. 80 to 100 breaths/min
    d. 120 to 140 breaths/min

21. The concentration of oxygen for positive-pressure ventilation of a newborn should be:

    a. 90% to 100%
    b. 50% to 60%
    c. 24% to 36%
    d. Never give oxygen to a newborn

22. Chest compressions in the newborn should be:

    a. One third of the anterior-posterior depth of the chest at a rate of 100 compressions/min
    b. One third of the anterior-posterior depth of the chest at a rate of 120 compressions/min
    c. Half of the anterior-posterior depth of the chest at a rate of 100 compressions/min
    d. Half of the anterior-posterior depth of the chest at a rate of 120 compressions/min

23. A newborn is breathing at birth, so you check the heart rate. It is 80 beats/min. Your next action would be to:

    a. Evaluate the baby's color
    b. Begin positive-pressure ventilation with 100% oxygen
    c. Begin cardiac compressions
    d. Give 100% free-flow oxygen

24. When resuscitating a newborn, cardiac compressions should be discontinued once the baby's heart rate is more than:

    a. 60 beats/min
    b. 80 beats/min
    c. 90 beats/min
    d. 100 beats/min

25. An infant born with a cleft palate:

    a. Will probably also be brain damaged
    b. Should not be allowed to nurse
    c. Should not be shown to the mother
    d. All the above

26. Allowing the newborn to become chilled can:

    a. Help establish respirations if the baby does not cry
    b. Cause hypoglycemia and acidosis
    c. Stimulate a more rapid heart rate as the baby tries to stay warm
    d. Help to keep the baby awake so that it can nurse

27. In general, the position for transport of a pregnant patient in her third trimester is:

    a. Supine
    b. Prone
    c. On her left side
    d. On her right side

28. The reason for transporting a pregnant woman in this position is:

    a. You always want to have the mother facing you in the ambulance
    b. Most babies are facing the mother's right side late in pregnancy, and pressure on the back of the baby's head can dangerously lower the heart rate
    c. To prevent damage to the liver
    d. The vena cava is right of the midline and you do not want to compress it between the spinal column and the weight of the baby

29. During normal pregnancy, the blood pressure:

    a. Should not change
    b. Becomes slightly higher than it was before pregnancy
    c. Becomes much higher than it was before pregnancy
    d. Becomes lower than it was before pregnancy

30. A baby born to a diabetic mother:

    a. Is prone to hypoglycemia after delivery
    b. Is prone to hyperglycemia after delivery
    c. Is not usually affected by the mother's disease
    d. Will probably be born with diabetes

31. A baby born to a diabetic mother is likely to be:

    a. Larger than normal
    b. Smaller than normal
    c. Average size

32. Maternal hypertension is defined as:

    a. Systolic greater than 180 or diastolic greater than 100 mm Hg
    b. Systolic greater than 160 or diastolic greater than 100 mm Hg
    c. Systolic greater than 150 or diastolic greater than 90 mm Hg
    d. Systolic greater than 140 or diastolic greater than 90 mm Hg

33. Preeclampsia becomes eclampsia when:

    a. Hypertension and edema are both present
    b. The blood pressure exceeds 180/100 mm Hg
    c. A seizure occurs
    d. All the above

34. If you examine a laboring patient and find the umbilical cord bulging out of the vagina, you should:

    a. Clamp and cut the cord so that the baby can be delivered
    b. Try to elevate the presenting part with a gloved hand so it does not compress the cord
    c. Gently place the cord back inside the vagina
    d. Place a moist pressure dressing over the vagina

35. Prolapsed cord is often associated with:

    a. Placenta previa
    b. Abruptio placentae
    c. Abnormal presentation, such as breech or shoulder
    d. Preeclampsia

36. You arrive at a call to find a patient who states she is approximately 32 weeks' pregnant, but she has not seen a doctor because she has no money. She awoke in the middle of the night and was very upset to find that she had passed a good deal of bright red blood from her vagina. She has no abdominal or pelvic tenderness but complains of mild low back pain. Her skin is pale, warm, and dry to the touch. Her vital signs are blood pressure 100/56 mm Hg, pulse 108 beats/min, and respirations 22 breaths/min. Your first action for this patient would be to:

    a. Do a gentle vaginal examination to see if the patient is about to deliver
    b. Place the patient on her left side and give high-concentration oxygen
    c. Insert a pressure dressing into the vagina to control the bleeding
    d. Massage the patient's uterus to control the bleeding

37. All the following are indications of imminent delivery *except*:

    a. Urge to move her bowels
    b. Bulging of the perineum
    c. Bloody show
    d. Rupture of membranes

38. You arrive at a call to find a woman who is 30 weeks' pregnant with her second child. She complains of labor pains but cannot say how far apart they are because the pain is almost constant. Her uterus feels hard and she is restless and crying with the pains. History reveals that she was in a motor vehicle accident yesterday, was seen in the emergency department and treated for sprained wrists, which she injured bracing herself against the dashboard. She was a front-seat passenger wearing a lap belt restraint. There is no vaginal bleeding or discharge. Her vital signs are blood pressure 130/80 mm Hg, pulse 114 beats/min, and respirations 24 breaths/min. Your best action for this patient would be to:

    a. Take out an obstetric kit and prepare for a premature delivery
    b. Place her on her left side, give oxygen, and transport immediately
    c. Do a vaginal examination to see if the cervix is dilated
    d. Use McRobert's maneuver

39. A patient complains of severe shoulder pain that came on suddenly. Physical examination reveals abdominal tenderness, and she is starting to have some vaginal bleeding. Her skin is pale, cool, and clammy. She missed her last period. This patient's symptoms are most likely caused by:

    a. Placenta previa
    b. Threatened abortion
    c. Ruptured ectopic pregnancy
    d. Breech presentation

Questions 40 and 41 refer to the following scenario.

You arrive at a call to find a patient in labor. She is very uncomfortable, with contractions occurring every 3 minutes and lasting 60 seconds. She is noisy and restless with contractions and loudly demands to go to the bathroom. Physical examination reveals a slight bulging of the perineum and rectum, but no presenting part is visible. There is a gush of fluid during a contraction, and you note that the fluid is meconium stained.

40. The meconium in the fluid alerts you to all the following *except:*

    a. The baby may be breech
    b. There is a 20% chance that the baby may have respiratory distress
    c. The fetus has had a bowel movement
    d. The mother probably has an infection

41. Your best action for this patient would be to:

    a. Explain that the urge to go to the bathroom is probably the baby coming, then have the woman lie on her bed and prepare for a delivery
    b. Allow her to go to the bathroom so that she will be more cooperative
    c. Explain that the urge to go to the bathroom is probably the baby coming, then get her to lie on the stretcher in the ambulance and prepare for a delivery en route to the hospital
    d. Put the mother in knee-chest position

Questions 42 and 43 refer to the following scenario.

You arrive at a call and find a 34-year-old woman who has just delivered her third child, a full-term girl. A survey of the newborn reveals a healthy infant with well-established respirations and no signs of distress. The placenta delivers spontaneously, and you are about to transport the patient when the vaginal bleeding becomes very heavy. The mother's blood pressure is 90/50 mm Hg, pulse is 118 beats/min, and respirations are 22 breaths/min. Her skin is cool, somewhat clammy, and pale.

42. The most common cause of early postpartum hemorrhage is:

    a. Perineal lacerations
    b. Uterine atony
    c. Ruptured uterus
    d. Prolapsed uterus

43. Your first action for this patient would be to:

    a. Apply direct pressure to the perineum
    b. Palpate and massage the uterus
    c. Elevate the patient's hips
    d. Apply an ice pack to the perineum

44. Postpartum hemorrhage is defined as a blood loss equal to or greater than

    a. 100 mL
    b. 500 mL
    c. 800 mL
    d. 1000 mL

Questions 45 and 46 refer to the following scenario.

You arrive at a call to find a 19-year-old woman who has been beaten and raped by a stranger. Her clothes are torn and bloodstained, and she is crying.

45. The best way to proceed in this situation is:

    a. Gently help the woman to change her clothes, wash up, and transport
    b. Gently assess for further injuries, treat as necessary, and transport
    c. Examine her perineum to assess for injuries
    d. Encourage her to douche before you go to the hospital to prevent infection

46. The best attitude to take with this patient is to:

    a. Minimize the event so that it does not seem so bad
    b. Be gentle, understanding, and compassionate
    c. Talk to her as little as possible
    d. Be authoritative because she needs to feel someone is in control

Questions 47 to 50 refer to the following scenario.

You have a patient whose chief complaints are epigastric pain, headache, and dizziness. She is about 30 weeks' pregnant and has marked puffiness in her hands, legs, and face. As you lift the stretcher, she starts to complain of blurred vision. Her vital signs are blood pressure 170/100 mm Hg, pulse 122 beats/min, and respirations 24 breaths/min.

47. This patient probably has:

    a. Diabetes
    b. Heart attack
    c. Preeclampsia
    d. Gastric ulcer

48. Your best action for this patient would be to:

    a. Put on lights and sirens and rush to the hospital
    b. Place her on her left side, give oxygen, have suction equipment ready, and proceed quietly to the hospital
    c. Ask her to push so you can deliver the baby
    d. Give her milk to drink to relieve the gastric acidity

49. The dizziness, blurred vision, and headache are probably caused by:

    a. Cerebral and retinal edema
    b. Gastric ulcer
    c. Hypoglycemia
    d. Shock

50. There is a good possibility that this patient may soon have a:

    a. Cardiac arrest
    b. Full gastric bleed
    c. Seizure
    d. Hypoglycemic reaction

Questions 51 to 56 refer to the following scenario.

> You arrive at an obstetric call to find that a breech delivery is in progress. The patient is a 28-year-old woman who tells you that this is her third pregnancy. The baby has been born up to the neck.

51. Which of the following is almost always present in a breech delivery?

    a. A premature baby
    b. Meconium fluid
    c. An umbilical cord around the neck
    d. Heavy vaginal bleeding

52. The mother is pushing uncontrollably, but the head will not deliver. To assist, you might:

    a. Twist the baby's body around until the head pops out
    b. Place your fingers on both sides of the baby's nose and flex the baby's chin on the chest
    c. Clamp and cut the umbilical cord
    d. Place the mother on her left side and ask her to stop pushing

53. The baby requires positive-pressure ventilation. The percentage of oxygen given during positive-pressure ventilation is:

    a. 100%
    b. 80%
    c. 50%
    d. 21%

54. After 30 seconds of positive-pressure ventilation, your partner checks the baby's heart rate. It is 50 beats/min. She should now:

    a. Discontinue positive-pressure ventilation
    b. Continue positive-pressure ventilation and begin chest compressions
    c. Stimulate the baby if it is breathing
    d. Suction the baby's mouth and nostrils

55. The baby has been successfully resuscitated. You notice that his right arm hangs limply at his side and there is no grasp reflex in the hand. This is probably caused by:

    a. Brain damage
    b. Damage to the brachial nerves
    c. Hypoglycemia
    d. Dislocation of the shoulder

56. Your best action at this time would be to:

    a. Reduce the dislocation by pulling the arm out and then up
    b. Immobilize the arm by wrapping the baby firmly in a blanket and handling it as little as possible
    c. Continue to stimulate the baby's hand until you can elicit a grasp reflex
    d. Wrap the baby loosely with the arm outside the blanket and ask the mother to nurse the baby

57. Proper body substance isolation procedures for a childbirth includes:

    a. Gloves only
    b. Gloves and goggles
    c. Gloves, goggles, and mask
    d. Gloves, goggles, and gown

58. All the following are components of a typical obstetrics kit *except*:

    a. Clamps
    b. Bag-valve-mask
    c. Surgical scissors or scalpel
    d. Bulb syringe

59. An explosive delivery is best prevented by:

    a. Applying gentle pressure to the crown of the baby's head during delivery
    b. Elevating the mother's hips during delivery
    c. McRobert's maneuver
    d. Applying gentle downward pressure on the shoulders

60. Premature babies are at very high risk for:

    a. Respiratory problems and hypothermia
    b. Meconium aspiration
    c. Ventricular fibrillation
    d. Cleft palate

61. As a general rule, how long should you wait before transport for the second baby to deliver in a mother who is expecting twins?

    a. 3 minutes
    b. 5 minutes
    c. 10 minutes
    d. 30 minutes

List the seven questions to ask the patient with an obstetric emergency.

62. ______________________________

63. ______________________________

64. ______________________________

65. ______________________________

66. ______________________________

67. ______________________________

68. ______________________________

Left shoulder pain with no history of trauma can be caused by:

69. ______________________________

70. ______________________________

71. The Apgar score is performed at 1 minute after birth and is repeated _________ after birth.

Signs of respiratory distress in the newborn include:

72. ______________________________

73. ______________________________

74. ______________________________

75. ______________________________

76. Approximately how far from the infant's nose should you hold the oxygen tubing when administering free-flow oxygen?

77. Approximately what volume of air do the lungs of a newborn hold?

The word *Apgar* is an acronym for the five criteria that are evaluated in the newborn. List the five components of the Apgar score.

78. A ______________________________

79. P ______________________________

80. G ______________________________

81. A ______________________________

82. R ______________________________

Questions 83 to 87 refer to the following scenario.

> You respond to a call at the shopping mall and encounter a 23-year-old woman who informs you that she is 32 weeks' pregnant with her second child. She was walking in the mall when her water broke and she immediately began to feel contractions. You place the patient out of public view and begin your evaluation. You perform a visual examination of the patient and notice that the baby's head is visible in the vagina with each contraction. The patient asks permission to use the bathroom because she has a strong urge to move her bowels.

83. Based on your examination you:

    a. Escort the patient to the bathroom
    b. Begin transport to the hospital and allow the patient to use a bedpan
    c. Prepare for imminent delivery of the baby
    d. Place the patient in the knee-chest position on the stretcher and begin rapid transport to the hospital

84. After your initial steps in treating the baby, you evaluate the baby and determine that the baby is not breathing. Your immediate response is to:

    a. Provide positive-pressure ventilations and cardiopulmonary resuscitation compressions
    b. Provide positive-pressure ventilations without cardiopulmonary resuscitation compressions
    c. Deliver supplemental oxygen with an infant oxygen mask
    d. Deliver supplemental oxygen with oxygen supply tubing

85. After 30 seconds of positive-pressure ventilations the infant starts to cry. Your next action is to:

    a. Check the heart rate and give free-flow oxygen
    b. Continue positive-pressure ventilations
    c. Start chest compressions
    d. Suction the infant

86. While you continue to treat the baby you notice that your partner delivers the placenta. The placenta delivers during the:

 a. First stage of labor
 b. Second stage of labor
 c. Third stage of labor
 d. Fourth stage of labor

87. After the placenta is delivered the patient continues to bleed heavily from the vagina. You evaluate the patient and you do not see any external tears in the perineum, but bleeding continues to come from the vagina. You should:

 a. Apply the pneumatic anti-shock garment and transport
 b. Massage the uterus
 c. Allow the baby to nurse, place the patient on her left side, and transport rapidly

Across

1. Feces found in amniotic fluid alerting to a stressed fetus
4. Home for the developing fetus
9. Condition characterized by high blood pressure and seizures
11. Absence or cessation of menstrual period
12. Pregnancy occurring outside the uterus
13. Appearance of the full diameter of fetal head through birth canal
14. _____ score is a system used to rapidly evaluate a newborn
16. Trumpet-shaped structures assisting with mature egg movement
19. Uterine _____ is a condition requiring replacement of the uterus into the vagina
21. Sign of respiratory distress in newborns
22. Vein that carries oxygenated blood to the fetus
23. Lowest segment of the uterus
24. An incision, made by the physician, to facilitate easier delivery
25. Presentation of buttocks first into the pelvis

Down

1. Maneuver used to assist in releasing a wedged anterior shoulder of baby during delivery
2. Nontraumatic, severe shoulder pain in a woman of childbearing age may be due to _____ _____
3. Hormone vital to menstruation and pregnancy
5. Loss of a pregnancy before 20 weeks' gestation
6. Watery liquid that protects the fetus
7. Afterbirth
8. Growth of placenta over part or all of the cervical opening
10. High blood pressure and edema during pregnancy
15. Uterine _____ may occur after a previous cesarean section or trauma
17. Loss of pregnancy after 20 weeks' gestation
18. Infant less than 5½ lbs or 37 weeks' gestation
20. Glands where eggs are produced

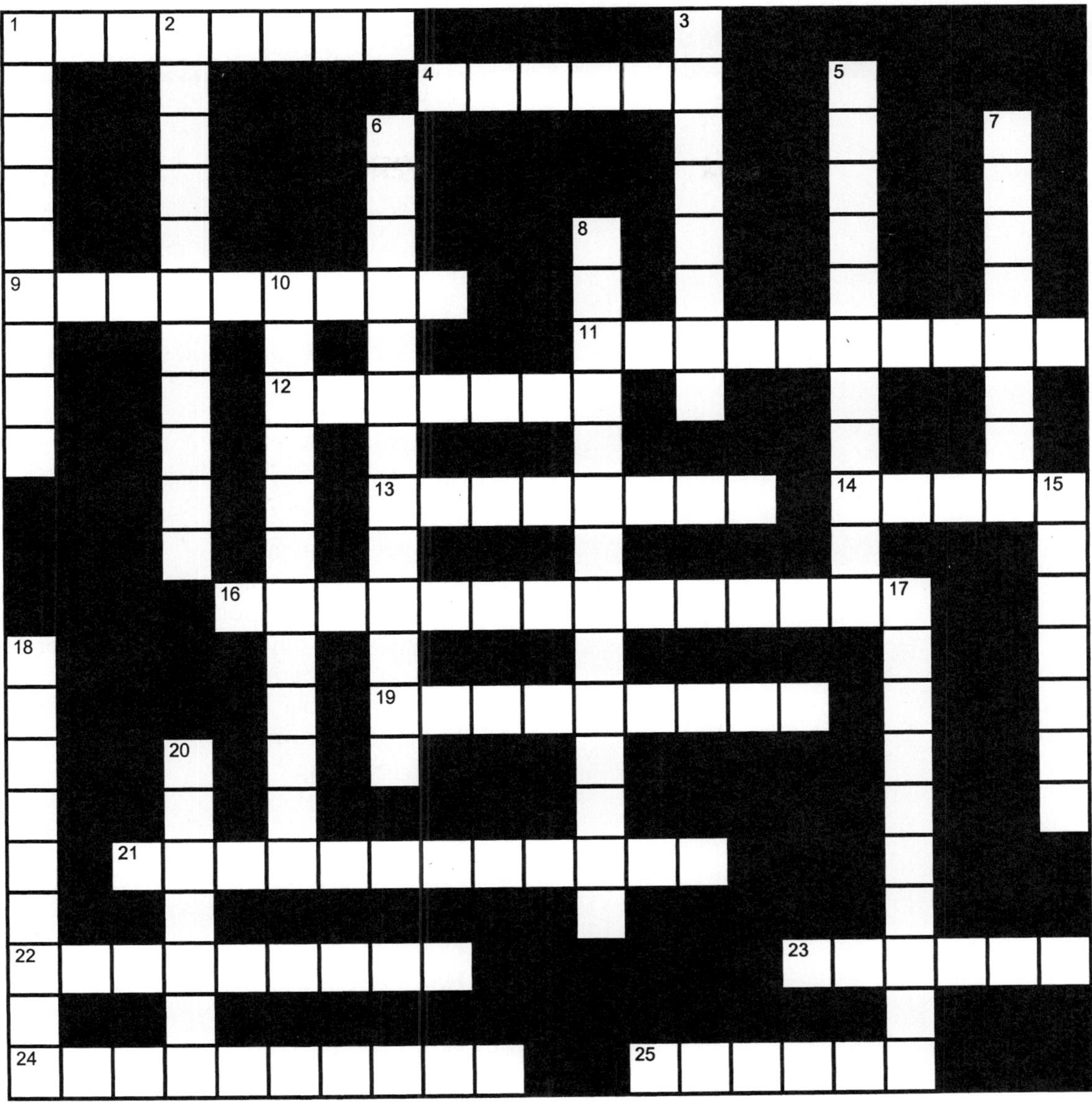
1
2
3
4
5
6
7
8
9
10
11
12
13
14
15
16
17
18
19
20
21
22
23
24
25

ANSWER KEY

1. a
2. c
3. b
4. b
5. b
6. b
7. b
8. a
9. b
10. b
11. c
12. b
13. b
14. c
15. b
16. b
17. b
18. c
19. b
20. b
21. a
22. b
23. b
24. a
25. b
26. b
27. c
28. d
29. d
30. a
31. a
32. d
33. c
34. b
35. c
36. b
37. d
38. b
39. c
40. d
41. c
42. b
43. b
44. b
45. b
46. b
47. c
48. b
49. a
50. c
51. b
52. b
53. a
54. b
55. b
56. b
57. d
58. b
59. a
60. a
61. c
62. Are you pregnant?
63. How long have you been pregnant?
64. Do you have any pain or contractions?
65. Do you have any vaginal bleeding or discharge?
66. Do you feel the need to push?
67. When was your last menstrual period?
68. Is the baby crowning?
69. Ruptured ectopic
70. Ruptured ovarian cyst
71. 5 Minutes
72. Retractions
73. Grunting
74. Nasal flaring
75. Cyanosis
76. Half inch
77. 20 to 30 mL
78. Appearance (color)
79. Pulse (heart rate)
80. Grimace (vigorous cry on stimulation)
81. Activity (extremities should have good tone and be flexed and moving)
82. Respirations
83. c
84. b
85. a
86. c
87. b

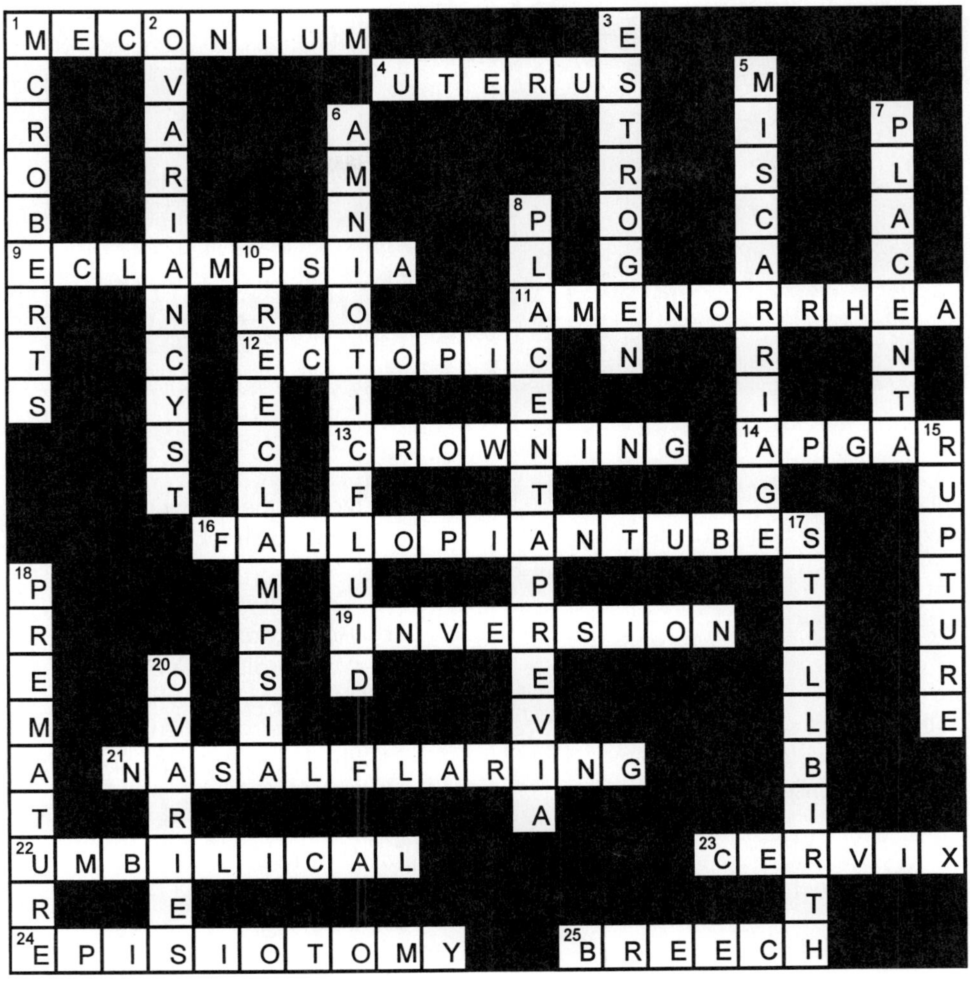

Chapter 25 Bleeding and Shock

1. Failure of the circulatory system to adequately perfuse and oxygenate the tissues of the body best defines:

   a. Respiratory failure
   b. Shock
   c. Heart failure
   d. Clinical death

2. The "fight or flight" response is mediated by:

   a. Atropine
   b. Epinephrine (adrenaline)
   c. Histamine
   d. Dopamine

3. Which of the following is an effect of epinephrine (adrenaline) release?

   a. Decreased heart rate
   b. Constriction of the pupils
   c. Increased force of heart contraction
   d. Decreased flow to the brain

4. Shock that occurs from a myocardial infarction (heart attack) is called:

   a. Cardiogenic shock
   b. Distributive shock
   c. Obstructive shock
   d. Hypovolemic shock

5. Which of the following is most likely to result in vasodilatory type shock?

   a. Anaphylaxis
   b. Hemorrhage
   c. Tension pneumothorax
   d. Heart attack

6. Which of the following conditions may cause obstructive shock?

   a. Coronary thrombosis
   b. Anaphylaxis
   c. Myocardial infarction
   d. Tension pneumothorax

7. All the following conditions may cause hypovolemic shock *except*:

   a. Diarrhea
   b. Burns
   c. Vomiting
   d. Fainting

8. A condition characterized by a low supply of hemoglobin is:

   a. Hypotensive syndrome
   b. Anemia
   c. Ischemia
   d. Hypovolemia

9. Bleeding characterized by pulsatile flow and bright red blood is:

   a. Capillary
   b. Venous
   c. Systemic
   d. Arterial

10. Which of the following is a characteristic of venous bleeding?

    a. Pulsatile flow
    b. Dark red color
    c. Occurs in deep wounds
    d. Always requires pressure point to control

11. The first step used to control bleeding is:

    a. Pressure point
    b. Tourniquet
    c. Air splint
    d. Direct pressure

12. Which of the following steps of bleeding control should be done as the final method?

    a. Direct pressure
    b. Tourniquet
    c. Pressure point
    d. Elevation

13. The pressure point for the upper extremity is located over the:

    a. Femoral artery
    b. Radial artery
    c. Ulnar artery
    d. Brachial artery

14. The pressure point for the lower extremity is located over the:

    a. Femoral artery
    b. Radial artery
    c. Ulnar artery
    d. Brachial artery

15. The first compensatory response of the body to acute blood loss (less than 15%) is:

    a. Venous constriction
    b. Hypotension
    c. Arterial constriction
    d. None of the above

16. Which of the following signs is the last to occur after acute blood loss?

    a. Pale skin
    b. Tachycardia
    c. Delayed capillary refill
    d. Hypotension

17. Which of the following best describes the sequence of the signs of hypovolemic shock?

    a. Altered mental status, rapid pulse, hypotension, delayed capillary refill
    b. Hypotension, rapid pulse, delayed capillary refill, altered mental status
    c. Rapid pulse, delayed capillary refill, hypotension, altered mental status
    d. Rapid pulse, altered mental status, hypotension, delayed capillary refill

18. Use of the abdominal section of the pneumatic anti-shock garment (PASG) is contraindicated in the presence of:

    a. Penetrating chest injury
    b. Suspected ruptured spleen
    c. Contusions on the abdominal wall
    d. Kidney injuries

19. The PASG is *primarily* used in the prehospital treatment of which form of shock:

    a. Cardiogenic shock
    b. Distributive shock
    c. Obstructive shock
    d. Hypovolemic shock

20. When removing the PASG in the hospital, you should:

    a. Remove them quickly starting with the legs
    b. Remove them quickly starting with the abdominal section
    c. Remove them slowly while monitoring blood pressure
    d. Remove them slowly while monitoring garment pressure

21. Which of the following is a possible effect of the PASG?

    a. Increases peripheral vascular resistance
    b. Tamponades bleeding in the chest
    c. Transfuses large amounts of blood to torso
    d. Shunts blood to the extremities

22. The upper margin of the abdominal section of the PASG should be placed no higher than the:

    a. Umbilicus
    b. Iliac crest of the pelvis
    c. Lower margin of the rib cage
    d. Suprapubic region

23. Which of the following is a contraindication to the use of the PASG?

    a. Intra-abdominal bleeding
    b. Pelvic injury
    c. Extremity bleeding
    d. Chest injury

Questions 24 to 26 refer to the following scenario.

> You respond to a call and find a 26-year-old man who was struck by an automobile. The initial assessment reveals that the patient is alert and oriented, is breathing, and has a carotid pulse. He has a wound on his right thigh that is spurting bright red blood. You attempt to control the bleeding with direct pressure and elevation but are unsuccessful.

24. Based on the description above the bleeding is most likely:

    a. Venous
    b. Capillary
    c. Arterial
    d. Venule

25. Your next action for treating the patient in the previous question is:

    a. Apply a tourniquet between the wound and heart
    b. Apply a pressure point over the popliteal artery
    c. Clamp the vessel with a hemostat
    d. Apply a pressure point over the femoral artery

26. If the above action is not successful, then, and only then, should you:

    a. Apply a tourniquet between the wound and heart
    b. Apply a pressure point over the popliteal artery
    c. Clamp the vessel with a hemostat
    d. Apply a pressure point over the femoral artery

Questions 27 to 30 refer to the following scenario.

> You respond to a call and find a 32-year-old woman who is the driver of a car involved in a front-end collision. She is alert and oriented and appears pale and sweaty with delayed capillary refill; her neck veins are flat. She is complaining of pain in her upper left quadrant of her abdomen and contusions on the left chest and abdominal walls. Her vital signs are respirations 26 breaths/min and shallow, pulse 120 beats/min and regular (at the carotids), and she has very weak radial pulses. Auscultation of her lungs reveals diminished breath sounds on the right side.

27. Based on the above signs, what percent of internal blood loss do you suspect has already occurred?

    a. Less than 10%
    b. 10% to 15%
    c. 20% to 25%
    d. More than 30%

28. The weak radial pulses in both arms are probably related to:

    a. Fractures
    b. Low blood pressure
    c. Blood clots
    d. Severed arteries in the arms

29. Based on these findings, which of the following oxygen delivery methods is appropriate?

    a. Venturi mask
    b. Nasal cannula
    c. Simple face mask
    d. Nonrebreather mask

30. If this patient had grossly distended neck veins, which of the following conditions would you search for?

    a. Cardiac contusion
    b. Tension pneumothorax
    c. Aortic aneurysm
    d. Arrhythmias

Questions 31 to 33 refer to the following scenario.

> You respond to a call and find a 30-year-old man who fainted after being robbed at gunpoint. His friend explains that during the stickup the patient fell unconscious for about 1 minute. The patient is now alert and oriented and has a perfectly normal physical examination. His vital signs are pulse 80 beats/min and regular, blood pressure 100/80 mm Hg, and respirations 18 breaths/min and of normal depth.

31. This patient most likely has a transient form of:

    a. Obstructive shock
    b. Vasodilatory shock
    c. Hypovolemic shock
    d. Cardiogenic shock

32. What action should his friend have taken to facilitate his recovery?

    a. Sit the patient up
    b. Administer ammonia capsules
    c. Elevate his legs while supine
    d. Administer glucose by mouth

33. This patient's primary cardiovascular problem was related to:

    a. A drop in blood pressure
    b. Tachycardia of the heart
    c. Vasoconstriction of the brain vessels
    d. Obstruction of blood flow through vessels

34. If a patient had severe bleeding in the face and mouth, your greatest immediate concern would be:

    a. Control of the airway
    b. Severe blood loss
    c. Brain injury
    d. Injury to the eyes

35. The appropriate body substance isolation procedures for a patient with a spurting wound would be:

    a. Gloves only
    b. Gloves and goggles only
    c. Gloves, goggles, and mask only
    d. Gloves, goggles, mask, and gown

36. The amount of blood pumped out of the heart with each beat is called the __________.

37. The amount of blood pumped by the heart each minute is called __________.

38. Stroke volume multiplied by _________ __________ equals cardiac output.

39. The force exerted by the blood volume on the walls of the vessels is called __________ __________.

TRUE OR FALSE

40. _____ The most effective treatment for cardiogenic shock is the use of the PASG.

41. _____ Infants and children may maintain their blood pressure until their blood volume is more than half gone.

42. _____ When we identify that the systolic blood pressure is 120, the number 120 refers to psi (pounds per square inch).

43. _____ The release of epinephrine causes the pupils to constrict.

44. _____ A patient with a closed fracture of the femur may lose approximately 1 L of blood at the injury site.

45. _____ A partially severed artery is most likely to clot because of the high volume of blood flowing through it.

46. _____ When controlling bleeding from the nose, the patient should be positioned sitting and leaning forward if there is no suspected neck or back injury.

Questions 47 to 52 refer to the following scenario.

> You respond to a call for a pedestrian struck by an automobile. You find an approximate 50-year-old woman lying on her left side on the ground. Bystanders state that the patient was thrown approximately 30 feet after being struck by a car traveling at a high rate of speed. Your initial assessment reveals a patient who does not respond to verbal or painful stimuli, she has a shard of glass in her cheek protruding into her mouth with moderate bleeding into her mouth, and you see gross deformity in both thighs. The patient also has a deep laceration to the medial aspect of the left lower leg with significant dark red colored bleeding that is not spurting. Vital signs are pulse 118 beats/min regular and weak, blood pressure 102/68 mm Hg, and respiratory rate 22 breaths/min and adequate.

47. Initial management of this patient's airway includes:

    a. Stabilizing the shard of glass in place
    b. Maintaining the patient on her side and transporting rapidly
    c. Removing the shard of glass and applying pressure to both sides of the laceration in the cheek
    d. Stabilizing the shard of glass in place, positioning the patient supine, and suctioning as needed

48. The appropriate position to transport this patient in is:

    a. Prone
    b. Left lateral recumbent
    c. In the position the patient was found
    d. Supine

49. The bleeding in the leg is probably:

    a. Capillary bleeding
    b. Venous bleeding
    c. Arterial bleeding
    d. Caused by an underlying fracture

50. The first method to control the bleeding in the leg is by:

    a. Elevation
    b. Compression of the pressure point in the leg
    c. Application of a tourniquet
    d. Direct pressure

51. If attempts to control bleeding are not working and you decide to apply compression to a pressure point, you would use a pressure point:

    a. Distal to the bleeding
    b. Proximal to the bleeding
    c. Directly over the wound
    d. At a point approximately 4 finger breadths below the injury

52. En route to the hospital you reevaluate your patient. The bleeding from the cheek and lower leg is controlled. Vital signs are now pulse 138 beats/min and weak, blood pressure 72/40 mm Hg, and respiratory rate 24 breaths/min. At this stage your patient is demonstrating signs of:

    a. Decompensated shock
    b. Compensated shock
    c. Obstructive shock
    d. Cardiogenic shock

Across

1. _____ is the last-resort method used to control bleeding because it completely obliterates blood flow
3. Vessels that carry blood back to the heart
5. The liquid portion of blood
6. A late sign of hypovolemic shock
8. Pressure in the arteries during a contraction
9. Very low blood volume
13. An emotional reaction that causes vasodilatory shock
15. The best and first way to control bleeding
18. Portion of blood that controls bleeding
20. Two receiving chambers of the heart
21. Amount of blood pumped by the heart each minute is the cardiac _____
23. Force exerted by the blood volume on the walls of the vessels
25. Pressure in the arteries during the relaxation period
27. The _____ _____ garment may be used to apply direct pressure over an extremity
29. The smallest vessels; gas exchanges take place here
31. Portion of blood that transports oxygen
32. _____ shock occurs when the cardiac output is inadequate to meet the body's needs

Down

2. Substance released by the body in response to stress
3. The total space within the arteries, veins, and capillaries
4. Hormone that regulates the utilization and storage of glucose
7. Capillary refill is delayed if the time it takes is more than _____ seconds
10. _____ shock may be caused by anaphylaxis and spinal cord injury
11. Portion of blood that fights infection
12. _____ _____ vomitus is a sign of internal bleeding
14. The blood, heart, and blood vessels are the three major components of the _____ system
16. To control bleeding from the extremities, use _____ in conjunction with direct pressure
17. The second method to control bleeding
19. _____ _____ isolation is a type of precaution taken to reduce the chances of disease transmission
22. The amount of blood pumped out of the heart with each beat is the _____ volume
24. _____ shock is caused by massive infection
26. Nosebleeds arise from the _____ portion of the nose
28. Patients who have a low supply of hemoglobin are said to be _____
30. Failure of the circulatory system to adequately perfuse and oxygenate the body tissues

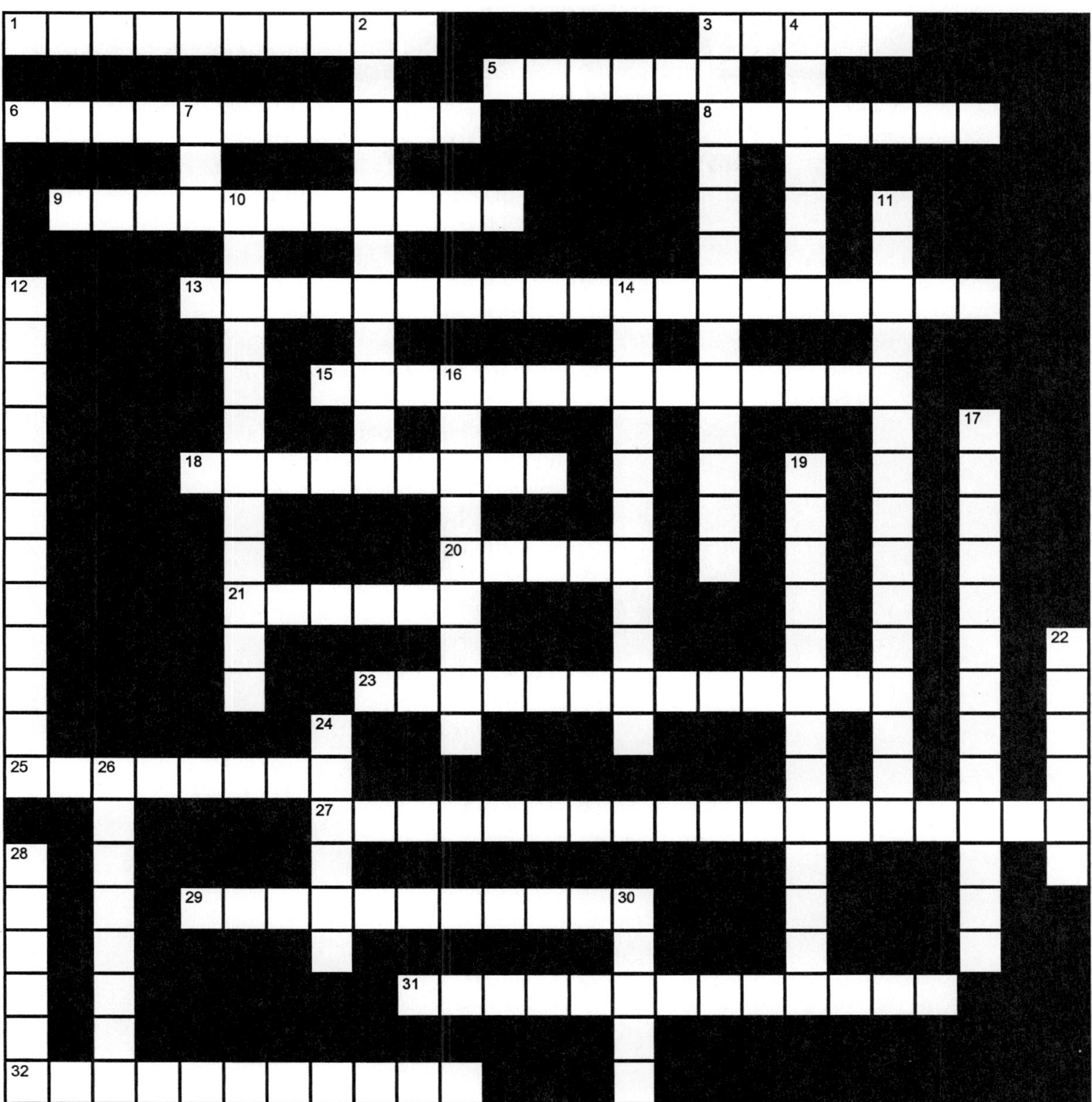
1
2
3
4
5
6
7
8
9
10
11
12
13
14
15
16
17
18
19
20
21
22
23
24
25
26
27
28
29
30
31
32

ANSWER KEY

1. b
2. b
3. c
4. a
5. a
6. d
7. d
8. b
9. d
10. b
11. d
12. b
13. d
14. a
15. a
16. d
17. c
18. a
19. d
20. c
21. a
22. c
23. d
24. c
25. d
26. a
27. c
28. b
29. d
30. b
31. b
32. c
33. a
34. a
35. d
36. Stroke volume
37. Cardiac output
38. Heart rate
39. Blood pressure
40. False
41. True
42. False
43. False
44. True
45. False
46. True
47. c
48. d
49. b
50. d
51. b
52. a

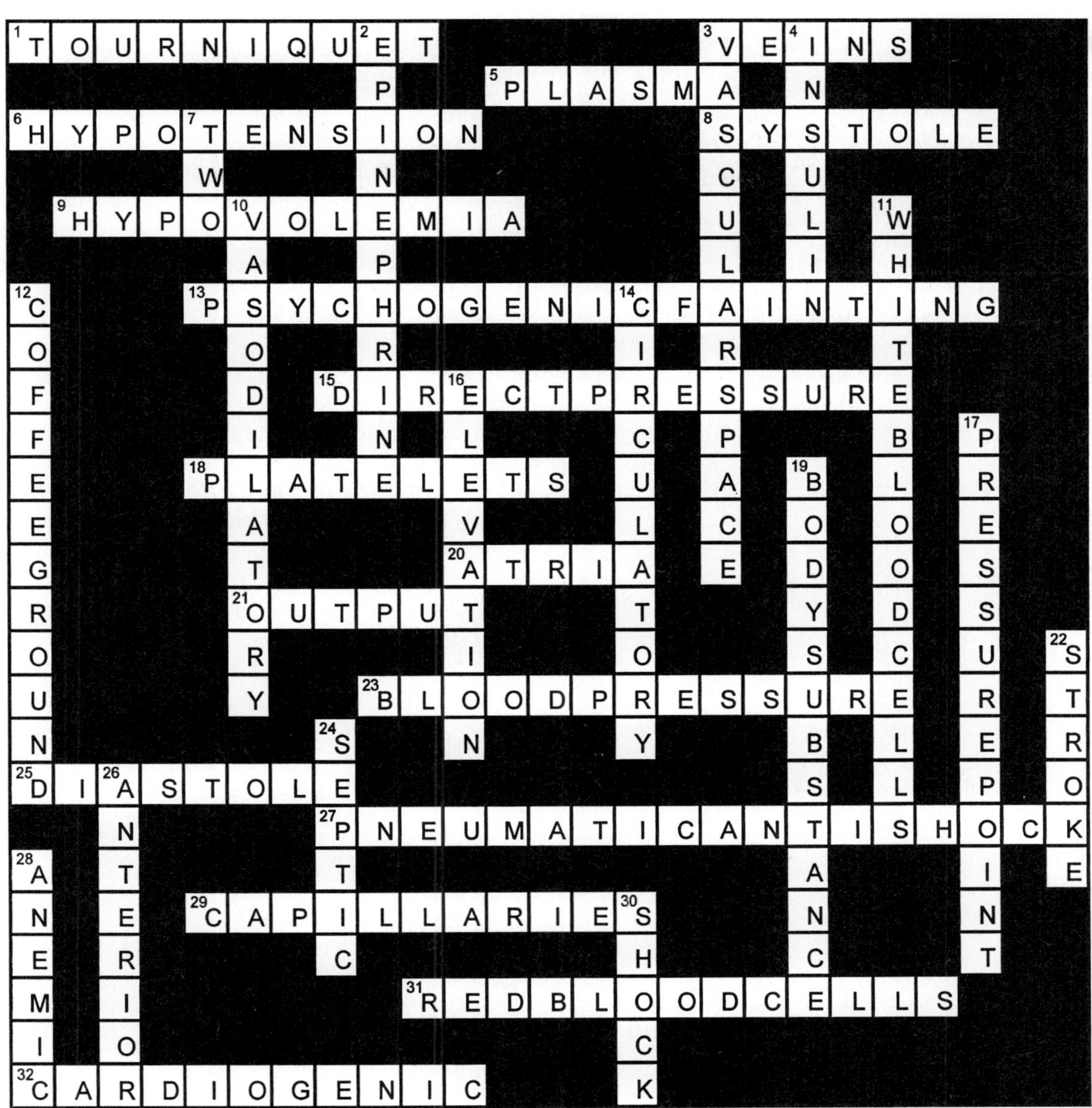
1 TOURNIQUET
3 VEINS
5 PLASMA
6 HYPOTENSION
8 SYSTOLE
9 HYPOVOLEMIA
13 PSYCHOGENICFAINTING
15 DIRECTPRESSURE
18 PLATELETS
20 ATRIA
21 OUTPUT
23 BLOODPRESSURE
25 DIASTOLE
27 PNEUMATICANTISHOCK
29 CAPILLARIES
31 REDBLOODCELLS
32 CARDIOGENIC

Chapter 26 Soft Tissue Injuries

1. The surface or outermost layer of the skin is called the:

   a. Subcutaneous layer
   b. Fascia
   c. Epidermis
   d. Dermis

2. The epidermis contains a special pigment that helps protect us from the sun's radiation and contributes to the color of the skin called:

   a. Melanin
   b. Keratin
   c. Surfactant
   d. Sebum

3. When blood flow to the skin is reduced (as a result of vasoconstriction in hypovolemic shock or in cold temperatures) the skin may appear:

   a. Red
   b. Cyanotic
   c. Pale
   d. Mottled

4. The layer of skin that is composed of dense connective tissue that contains the nerves, blood vessels, sweat and sebaceous glands, and hair follicles is called:

   a. Subcutaneous layer
   b. Fascia
   c. Epidermis
   d. Dermis

5. What will be the nature of sensory perception if the dermis is completely damaged, as in a full-thickness burn?

   a. Increased sensory function
   b. Extreme pain
   c. No sensory function
   d. Tingling sensation

6. Beneath the skin is a layer of fat and connective tissue called the:

   a. Mucosa
   b. Subcutaneous layer
   c. Subdermal layer
   d. Peritoneum

Match the type of wound in column A with the description in column B

Column A	Column B
7. _____ Contusion	a. Tearing away of the skin's surface
8. _____ Abrasion	b. Wound caused by a sharp instrument being driven through the skin
9. _____ Laceration	c. Scraping of the surface of the skin or mucous membrane
10. _____ Avulsion	d. Tearing of the skin or other soft tissues
11. _____ Puncture	e. Bruising of the skin

12. In general, impaled objects should be:

    a. Stabilized in place
    b. Carefully removed
    c. Repositioned to facilitate bandaging
    d. Left alone

13. Objects impaled in the cheek should be:

    a. Stabilized in place
    b. Carefully removed
    c. Repositioned to facilitate bandaging
    d. Left alone

14. What vessels are likely to promote air embolism when severed?

    a. Arteries in the head
    b. Veins in the neck and upper chest
    c. Capillaries in the chest
    d. Arteries in the chest

15. When a neck vein is severed, you should:

    a. Apply a gauze dressing and sit the patient upright
    b. Apply an air-tight dressing and place the patient in the head-down position
    c. Apply a saline dressing and place the patient on his or her side
    d. Apply a multitrauma dressing and place the patient prone

Match the type of bandage or dressing in column A with the description in column B.

Column A	Column B
16. _____ Multitrauma	a. Used as a sling or cravat bandage
17. _____ Triangular	b. Aluminum foil, plastic wrap, or petroleum gauze
18. _____ Self-adherent	c. Large dressing, used for massive abrasions or burns
19. _____ Occlusive	d. Allows elastic pressure for arterial bleeding

20. The first concern for a patient with injuries to the face and neck is the:

    a. Cervical spine
    b. Airway
    c. Eye
    d. Brain

21. Which of the following is a common effect of an improperly applied bandage?

    a. Obstruction of distal blood flow
    b. Damage to cartilage
    c. Obstruction of bowel function
    d. Tearing of muscles

22. The eye is a globular structure filled with gel-like fluid called the:

    a. Vitreous humor
    b. Mucus
    c. Peritoneal fluid
    d. Plasma

23. The collection of bones that surround the eye is (are) commonly called the:

    a. Ocular bones
    b. Orbit
    c. Periocular bones
    d. Acetabular

24. The white outer layer of the eye, which is composed of a tough, fibrous, and opaque (not transparent to light) protective membrane is called the:

    a. Cornea
    b. Retina
    c. Lens
    d. Sclera

25. The pigmented or colored portion of the eye that regulates the diameter of the pupil is called the:

    a. Retina
    b. Iris
    c. Cornea
    d. Macula

26. Anatomically, the eye can be divided into an anterior and posterior chamber by the:

    a. Lens
    b. Conjunctiva
    c. Retina
    d. Macula

27. When drainage of the aqueous humor is obstructed, pressure builds up and causes a condition known as:

    a. Retinitis
    b. Glaucoma
    c. Cataracts
    d. Aqueous tension

28. Tears are secreted from the:

    a. Mucous cells
    b. Ocular ducts
    c. Lacrimal glands
    d. Cornea

29. General principles for treating eye injuries include:

    a. Always irrigate and apply firm pressure
    b. Avoid pressure and cover both eyes
    c. Never treat in the field
    d. Use petroleum gauze and never cover both eyes

30. The best method for removing foreign bodies of the eye in the field is:

    a. With the use of suction cups
    b. Irrigation
    c. With the use of a cotton tip applicator
    d. With rapid eye movement

31. Impaled objects in the eyeball should be treated by:

    a. Pulling them out with a gloved hand
    b. Repositioning them to facilitate bandaging
    c. Stabilizing them in place
    d. Leaving them alone

32. Chemical burns to the eye are treated by:

    a. Bandaging the affected eye
    b. Irrigating with water or sterile saline
    c. Irrigating with an alkaline solution
    d. Rapid transport without field treatment

33. Light injuries caused by overexposure to infrared light from the sun or to ultraviolet light from arc welding are treated by:

    a. Placing moist patches over the eyes
    b. Taping the eyes closed
    c. Placing a cup over the eyes
    d. Irrigating the eyes

34. An extruded eyeball should be managed by:

    a. Replacing it in the eye socket
    b. Covering it with dry 4 × 4 bandage and a patch
    c. Covering it with a moist dressing and a cup
    d. Irrigation during transport

35. The outer visible flap of the ear is called the:

    a. Pinna
    b. Malleus
    c. Nares
    d. Vestibule

36. The middle ear communicates with the nasopharynx by the:

    a. Semicircular canal
    b. Cochlea
    c. Eustachian tube
    d. Vestibule

37. Other than hearing, the inner ear also contributes to control of:

    a. Voice transmission
    b. Heat exchange
    c. Balance and position
    d. Fluid exchange

38. Incomplete avulsed parts of the ear are treated by:

    a. Replacing them in anatomic position and bandaging them
    b. Removing them and storing them in saline solution
    c. Placing an ice pack over the site and transporting
    d. Irrigating with Betadine and alcohol solution

39. The rupture of the eardrum caused by changes in altitude and pressure is a type of:

    a. Tympanic syndrome
    b. Barotrauma
    c. The bends
    d. Pneumotympanic rupture

Questions 40 and 41 refer to the following scenario.

> You find a 28-year-old man lying on the living room floor of his apartment and bleeding profusely from the face. His wife states that he tripped and fell on a glass coffee table. You note on examination that he is in severe respiratory distress and has a large fragment of glass impaled in his left cheek that projects into his oral cavity.

40. The greatest immediate risk with this patient is:

    a. Aspiration and airway obstruction
    b. Bleeding and death
    c. Neurogenic shock from panic
    d. Severe infection

41. Your first action for the above patient should be to:

    a. Stabilize the glass with a stacked dressing and transport immediately
    b. Turn the patient into the prone position and transport immediately
    c. Remove the glass and hold direct pressure on the inside and outside of the wound
    d. Place a suction catheter in the mouth and continuously suction during transport

Questions 42 and 43 refer to the following scenario.

> You respond to a construction site and find a 40-year-old man in severe pain and holding his hand over his eye. Bystanders state that he was inadvertently stabbed in the eye socket with a sharp pipe. On close examination you note that his left eye is completely avulsed and hanging approximately 3 inches out of the socket.

42. The immediate care of the eye should consist of:

    a. Dry 4 × 4 dressing
    b. Moist dressing
    c. Petroleum dressing
    d. Betadine-soaked dressing

43. After applying the dressing, the eyeball can be stabilized with:

    a. Adhesive tape
    b. A cup and bandage
    c. An elastic bandage
    d. A stacked bandage

44. Amputated parts should be managed by:

    a. Placing them in a plastic bag and then placing the bag on ice
    b. Soaking them in saline solution and placing them directly on ice
    c. Wrapping them in an occlusive dressing to maintain moisture
    d. Wrapping them in a multitrauma dressing to maintain sterility

45. All the following are purposes of a triangular or cravat bandage *except*:

    a. Serve as a sling for an injured arm
    b. Serve as material for a tourniquet
    c. Directly cover a wound
    d. Hold a dressing in place

46. When applying a pressure bandage you should use enough pressure to:

    a. Occlude distal flow
    b. Cause venous distention
    c. Cause tingling in the affected part
    d. Control bleeding

Questions 47 to 49 refer to the following scenario.

> A 14-year-old boy is found at the bottom of a stairwell with a large avulsion of the scalp. The 6-inch flap of skin is folded posterior, exposing a large area of subcutaneous tissue. It is attached to the remaining skin with a 1-inch segment of tissue. The patient is alert and oriented and has no disability finding, but you note clear liquid escaping from the ear.

47. The management of the avulsed part should include:

    a. Disconnecting the flap from the skin and storing it in a bag of ice
    b. Rinsing the tissue and placing it in the normal anatomical position
    c. Bandaging it as it is found with an elastic bandage
    d. Placing an ice pack on the scalp and bandaging it in place

48. The clear liquid escaping from the ear suggests the possibility of a(n):

    a. Basilar skull fracture
    b. Eardrum rupture
    c. Wound infection
    d. Brainstem laceration

49. The leaking fluid should be managed by:

    a. Applying ice over the ear
    b. Packing the ear with gauze
    c. Applying a loose sterile dressing
    d. Applying a cup over the ear

Questions 50 and 51 refer to the following scenario.

> A scuba diver complains of severe earache after descending to 50 feet below the surface. He states that he had a slight cold and congestion for 3 days before the dive.

50. Based on the history, what injury do you suspect?

    a. The bends
    b. Barotrauma to the eardrum
    c. Ruptured cochlea
    d. Severe middle ear infection

51. This problem is caused by a clogged:

    a. External ear
    b. Middle ear
    c. Eustachian tube
    d. Cochlea

52. The two most critical variables in thermal burn injuries are:

    a. Degree of heat and length of exposure
    b. Type of heat and thickness of skin
    c. Distance from patient and pigment of skin
    d. Age of patient and pigment of skin

53. Skin that is blistered, red, blotchy, swollen, and very painful best describes a:

    a. Superficial or first-degree burn
    b. Partial-thickness or second-degree burn
    c. Full-thickness or third-degree burn
    d. Complete-thickness or fourth-degree burn

54. Which layer of the skin is injured in a superficial burn?

    a. The dermis
    b. The subcutaneous
    c. The epidermis
    d. The fascia

55. The most common cause of a superficial burn is:

    a. Scalding injury
    b. Sunburn
    c. Electrical injury
    c. Chemical injury

56. Which of the following burn types is likely to be most painful?

    a. Superficial
    b. Partial-thickness
    c. Full-thickness
    d. Fourth-degree

57. Skin that appears charred, yellow brown, dark red, or white and translucent with thrombosed veins that are visible is probably related to a:

    a. Superficial burn
    b. Partial-thickness burn
    c. Full thickness burn
    d. Partial-thickness chemical burn

58. A major complication of circumferential burns completely around a body part such as the arm is that they can:

    a. Increase lactic acid production
    b. Obstruct blood flow to the part
    c. Increase heat to the cells beneath
    d. Kill all superficial nerves

Match the correct percentage in column A with the burned body parts in column B.

Column A		Column B
59. _____	27%	a. A baby's entire head
		b. One leg and one arm of an adult
60. _____	36%	c. Both arms (anterior and posterior) and the anterior surface of both legs in an adult
61. _____	18%	
62. _____	9%	d. The entire anterior surface of an adult
63. _____	46%	e. Both legs, the groin, and one arm of an adult
64. _____	50%	f. An adult's entire head

65. Which of the following body areas is considered critical when evaluating a burn patient?

    a. Armpits
    b. Scalp
    c. Groin (perineum)
    d. Thigh

66. Charring around the mouth and nose, black sputum, and singed nasal hairs and eyebrows are considered critical signs of:

    a. Respiratory burn injuries
    b. Eye injuries
    c. Chemical burn injuries
    d. Electrical injuries

67. All the following are considered complicating factors in a burn patient *except*:

    a. Lighter skin pigment
    b. Elderly patients
    c. Preexisting cardiac and pulmonary disease
    d. Small children

List the following burn management steps in chronological order by assigning the numbers 1 through 5 to the treatment steps.

68. _____ Apply sterile dressing

69. _____ Administer high-concentration oxygen

70. _____ Open the airway

71. _____ Remove rings and bracelets

72. _____ Stop the burning process

73. The best dressing for a large thermal burn is:

    a. Petroleum gauze
    b. Dry sterile wrap
    c. Plastic wrap
    d. Moist sterile

74. A common major complication of large surface area burns is:

    a. Cardiac arrhythmias
    b. Hypothermia
    c. Pulmonary embolus
    d. Bone infections

75. The most common cause of death from fires is:

    a. Fluid loss
    b. Infection
    c. Airway obstruction
    d. Smoke inhalation

76. The most common toxic gas that is inhaled in a fire is:

    a. Phosgene
    b. Carbon dioxide
    c. Carbon monoxide
    d. Cyanide

77. An early complication of direct heat transfer and burns to the respiratory tract is:

    a. Pulmonary fibrosis
    b. Bronchitis from mucus production
    c. Airway obstruction
    d. Pulmonary embolus

78. Carbon monoxide is a particularly toxic gas because it has a 200 times greater affinity for

    __________ than does oxygen.

    a. Diffusion
    b. Inhalation
    c. Hemoglobin
    d. Cell bonding

79. In burn patients, stridor and hoarseness may suggest:

    a. Bronchiolar injury
    b. Alveolar irritation
    c. Airway obstruction
    d. Nasal burns

80. In general, the most effective treatment for chemical burn injuries is:

    a. Application of cold packs on the affected area
    b. Irrigation with copious amounts of water
    c. Application of sterile dressing
    d. Application of gels to smother the burning process

81. Treatment of chemical burns requires:

    a. Application of a neutralizing agent
    b. Irrigation for 20 to 30 minutes
    c. Submersion in a small tub of water
    d. Rapid transport only

82. The force with which the movement of electrical current occurs is:

    a. Amperage
    b. Voltage
    c. Resistance
    d. Wattage

83. The number or volume of flowing electrons is called:

    a. Amperage
    b. Voltage
    c. Resistance
    d. Wattage

84. The degree of hindrance to electron flow is called:

    a. Amperage
    b. Voltage
    c. Resistance
    d. Wattage

85. Generally speaking, voltage:

 a. Causes more injury as it increases
 b. Causes less injury as it increases
 c. Does not affect the degree of injury
 d. Cannot cause death when less than 60 cycles per second

86. If electrical current passes through the brain, the primary complication is most likely to be:

 a. Cardiac arrest
 b. Cardiac arrhythmias
 c. Respiratory arrest
 d. Coronary thrombosis

87. Which of the following materials provides the greatest degree of resistance to electrical flow?

 a. Water
 b. Rubber
 c. Copper
 d. Steel

88. A large conducting body, such as the earth, that is used as a common return for an electrical circuit and an arbitrary zero of potential best describes:

 a. Current
 b. Voltage
 c. Flow
 d. Ground

89. The best action to take when a downed power line is in contact with the car you occupy is to:

 a. Step out of the car quickly
 b. Step out of the car if you have rubber soles
 c. Stay in the car until the power experts arrive
 d. Step out of the car slowly

90. Wet skin offers __________ resistance to electricity.

 a. Low
 b. High
 c. Very high
 d. No

91. High voltage traveling through air and generating intense heat that can cause thermal burns is

 called a(an) _________ burn:

 a. Air
 b. Jump
 c. Light
 d. Arc

92. Which of the following is a complication of electrical current flowing through skeletal muscle?

 a. Fat tumors because of the release of lipoproteins
 b. Hyperglycemia from glucagon release
 c. Contractions preventing release of a grasped electrical source
 d. Explosion of the muscle and skin

Questions 93 to 95 refer to the following scenario.

> You respond to a chemical manufacturing plant and find a 42-year-old woman who has received an entire body splash with an acid solution. She is alert and oriented and is in severe pain.

93. Your immediate action should be to:

 a. Provide rapid transport while irrigating with an intravenous solution en route
 b. Have the patient remove all her clothing and place her in a shower to irrigate
 c. Rinse the patient with an alkali solution to neutralize the acid
 d. Irrigate with a mild acid solution (e.g., orange juice) to avoid a chemical reaction

94. This patient's skin should be irrigated for a minimum of:

 a. 5 to 10 minutes
 b. 10 to 15 minutes
 c. 15 to 20 minutes
 d. 20 to 30 minutes

95. If this substance were a dry chemical, what actions would you take before irrigating?

 a. Neutralizing the substance
 b. Brushing the substance off skin
 c. Blowing the substance off skin
 d. Rubbing the substance off skin

Questions 96 to 99 refer to the following scenario.

> A 42-year-old man fell asleep while smoking in his den. His chair caught fire, and soon the house was in flames. The firefighters bring the man out of the burning house to your ambulance. The patient has blistering burns on his head and entire neck (completely around), his anterior chest and abdomen, and his groin. He has singed nasal hairs and eyebrows, and there is soot within the nostrils. His voice is very hoarse, and he is exhibiting stridor. He is alert, and his vital signs are respirations 20 breaths/min and regular, pulse 100 beats/min and regular, and blood pressure 140/70 mm Hg.

96. What percentage of his body do you estimate is burned?

 a. 15%
 b. 21%
 c. 28%
 d. 35%

97. The burned areas of the patient in the previous question are probably:

 a. Superficial
 b. Partial-thickness
 c. Full-thickness
 d. Fourth-degree

98. What is your greatest concern regarding this patient?

 a. Hypovolemic shock from fluid loss
 b. Airway obstruction from respiratory burns
 c. Massive infection from surface area
 d. Neurogenic distributive shock from pain

99. How should oxygen be provided?

 a. By nasal cannula
 b. By high-concentration nonrebreather mask, humidified if possible
 c. By bag-valve-mask
 d. By manually triggered resuscitator mask

Questions 100 to 103 refer to the following scenario.

> You respond to a call and find a 2-year-old boy who has bitten into an electrical wire and appears to be having a grand mal seizure. His father is in a panic and is unable to provide a history of what happened. The child appears to still be biting the wire.

100. The child is probably still in contact with the wire because:

 a. He is having sustained contractions of the jaw
 b. The wire had adhered to the mucosa
 c. He has aspirated the wire into his pharynx
 d. The wire has looped around his teeth

101. Your immediate action would be to:

 a. Call the power company to disconnect the electricity
 b. Find the fuse box and disconnect the fuse
 c. Pull the plug from the outlet
 d. Hit the child with a piece of wood to disconnect him from the wire

102. Of the following, which offers the least resistance to electricity?

 a. Muscles
 b. Nerves
 c. Bone
 d. Fatty tissue

103. Once the child was disconnected from the wire, your first concern should be:

 a. Severe internal burns
 b. Destruction of the skeletal muscles
 c. Respiratory status
 d. Eye injuries from burns

List five physical signs that should raise suspicion of inhalation injury.

104. ______________________________

105. ______________________________

106. ______________________________

107. ______________________________

108. ______________________________

109. Generally, adults older than _____ years are considered at increased risk of burn severity.

110. Generally, children younger than _____ years are considered at increased risk of burn severity.

111. Which type of burn is not included in estimating the extent of burn injury?

 a. First-degree burns
 b. Second-degree burns
 c. Third-degree burns
 d. Burns involving the bones, sometimes referred to as fourth-degree burns

Across

1. Scraping of the skin surface
3. Sunburn is an example of a _____ -degree burn
8. _____ glands are important in the regulation of body temperature
10. The second of the three tiny bones in the ear, also known as the anvil
11. The external ear
12. The third of the three tiny bones in the ear, also known as the stirrup
14. A burn characterized by blisters is a _____ -degree burn
17. Powdered or dried chemicals should be _____ off
20. A measure of the decrease of electrical flow through a given material
22. The outer layer over most of the eye
23. Your first concern for a patient with facial injuries is the patient's _____
25. The colored portion of the eye
26. A physical sign of an inhalation burn is _____ nasal hair
27. The outermost layer of the skin
29. Material used to secure a wound covering in place
30. A topical anesthetic solution used to assist patients in holding their eyes open during an eye irrigation process
31. A full-thickness burn is characterized as a _____-degree burn
33. _____ sputum contains black particles
35. The _____ constricts in response to bright light
36. Pigment of the skin that protects the body from the sun's radiation
37. A sign of airway compromise and respiratory distress
38. Glands that secrete tears
39. _____ membranes line the internal surface of the body

Down

1. Watery fluid in the anterior chamber of the eye
2. _____ objects should be stabilized in place unless they are in the cheek
3. A burn to the _____ is more critical because of the tendency for respiratory involvement
4. Posterior wall of the eye
5. Injury caused by compression force
6. The chest cavity is unique because it contains the pleural space that maintains _____ _____
7. Filters that prevent small particles from entering the eye
9. A burn that circles a limb or the torso is called a _____ burn
13. Depth, extent, and location of the burn are used to assess the ____ of the burn
15. Bruise
16. The cutting away of a limb or protruding structure from the body
18. The largest organ of the body
19. Classification of burn depth is spoken of in terms of _____
21. A tearing of the skin, usually from a sharp object
24. Blood collection in a pocket beneath the skin
26. _____ glands help moisturize the skin
28. One of the bones that protects the eye
30. _____ burns are those associated with heat
32. The layer of skin composed of dense connective tissue that plays a role in temperature regulation
34. A high-voltage current traveling through the air

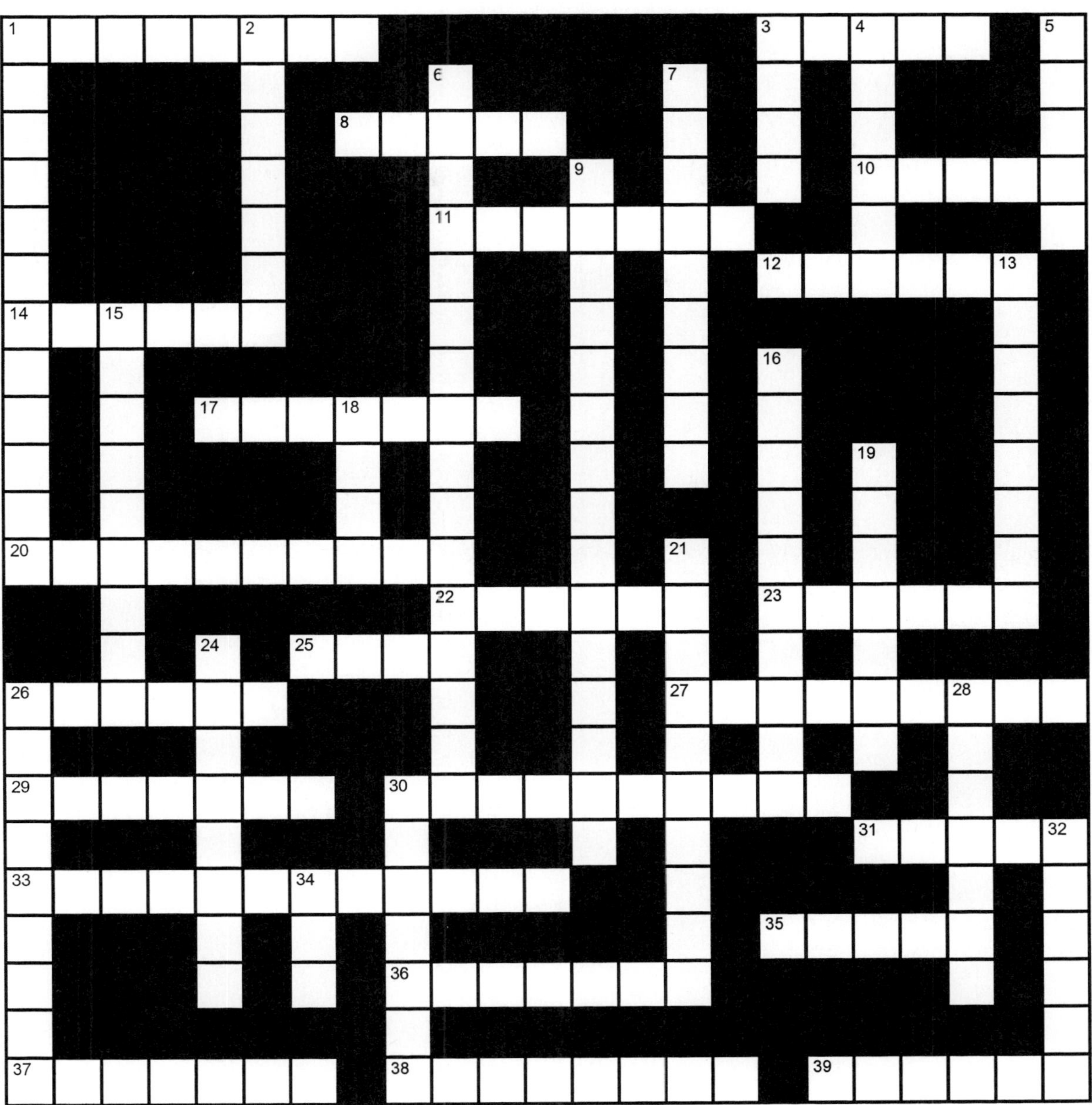

ANSWER KEY

1. c
2. a
3. c
4. d
5. c
6. b
7. e
8. c
9. d
10. a
11. b
12. a
13. b
14. b
15. b
16. c
17. a
18. d
19. b
20. b
21. a
22. a
23. b
24. d
25. b
26. a
27. b
28. c
29. b
30. b
31. c
32. b
33. a
34. c
35. a
36. c
37. c
38. a
39. b
40. a
41. c
42. b
43. b
44. a
45. c
45. d
47. b
48. a
49. c
50. b
51. c
52. a
53. b
54. c
55. b
56. b
57. c
58. b
59. b
60. c
61. a
62. f
63. e
64. d
65. c
66. a
67. a
68. 5
69. 3
70. 2
71. 4
72. 1
73. b
74. b
75. d
76. c
77. c
78. c
79. c
80. b
81. b
82. b
83. a
84. c
85. a
86. c
87. b
88. d
89. c
90. a
91. d
92. c
93. b
94. d
95. b
96. c
97. b
98. b
99. b
100. a
101. c
102. b
103. c
104. Singed nasal hairs
105. Sputum with black particles (carbonaceous sputum)
106. Burns around the mouth and nose
107. Hoarseness of the voice
108. Respiratory distress
109. 65 years
110. 5 years
111. a

1 A	B	R	A	S	2 I	O	N									3 F	I	4 R	S	T		5 C
Q					M				6 N					7 E		A		E				R
U					P		8 S	W	E	A	T			Y		C		T				U
E					A				G			9 C		E		E		10 I	N	C	U	S
O					L				11 A	U	R	I	C	L	E			N				H
U					E				T			R		A		12 S	T	A	P	E	13 S	
14 S	E	15 C	O	N	D				I			C		S							E	
H		O							V			U		H		16 A					V	
U		N		17 B	R	U	18 S	H	E	D		M		E		M					E	
M		T					K		P			F		S		P		19 D			R	
O		U					I		R			E				U		E			I	
20 R	E	S	I	S	T	A	N	C	E			R		21 L		T		G			T	
		I							22 S	C	L	E	R	A		23 A	I	R	W	A	Y	
		O		24 H		25 I	R	I	S			N		C		T		E				
26 S	I	N	G	E	D				U			T		27 E	P	I	D	E	R	28 M	I	S
E				M					R			I		R		O		S		A		
29 B	A	N	D	A	G	E		30 T	E	T	R	A	C	A	I	N	E			X		
A				T				H				L		T				31 T	H	I	R	32 D
33 C	A	R	B	O	N	34 A	C	E	O	U	S			I						L		E
E				M		R		R						O		35 P	U	P	I	L		R
O				A		C		36 M	E	L	A	N	I	N						A		M
U								A														I
37 S	T	R	I	D	O	R		38 L	A	C	R	I	M	A	L		39 M	U	C	O	U	S

Chapter 27 Chest and Abdominal Trauma

1. The thoracic cavity begins just below the neck and extends down to:

   a. The umbilicus
   b. The pelvic girdle
   c. The diaphragm
   d. The xiphoid process

2. There are a total of how many pairs of ribs?

   a. 10
   b. 11
   c. 12
   d. 13

3. The lowest two pairs of ribs are called:

   a. Inferior ribs
   b. Floating ribs
   c. Thoracic ribs
   d. Superior ribs

4. The upper part of the sternum is called the:

   a. Manubrium
   b. Middle body
   c. Superior body
   d. Xiphoid process

5. During inspiration the diaphragm:

   a. Relaxes and pushes downward into the abdomen
   b. Contracts and pushes downward into the abdomen
   c. Relaxes and rises into the thoracic cavity
   d. Contracts and rises into the thoracic cavity

6. During expiration the diaphragm:

   a. Relaxes and pushes downward into the abdomen
   b. Contracts and pushes downward into the abdomen
   c. Relaxes and rises into the thoracic cavity
   d. Contracts and rises into the thoracic cavity

7. During forced exhalation the upper portion of the right diaphragm can extend as high as the:

   a. Fourth costal cartilage anteriorly and to the eighth rib posteriorly
   b. Fourth costal cartilage anteriorly and to the tenth rib posteriorly
   c. Fifth costal cartilage anteriorly and to the eighth rib posteriorly
   d. Fifth costal cartilage anteriorly and to the tenth rib posteriorly

8. Which of the following structures are contained within the mediastinum?

   a. Heart, lungs, esophagus, and trachea
   b. Main stem bronchi, carotid arteries, heart, and lungs
   c. Heart, esophagus, main stem bronchus, and trachea
   d. Lungs, trachea, great vessels, and esophagus

9. The diaphragm connects to the ribs at what level?

   a. At the lower fifth pair of ribs
   b. At the lower sixth pair of ribs
   c. At the lower seventh pair of ribs
   d. At the lower eighth pair of ribs

10. __________ is the major vein that returns blood to the heart from the body.

11. _________ is the major artery that delivers blood from the heart to the body.

12. _________ is the "food pipe" that brings food from the mouth to the stomach.

13. _________ is the lowest portion of the sternum.

14. The major cause of severe blunt trauma injury to the chest is:

a. Falls
b. Gunshot wounds
c. Industrial accidents
d. Motor vehicle crashes

15. This type of mechanism of injury is primarily responsible for tears of major vessels, especially the aorta: ______________.

16. Air in the pleural space is called a:

a. Hydrothorax
b. Hemothorax
c. Pneumothorax
d. Flail chest

17. Bleeding in the pleural space is called a:

a. Hydrothorax
b. Hemothorax
c. Pneumothorax
d. Flail chest

TRUE OR FALSE

18. _____ Penetrating gunshot wounds to the neck may cause severe chest injuries.

19. _____ The lower ribs protect the abdominal organs, and blunt trauma to the lower chest will not result in injuries to these organs.

20. _____ A pneumothorax can be corrected in the field by positioning the patient supine with the patient's legs elevated.

21. _____ A flail chest is when two or more ribs are broken in two or more places.

22. _____ A common cause of a flail chest is a gunshot wound.

23. _____ One method to stabilize a flail segment, in the patient without suspected neck or spinal injury, is to position the patient with the injured side down.

24. A flail portion of the chest wall is pulled inward by:

a. Positive pressure during inhalation
b. Positive pressure during exhalation
c. Negative pressure during inhalation
d. Negative pressure during exhalation

Questions 25 to 29 are based on the following scenario.

> You are called to the scene of a motor vehicle accident and find a patient behind the steering wheel complaining of chest pain and difficulty breathing. You notice that the air bag has deployed but you "lift and look" and determine that the steering wheel has been deformed. The patient is alert and oriented, has significant bruising to the anterior chest wall, has a blood pressure of 90/62 mm Hg, pulse of 136 beats/min, respiratory rate of 32 breaths/min and shallow, and has pale, cool, and moist skin. Your physical examination of the chest reveals a segment of the chest wall that is moving in the direction opposite the remaining chest wall and there are diminished breath sounds on the left with normal breath sounds on the right.

25. Based on the chest wall movement you suspect that this patient may have sustained a _________ injury.

26. This physical finding, characterized by the segment of chest wall moving in the direction opposite the remaining chest wall, is termed ____________.

27. The breath sounds in the patient indicate the possible presence of ___________.

28. You work with your partner and determine that the best method to use to extricate the patient from the car is the ______________.

29. The two major objectives in treating this patient's chest injury are ____________ and ______________.

30. A patient presenting with severe swelling and ecchymosis of the neck and face after a heavy weight falling on his chest has:

a. Cardiac tamponade
b. Sucking chest wound
c. Pneumothorax
d. Traumatic asphyxia

31. A penetrating wound to the chest should be treated with:

    a. Supplemental oxygen and a 4 × 4 gauze taped on 3 sides over the wound
    b. Supplemental oxygen and a 4 × 4 gauze taped on all 4 sides over the wound
    c. Supplemental oxygen and an occlusive dressing taped on 3 sides over the wound
    d. Supplemental oxygen and an occlusive dressing taped on all 4 sides over the wound

Questions 32 to 35 are based on the following scenario.

> You are called to the scene of a motor vehicle crash and find a 35-year-old woman who was the driver of the car lying supine next to the car. Bystanders inform you that the driver lost control of the car and went off the road and struck a tree at approximately 30 mph. You look in the car and identify that this older model vehicle does not have an airbag. The patient was not wearing a seat belt. Your evaluation of the patient reveals a significant contusion on the chest wall consistent with striking the steering wheel. Your patient has a blood pressure of 82/60 mm Hg, heart rate of 132 beats/min, respiratory rate of 28 breaths/min, absent breath sounds on the right, good breath sounds on the left, distended neck veins, and the trachea shifted to the left.

32. Based on your evaluation of the patient you suspect that the patient may have a:

    a. Pneumothorax
    b. Hemothorax
    c. Cardiac tamponade
    d. Tension pneumothorax

33. The best position to transport this patient is:

    a. Left lateral recumbent
    b. Supine with the head elevated
    c. Supine on a spine board with the neck and spine immobilized
    d. In the position of comfort

34. The tracheal shift in this patient is caused by:

    a. Blunt trauma to the neck
    b. A possible tension pneumothorax
    c. A possible pneumothorax
    d. A possible hemothorax

35. The distended neck veins are caused by:

    a. The obstruction of blood returning to the heart through the large veins
    b. The obstruction of blood leaving the heart through the aorta
    c. The increased heart rate
    d. The patient's low blood pressure

List four signs of a tension pneumothorax.

36. ______________________________

37. ______________________________

38. ______________________________

39. ______________________________

TRUE OR FALSE

40. ______ A patient with cardiac tamponade will usually present with tracheal shift and distended neck veins.

41. ______ Blood in the mediastinum compresses the chambers of the heart in a patient with cardiac tamponade.

42. ______ An aortic tear is most common at the point where mobile and attached portions of the aorta meet.

43. ______ Eighty percent of patients with an aortic tear die at the scene.

44. ______ If a patient develops signs of a tension pneumothorax after an appropriate bandage has been applied to an open chest wound, you should immediately remove the dressing and reseal it after the release of the tension, which is at the end of a forced exhalation.

45. ______ Penetrating wounds to the lower chest cannot enter the abdominal cavity.

46. ______ The pelvic cavity is the lowermost portion of the abdominal cavity.

47. Which organs are considered to be solid organs?

    a. Liver, spleen, and kidneys
    b. Stomach, pancreas, and liver
    c. Kidneys, bladder, and spleen
    d. Liver, bladder, and kidneys

48. The pelvic girdle is formed by all these bones *except*:

    a. Sacrum
    b. Ilium
    c. Ischium
    d. Coccyx

49. The ___________ peritoneum lines the abdominal and pelvic walls.

50. The ___________ peritoneum covers most of the intra-abdominal organs.

51. ___________ is the term for inflammation of the peritoneum.

52. The abdomen is divided into quadrants by two imaginary lines that intersect at the ___________.

Identify the two distinct pathways that abdominal pain may be transmitted by.

53. ______________________________

54. ______________________________

55. The pathway that allows pain to be localized anatomically near the affected organ is the _________ pathway.

List three common characteristics of how the patient may describe visceral pain.

56. ______________________________

57. ______________________________

58. ______________________________

TRUE OR FALSE

59. _____ Distention of the abdomen may not be apparent, even after significant abdominal bleeding.

60. _____ The primary goal of prehospital care for a patient with abdominal injuries is to summon advanced life support to the scene to stabilize the patient in the field.

61. _____ Blunt abdominal trauma may result from compression-type forces or from knife wounds.

62. _____ An injury to a hollow organ can commonly cause profuse bleeding, causing hypovolemic shock.

63. _____ A properly worn seat belt cannot cause deceleration force injuries on internal organs.

During the focused history and physical examination the chest and abdomen are examined for DCAP/BTLS. What does this mnemonic stand for?

64. D ______________________________

65. C ______________________________

66. A ______________________________

67. P ______________________________

68. B ______________________________

69. T ______________________________

70. L ______________________________

71. S ______________________________

72. The presence of intestines protruding through a laceration in the abdominal wall is termed a (an) _________.

73. The proper treatment for this type of injury is:

    a. The application of a dry, sterile dressing
    b. Replacing the intestines in the abdominal cavity
    c. The application of a moist, sterile dressing
    d. The pneumatic anti-shock garment

List four possible findings that may be present in a patient who presents with an acute abdomen.

74. ______________________________

75. ______________________________

76. ______________________________

77. ______________________________

78. Treatment of the patient with an acute abdomen includes the administration of _____.

79. During your physical examination you should begin palpation _____ from the quadrant where the patient identifies the pain is located.

Across

1. _____ occurs when the diaphragm relaxes
5. A _____ chest wound results from air drawn into the pleural space during inspiration
9. Shoulder blades
11. Top of the ilium bone
13. The cavity bordered by the diaphragm and the pelvis
14. The reduced movement of the chest wall to avoid pain caused by broken or bruised ribs
15. _____ pneumothorax is a condition in which air entering the chest cavity cannot escape
17. Collapse of a lung from air in the pleural space
20. Pain perceived in a location distant from the actual site
21. A single, large, triangular bone of the pelvis
23. The uppermost portion of the sternum
24. Bleeding in the pleural space
26. The lowest portion of the sternum is called the _____ process
27. Motor vehicle crashes are the major cause of severe _____ _____ to the chest
29. Mechanism of injury that causes a tear of an organ or vessel from a point of attachment
30. The center of the thoracic cavity

Down

2. Major artery leaving the heart
3. _____ occurs when the diaphragm contracts
4. Nerve pathway with imprecise perceptions to quality and location of pain
5. Nerve pathway perceiving clear quality of pain
6. Collarbones
7. Entrapment of air beneath the skin
8. Ribs are attached to the sternum by _____ cartilage
10. Bruises to the flank are often associated with injuries to the _____
12. Most common breath sound associated with pneumothorax
16. Protection is provided for the pelvic organs by the pelvic _____
17. A sign of flail chest, exhibited by the opposing motion of the chest wall motion
18. Bony tip of the shoulder
19. Lining of the inner abdominal cavity
22. Respiratory muscle that separates the thorax and abdomen
25. Black or tarry stool
28. Cavity that is the lowermost portion of the abdomen

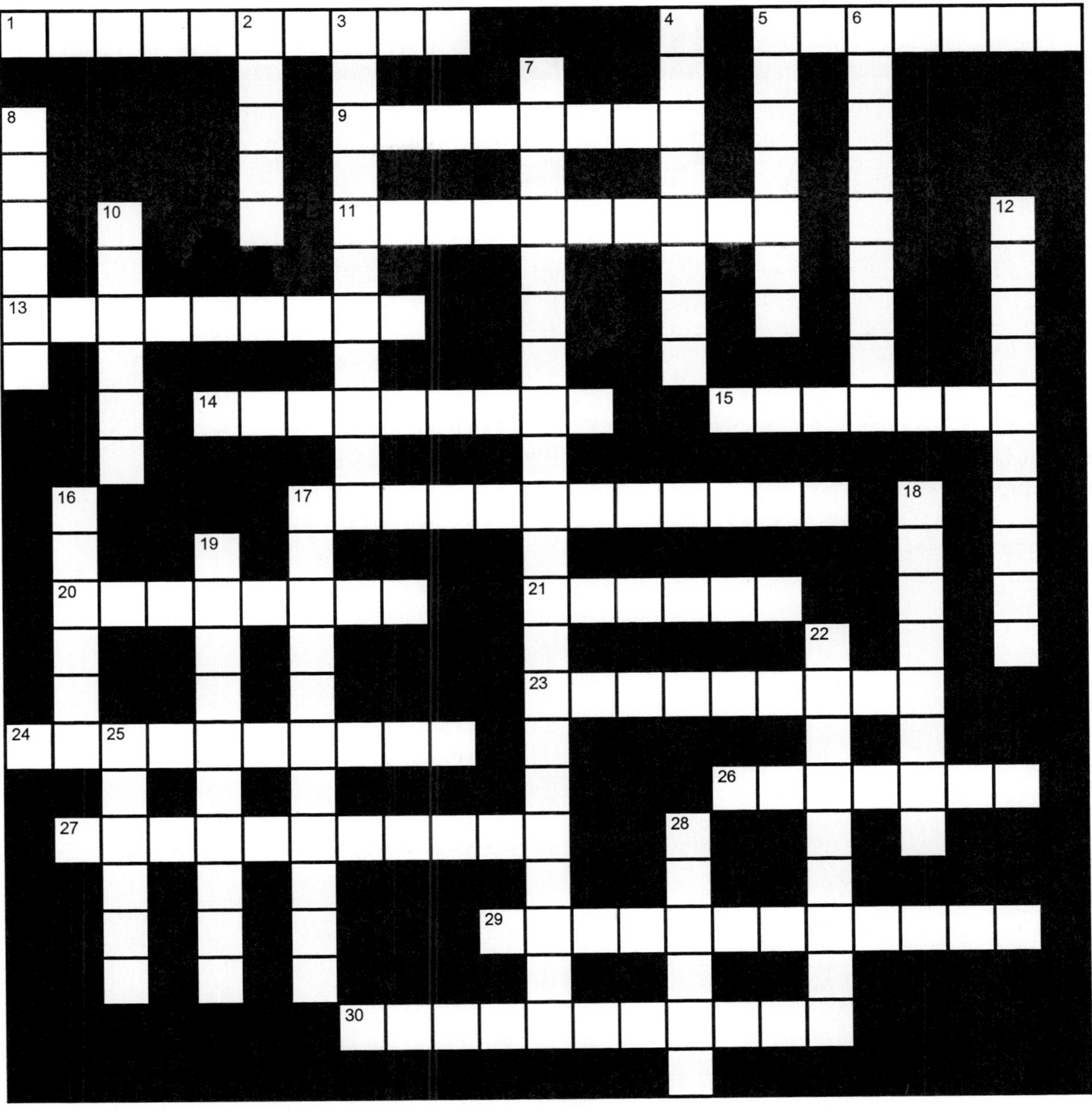
1
2
3
4
5
6
7
8
9
10
11
12
13
14
15
16
17
18
19
20
21
22
23
24
25
26
27
28
29
30

ANSWER KEY

1. c
2. c
3. b
4. a
5. b
6. c
7. a
8. c
9. b
10. Vena cava
11. Aorta
12. Esophagus
13. Xiphoid process
14. d
15. Deceleration injuries
16. c
17. b
18. True
19. False
20. False
21. True
22. False
23. True
24. c
25. Flail chest
26. Paradoxic movement
27. Pneumothorax or hemothorax
28. Rapid extrication
29. a. Supplemental oxygen
    b. Stabilization of the flail segment
30. d
31. c
32. d
33. c
34. b
35. a
36. Breath sounds absent on the affected side
37. Distended neck veins
38. Other signs of shock
39. Shifting of the trachea away from the affected side
40. False
41. False
42. True
43. True
44. True
45. False
46. True
47. a
48. d
49. Parietal
50. Visceral
51. Peritonitis
52. Umbilicus (navel)
53. Visceral pathway
54. Somatic pathway
55. Somatic
56. Diffuse
57. Cramping
58. Aching
59. True
60. False
61. False
62. False
63. False
64. Deformities
65. Contusions
66. Abrasions
67. Punctures or penetrations
68. Burns
69. Tenderness
70. Lacerations
71. Swelling
72. Evisceration
73. c
74. Patient positioned to minimize any movement of the abdomen, commonly supine with knees raised and shallow breathing
75. A distended and tense abdomen
76. Abdominal tenderness
77. Abdominal guarding
78. Oxygen
79. Away

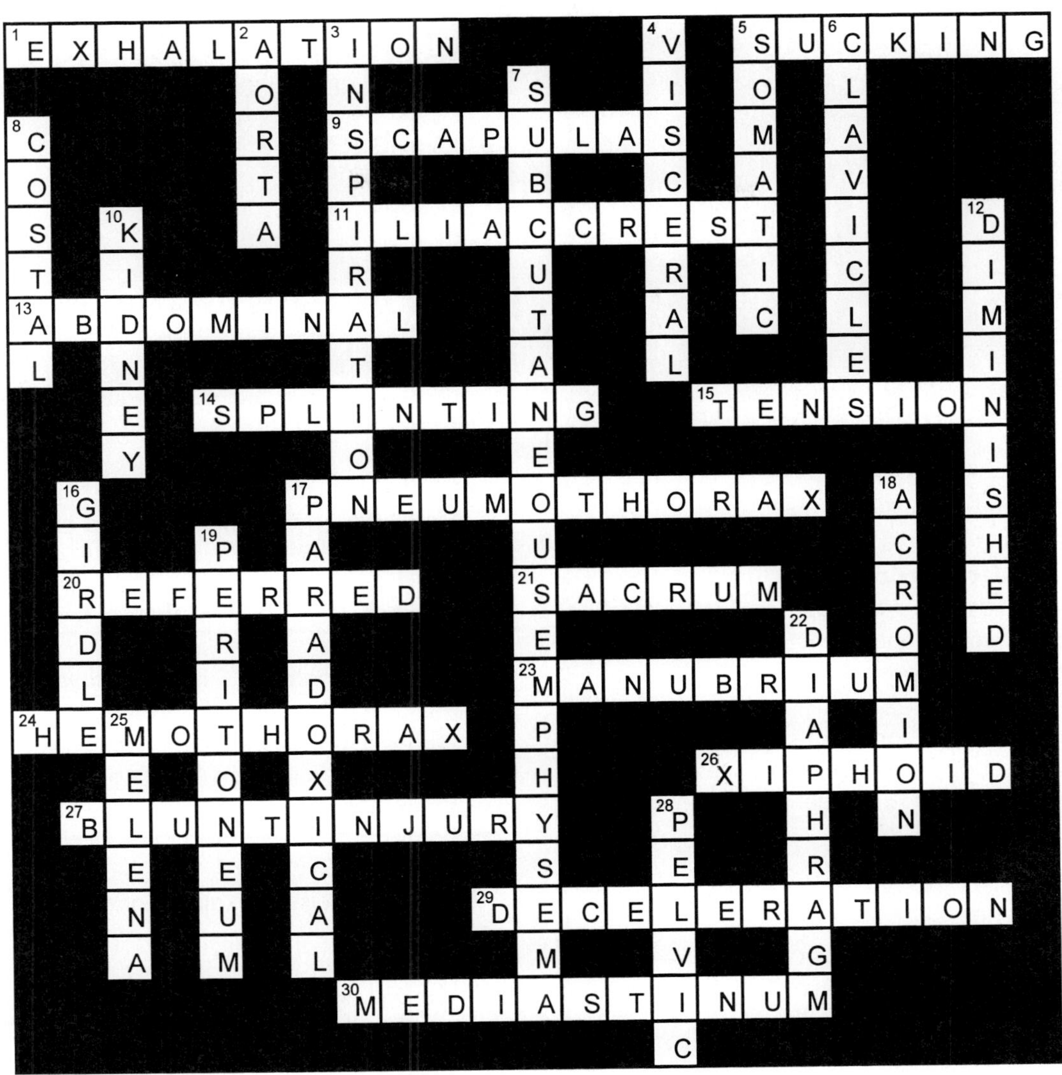
1 EXHALATION
2 AORTA
3 INSPIRATION
4 VISCERAL
5 SUCKING
5 SOMATIC
6 CLAVICLE
7 SUBCUTANEOUS EMPHYSEMA
8 COSTAL
9 SCAPULAS
10 KIDNEY
11 ILIAC CREST
12 DIMINISHED
13 ABDOMINAL
14 SPLINTING
15 TENSION
16 GIRDLE
17 PNEUMOTHORAX
17 PARADOXICAL
18 ACROMION
19 PERITONEUM
20 REFERRED
21 SACRUM
22 DIAPHRAGM
23 MANUBRIUM
24 HEMOTHORAX
25 MELENA
26 XIPHOID
27 BLUNT INJURY
28 PELVIC
29 DECELERATION
30 MEDIASTINUM

Chapter 28 Musculoskeletal Care

1. The axial skeleton consists of the:

   a. Skull, spine, ribs, and sternum
   b. Pelvis and lower extremities
   c. Upper extremities and clavicles
   d. The joints of the body

2. A softer precursor of bone that is present throughout the body and persists at sites of bone growth and at joints to provide a smooth, friction-free surface is called:

   a. Ligament
   b. Tendon
   c. Cartilage
   d. Fascia

3. Connective bands of tissue that attach bone to bone and maintain the stability of joints are called:

   a. Ligaments
   b. Tendons
   c. Cartilage
   d. Fascia

4. Thin bands of tissue that attach muscle to bone and initiate movement of joints are called:

   a. Ligaments
   b. Tendons
   c. Cartilage
   d. Fascia

5. The portion of bone responsible for the production of red blood cells is:

   a. Spongy bone
   b. Periosteum
   c. Red marrow
   d. Epiphysis

Match the appropriate muscle in column A with the structures in column B.

Column A	Column B
6. _____ Smooth	a. Blood vessel
	b. Biceps
7. _____ Cardiac	c. Heart
8. _____ Skeletal	

9. The elbow is an example of a:

   a. Hinged joint
   b. Ball and socket joint
   c. Fused joint
   d. Gliding joint

10. Displacement of bones in a joint from their normal anatomic position is called a:

    a. Compression injury
    b. Dislocation
    c. Sprain
    d. Strain

11. The stretching or tearing of a ligament is called a:

    a. Compression injury
    b. Dislocation
    c. Sprain
    d. Strain

12. The term used to describe the sensation felt during palpation that is created by the grating of bone ends together is:

    a. Friction rub
    b. Homan's sign
    c. Rhonchi
    d. Crepitus

13. A joint locked in a deformed position after an injury is highly suggestive of a:

    a. Sprain
    b. Dislocation
    c. Strain
    d. Spiral fracture

14. The five Ps that may indicate vascular or nerve injury in a fractured extremity include pain, pulselessness, pallor, paresthesia (numbness or tingling), and:

    a. Paralysis
    b. Priapism
    c. Purple skin
    d. Palpitations

15. Bladder, rectal, and urethral injuries are commonly associated with fracture of the:

    a. Femur
    b. Lumbar spine
    c. Pelvis
    d. Hip

Match the appropriate mechanism of injury in column A with the type of force in column B.

Column A	Column B
16. _____ Bumper striking a tibia causing a transverse fracture at the site of impact	a. Twisting force
17. _____ An ice skater fracturing the tibia during a spin when the blade gets stuck in the ice	b. Indirect for along bone's axis
18. _____ A humerus fracture after a fall on an outstretched hand	c. Direct force

19. The most common sign or symptom of a fracture is:

    a. Discoloration
    b. Deformity
    c. Pain
    d. Swelling

20. Which of the following is a major cause of deformity after a fracture?

    a. The pulling force of opposing muscles
    b. Ecchymosis at the site of injury
    c. Obstruction of an artery
    d. Nerve paralysis in the extremity

21. Absence of capillary refill in a single extremity is highly suggestive of:

    a. Hypovolemic shock caused by severe blood loss and vasoconstriction
    b. Vascular compromise from a fracture or dislocation
    c. Spinal shock causing vasoconstriction to one side of the body
    d. Cardiac tamponade causing poor cardiac output through the aorta

22. A primary rule of fracture management is to splint the fracture site and the:

    a. Surrounding tissues
    b. Distal extremity
    c. Adjacent joints
    d. Proximal extremity

Match descriptions in column A with the type of splint in column B.

Column A	Column B
23. _____ Made of padded cardboard, wood, metal, or plastic	a. Traction splint
24. _____ Environmental temperature can impair function	b. Pillow splint
25. _____ Best splint for femur fracture	c. Rigid splint
26. _____ Best ankle splint	d. Sling and swathe
27. _____ Can be made from triangular bandages	e. Air splint

28. The bone that can be palpated on the anterior upper chest region that extends from the sternum to the shoulder region is called the:

    a. Scapula
    b. Glenoid
    c. Olecranon
    d. Clavicle

29. Injuries to the shoulder, humerus, scapula, and clavicle are best treated with a(n)

    a. Pillow splint
    b. Sling and swathe
    c. Rigid splint
    d. Air splint

30. The most common mechanism of injury for the upper extremity is a:

    a. Direct blow
    b. Fall on an outstretched hand
    c. Twisting force
    d. Hyperextension injury

31. Shoulder dislocations are commonly caused by a:

    a. Blow to the scapula
    b. Fall on an outstretched arm
    c. Tugging force applied to the arm
    d. Blow to the clavicle

32. Vascular compromise resulting from shoulder dislocations can be evaluated by palpating the:

    a. Popliteal artery
    b. Dorsalis pedis artery
    c. Radial artery
    d. Humeral artery

33. The longest and strongest bone of the body is the:

    a. Humerus
    b. Tibia
    c. Fibula
    d. Femur

34. A patient who has an extremity with a good pulse with no feeling or movement has probably injured a (an):

    a. Ligament
    b. Growth plate
    c. Artery
    d. Nerve

35. Angulated elbow fractures or dislocations are best immobilized by a(n):

    a. Pillow splint on the medial side of the arm
    b. Sling and swathe
    c. Rigid splint, sling and swathe
    d. Air splint extending from the wrist to the axilla

36. The bones of the forearm include the radius and the:

    a. Humerus
    b. Fibula
    c. Manubrium
    d. Ulna

37. Using the basic rules of splinting, fractures of the wrist should be immobilized from the finger to the:

    a. Mid-forearm
    b. Wrist
    c. Shoulder
    d. Humerus

38. Placing a roller bandage in the hand before splinting fractures places the hand in the position of:

    a. Extension
    b. Rotation
    c. Function
    d. Articulation

Match the fracture or dislocation in column A with the splinting method in Column B.

Column A	Column B
39. _____ Dislocated shoulder	a. Traction splint
40. _____ Fractured ankle	b. 3-foot and 5-foot splint
41. _____ Fractured hand	c. Sling and swathe
42. _____ Fractured tibia	d. Tongue blade splint
43. _____ Fractured finger	e. Pillow splint
44. _____ Fractured femur	f. Rigid 9-inch splint

45. Multiple fractures of the pelvis associated with hypovolemic shock are best treated by application of:

    a. A traction splint
    b. Pneumatic anti-shock garment (PASG)
    c. 3- and 5-foot rigid splint
    d. Tying the legs together

46. The lower leg bone that can be palpated on the anterior lower leg is the:

    a. Fibula
    b. Radius
    c. Tibia
    d. Talus

47. Which of the following fractures is commonly associated with spine injuries?

    a. Patella
    b. Calcaneus
    c. Metatarsal
    d. Hip

48. Pelvic fractures in stable patients are best splinted by:

    a. Rigid 3- and 5-foot splints
    b. Securing patient to long spine board
    c. Traction splint application
    d. PASG application

Questions 49 to 51 refer to the following scenario.

> You respond to a call and find 83-year-old woman complaining of pain in the mid-thigh region. She states that she fell from a ladder and landed on her foot and heel. The leg feels quite stable and she is able to walk on it.

49. Based on the history, what type of fracture might this patient most likely have sustained?

    a. A stable femur fracture
    b. An open femur fracture
    c. A dislocated hip
    d. A fractured hip

50. The mechanism of injury for this patient is best described as:

    a. Direct
    b. Twisting
    c. Indirect
    d. Rotational

51. The splint of choice for this patient is:

    a. Traction
    b. Pillow
    c. 3-inch lateral splints
    d. Long spine board

Questions 52 to 54 refer to the following scenario.

> You respond to a call and find a 24-year-old ice skater who fell on an outstretched arm and is complaining of shoulder pain. She is supporting her forearm with her opposite hand, and her upper arm is positioned slightly away from her chest wall on the injured side. You note deformity and tenderness in the shoulder region.

52. Based on the history and physical exam, you suspect a(n):

    a. Fracture shaft of the humerus
    b. Anterior shoulder dislocation
    c. Fracture of the scapula
    d. Fracture of the olecranon

53. The splint of choice for this patient is a(n):

    a. Rigid board splint
    b. Air splint
    c. Pillow splint
    d. Sling and swathe

54. Given the site and nature of this injury, what complication are you most concerned about in this patient?

    a. Hemorrhage at the site of injury
    b. Fat embolism
    c. Neurovascular compromise
    d. Poor healing

Questions 55 to 57 refer to the following scenario.

> You respond to a call and find a 74-year-old man complaining of hip pain. He states that he simply stepped off a high curb and planted his foot forcefully on the ground and felt severe pain in his hip. He is lying on the ground, and his leg appears externally rotated and shortened.

55. Based on the history and physical examination, you suspect a:

    a. Minor muscle injury
    b. Dislocation of the hip
    c. Fracture of the hip
    d. Pelvic fracture

56. Given the minor nature of the mechanism of injury, what preexisting condition might explain this injury?

    a. Osteoporosis
    b. Arteriosclerosis
    c. Hypercalcemia
    d. Stress injury

57. The best method to transport this patient will be:

    a. Prone on the ambulance stretcher
    b. In the left lateral recumbent position
    c. Supine with knees flexed
    d. Supine on a long back board with the patient secured to the board

Questions 58 to 60 refer to the following scenario.

> A 45-year-old construction worker fell from a 20-foot scaffold and landed on his feet. He is found lying on his left side. He is pale, sweaty, and has delayed capillary refill. His blood pressure is 80/60 mm Hg and his pulse is 140 beats/min and regular. You note that his left leg is deformed at the mid-thigh region and at the mid lower leg. His right leg appears normal, but he has no dorsalis pedis or posterior tibial pulses in either leg.

58. Based on the above history and physical exam, your immediate concern is:

    a. Losing the extremities because of poor blood supply
    b. Decompensated hypovolemic shock
    c. Causing open fractures during transport
    d. Paralysis of the right leg

59. The absence of pulses in both legs is probably related to:

    a. The vasoconstriction response of shock
    b. Compression of an artery because of fractures
    c. Swelling in the thighs
    d. Peripheral nerve injury

60. Treatment for this patient includes:

    a. Spinal immobilization and high-concentration oxygen
    b. Application of the PASG with inflation of the abdominal section only
    c. High-concentration oxygen and securing the patient to the long board in the left lateral recumbent position
    d. Rapid transport with the neck immobilized in a cervical collar and the patient positioned supine on the stretcher with his head elevated

Questions 61 and 62 refer to the following scenario.

> A 40-year-old female pedestrian is struck in the left knee region by an automobile. You note the leg is grossly angulated at the left knee, and pulses are absent on the injured side. The patient also has a deformity in her right wrist. Otherwise the patient is stable and has no other obvious injuries.

61. Based on the above finding you should:

    a. Splint the leg as you found it
    b. Attempt gentle straightening to regain pulse
    c. Apply traction with a hare or Sager splint
    d. Elevate the limb in the angulated position

62. The hand and wrist should be placed in the position of function and splinted with a:

    a. Traction splint
    b. Rigid splint
    c. Pillow splint
    d. Sling and swathe

63. Numbness or tingling is also called ________.

64. When applying the Sager traction splint, mechanical traction should be applied by using

    _____ % of the patient's body weight, not to

    exceed _____ lbs of traction.

65. When applying a Hare traction splint, the

    ________ strap should be applied first.

66. When applying a splint that encompasses the hand, the hand should be splinted in the

    ___________.

67. The __________ is the major weight-bearing bone of the lower leg.

List the two goals of management for patients with extremity injuries.

68. ______________________________

69. ______________________________

List the four signs and symptoms of nerve injury.

70. ______________________________

71. ______________________________

72. ______________________________

73. ______________________________

Across

5. Force usually transmitted along the axis of bone resulting in injury to a point other than site of impact
8. _____ splints are made of cardboard, wood, metal, or plastic
9. Ankle bones
11. A bandage used to bind the upper arm to the chest wall
13. Serves as a cushion at the sites of two or more bones
14. Injury to ligaments
16. An open or _____ fracture communicates with the outside environment
19. A _____ fracture has no break in skin over the site
20. Kneecap
21. Major weight-bearing bone of the lower leg
22. Pneumatic or _____ splints provide circumferential support to an extremity
24. Skeleton that supports and protects the internal organs
26. A shortened and externally rotated leg is an indication of a _____ fracture
27. Triangle-shaped bandage used to support the weight of the arm
29. Winglike bone forming the superior lateral aspect of the pelvis
30. Calcified connective tissues that give strength to the skeleton
32. Eight small bones of the wrist
33. The knee is an example of a _____ joint
34. Long bone that runs parallel to the tibia

Down

1. Involuntary or _____ muscles contract automatically and are not under the individual's control
2. Longest and strongest bone in the body
3. Pain, abnormal sensation, and loss of movement are signs of _____ injury
4. Muscle that is similar in structure to voluntary muscle but is directed by the involuntary nervous system
6. To flex upward
7. Tough connective tissue that binds bone to bone
10. The _____ skeleton is primarily concerned with movement and support of the erect body
11. Injury to muscle or tendon
12. Inside of bone that is the source of blood cells
14. Framework of the body
15. Five bones from the wrist to the knuckles
17. Finger or toe bones
18. Bone located along the medial length of the forearm
23. Bone on the lateral aspect of the arm
25. The most common symptom of bone or joint injury
26. Long bone of the arm
28. Posterior portion of the pelvic ring along with the sacrum
31. An obvious sign of an _____ fracture is a bone protruding through the skin

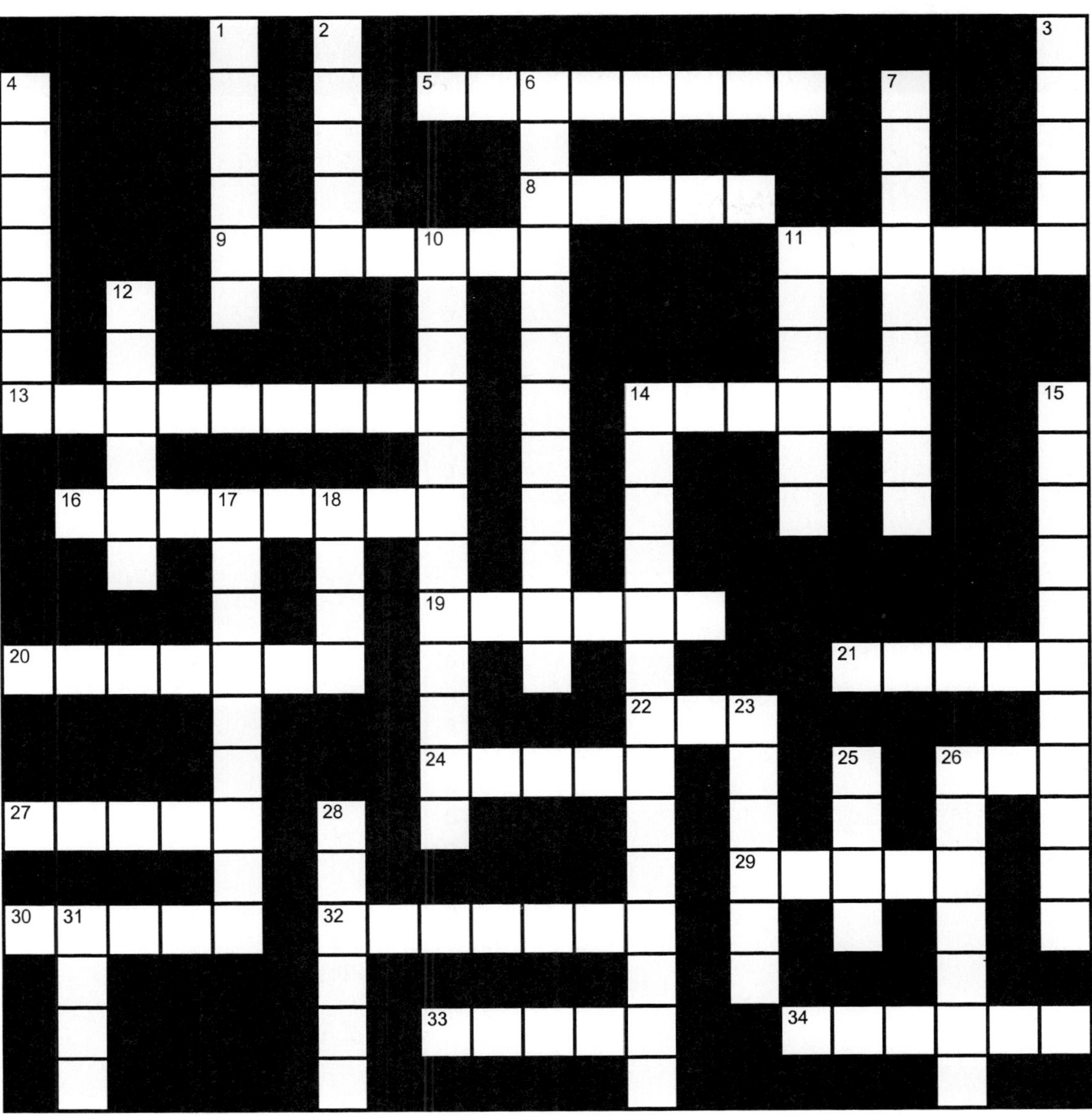

ANSWER KEY

1. a
2. c
3. a
4. b
5. c
6. a
7. c
8. b
9. a
10. b
11. c
12. d
13. b
14. a
15. c
16. c
17. a
18. b
19. c
20. a
21. b
22. c
23. c
24. e
25. a
26. b
27. d
28. d
29. b
30. b
31. b
32. c
33. d
34. d
35. c
36. d
37. a
38. c
39. c
40. e
41. f
42. b
43. d
44. a
45. b
46. c
47. b
48. b
49. a
50. c
51. a
52. b
53. d
54. c
55. c
56. a
57. d
58. b
59. a
60. a
61. b
62. b
63. Paresthesia
64. 10%, 15 lbs
65. Ischial
66. Position of function
67. Tibia
68. Reduced pain
69. Prevent further injury
70. Numbness
71. Pain
72. Abnormal sensation
73. Loss of motor ability

				1 S		2 F														3 N
4 C				M		E		5 I	N	6 D	I	R	E	C	T		7 L			E
A				O		M				O							I			R
R				O		U				8 R	I	G	I	D			G			V
D				9 T	A	R	S	10 A	L	S					11 S	W	A	T	H	E
I		12 M		H				P		I					T		M			
A		A						P		F					R		E			
13 C	A	R	T	I	L	A	G	E		L		14 S	P	R	A	I	N			15 M
		R						N		E		K			I		T			E
	16 C	O	M	17 P	O	18 U	N	D		X		E			N		S			T
		W		H		L		I		I		L								A
				A		N		19 C	L	O	S	E	D							C
20 P	A	T	E	L	L	A		U		N		T				21 T	I	B	I	A
				A				L				22 A	I	23 R						R
				N				24 A	X	I	A	L		A		25 P		26 H	I	P
27 S	L	I	N	G		28 C		R				S		D		A		U		A
				E		O						Y		29 I	L	I	U	M		L
30 B	31 O	N	E	S		32 C	A	R	P	A	L	S		U		N		E		S
	P					C						T		S				R		
	E					Y		33 H	I	N	G	E			34 F	I	B	U	L	A
	N					X						M						S		

Chapter 29 Injuries to the Head and Spine

1. The nervous system is structurally divided into two main divisions: the central nervous system and the:

   a. Peripheral nervous system
   b. Ganglionic nervous system
   c. Proximal nervous system
   d. Core nervous system

2. The central nervous system is made up of the brain, the brainstem, and the:

   a. Afferent nerves
   b. Peripheral nerves
   c. Dermatomes
   d. Spinal cord

3. The nervous system can also be divided by function, creating the voluntary division and:

   a. Paravoluntary division
   b. Autonomic division
   c. Reflex division
   d. Ganglionic division

4. Willful activities such as running to catch a train, reaching for an object, or buttoning a shirt are examples of functions mediated through the:

   a. Autonomic division
   b. Reflex division
   c. Spinal division
   d. Voluntary division

5. The control of the heart, the glands, and smooth muscles within organs such as the digestive tract is mediated through the:

   a. Autonomic division
   b. Reflex division
   c. Spinal division
   d. Voluntary division

6. There are two main divisions of the autonomic nervous system: the parasympathetic and the:

   a. Paraspinal
   b. Parasympathomimetic
   c. Sympathetic
   d. Sympathomimetic

7. Which of the following is mediated through the parasympathetic nervous system?

   a. Sweating
   b. Constriction of pupils
   c. Increasing the heart rate
   d. Vasoconstriction

8. If complete cessation of oxygen delivery occurs, as in cardiac arrest, the patient will become unconscious in about:

   a. 5 seconds
   b. 1 minute
   c. 4 to 6 minutes
   d. 10 minutes

9. Approximately how long will it take for irreversible brain damage to occur when the brain is totally deprived of oxygen?

   a. 5 to 10 seconds
   b. 1 to 2 minutes
   c. 2 to 3 minutes
   d. 4 to 6 minutes

10. The most sensitive indicator of inadequate oxygenation of the brain is:

    a. Alteration of mental status
    b. Motor function
    c. Sensory function
    d. Heart rate

Match the bones in column A with their related regions of the skull in column B. You can use the column B selections more than once.

Column A	Column B
11. _____ Mandible	a. Cranium b. Face
12. _____ Parietal	
13. _____ Maxilla	
14. _____ Temporal	
15. _____ Occipital	

16. The brainstem exits the lower skull through an opening called the:

    a. Foramen arteriosum
    b. Foramen magnum
    c. Foramen ovale
    d. Foramen minor

17. The space within the adult cranium has about a:

    a. 0.5 L capacity
    b. 1.0 L capacity
    c. 2.0 L capacity
    d. 3.0 L capacity

18. If the pressure within the cranium becomes severe, the brain may be forced down through the opening in the base of the skull. This dire emergency is called:

    a. Displacement
    b. Herniation
    c. Pressure syndrome
    d. Compression syndrome

Match the type of vertebrae in column A with the number of vertebrae in column B.

Column A	Column B
19. _____ Cervical	a. 5 (mobile) b. 4 (fused)
20. _____ Lumbar	c. 12 d. 5 (fused)
21. _____ Coccyx	e. 7
22. _____ Sacral	
23. _____ Thoracic	

24. Most vertebrae are held together by ligaments and separated by:

    a. Disks
    b. Nerves
    c. Bone
    d. Tendons

25. The three layered membranous coverings of the brain and spinal cord that serve to protect the central nervous system are called the:

    a. Pleura
    b. Periosteum
    c. Myelin sheath
    d. Meninges

Match the appropriate membranous layer in column A with the description in column B.

Column A	Column B
26. _____ Pia mater	a. Tough, leathery outer layer
27. _____ Arachnoid	b. Middle layer c. Inner layer
28. _____ Dura mater	

29. The largest and most superior portion of the brain is called the:

    a. Cerebrum
    b. Brainstem
    c. Cerebellum
    d. Diencephalon

30. The lower part of the brain that is made up of bundles and tracts of nerves traveling down to the spinal cord and has distinct nerve cell centers of its own is called the:

    a. Cerebrum
    b. Brainstem
    c. Cerebellum
    d. Diencephalon

31. The posterior outpocketing of the brain that is primarily concerned with coordination of movement and balance is called the:

    a. Cerebrum
    b. Brainstem
    c. Cerebellum
    d. Diencephalon

Match the category in column A with the type of action mediated by the central nervous system in column B.

Column A	Column B
32. _____ Automatic	a. Withdrawal from hot candle
33. _____ Reflex	b. Breathing, heart rate, etc.
	c. Lifting a box
34. _____ Conscious	

35. Most of the blood supply to the brain (80%) is provided through the:

    a. Vertebral arteries
    b. Subleasing arteries
    c. Middle meningeal arteries
    d. Carotid arteries

Match the area of the brain in column A with its functions in column B.

Column A	Column B
36. _____ Frontal lobe	a. Vision
	b. Intelligence, motor function
37. _____ Parietal lobe function	c. Respiratory function
	d. Sensory function
38. _____ Occipital lobe	e. Hearing, smell
39. _____ Brainstem	
40. _____ Temporal lobe	

41. Injuries that cause disruption of specific sections of brain tissue or nerves (e.g., gunshot wounds) and result in loss of specific functions are called:

    a. Metabolic
    b. Secondary
    c. Structural
    d. Contained

42. Problems that affect all of the brain cells equally, such as hypoxia, low blood sugar, shock and poisoning, are called:

    a. Metabolic
    b. Secondary
    c. Structural
    d. Contained

43. Hypoxia, hypotension, hypoglycemia, infections, and increased intracranial pressure are all examples of:

    a. Secondary brain injuries
    b. Primary brain injuries
    c. Modifying brain injuries
    d. Complicating brain injuries

44. Injuries that occur on the opposite side of the brain from the site of the blow (due to the dynamic movement of the brain after initial impact) are called:

    a. Compression
    b. Deceleration
    c. Contrecoup
    d. Ipsilateral contusion

Match the type of skull fracture in column A with the description in column B.

Column A	Column B
45. _____ Basilar	a. A crack in the floor of the skull
46. _____ Depressed	b. Bone fragments that are pressed downward toward the brain

47. Cerebrospinal fluid leaking from the ear should be treated by:

    a. Packing the ear to contain fluid
    b. Attaching a loose sterile dressing over the ear
    c. Doing nothing
    d. Placing the patient on the affected side

48. Raccoon eyes, Battle's sign, and cerebrospinal fluid leakage from the nose or ear are all signs of:

    a. Brain laceration
    b. Epidural hematoma
    c. Basilar skull fracture
    d. Increased intracranial pressure

49. A transient loss of consciousness or neurologic function from a blow to the brain is called a:

    a. Contusion
    b. Concussion
    c. Compression
    d. Contortion

50. Headaches, nausea, and vomiting (sometimes projectile) are common signs of:

   a. Skull fracture
   b. Brain contusion
   c. Increased intracranial pressure
   d. Infection

51. Which of the following vital sign presentations may signify an increase in intracranial pressure?

   a. Decreased pulse rate, increased blood pressure
   b. Increased pulse rate, decreased blood pressure
   c. Decreased pulse rate, decreased blood pressure
   d. Increased pulse rate, increased blood pressure

52. Epidural hematomas are caused by:

   a. Arterial bleeding
   b. Capillary bleeding
   c. Venous bleeding
   d. Venule bleeding

53. Subdural hematomas are caused by:

   a. Arterial bleeding
   b. Capillary bleeding
   c. Venous bleeding
   d. Venule bleeding

54. All the following are potential implications of poor spinal immobilization for a high cervical spine injury (C1, C2) *except*:

   a. Respiratory arrest
   b. Diaphragmatic breathing only
   c. Spinal shock
   d. Complete paralysis

55. The manual airway maneuver of choice for the head-injured patient is:

   a. Head tilt/chin lift
   b. Head tilt/neck lift
   c. Jaw thrust without head tilt
   d. Triple airway maneuver

56. What effect does increased levels of carbon dioxide have on cerebral vessels?

   a. Constriction
   b. Dilation
   c. Spasm
   d. Obstruction

57. The Glasgow Coma Scale score for a patient who has no verbalizations, does not open his eyes, and who is decorticate (has abnormal flexion) to painful stimuli is:

   a. 4
   b. 5
   c. 7
   d. 9

58. The first priority in the management of a patient with a severe head trauma is:

   a. Performing a neurologic exam
   b. Establishing an airway and adequate ventilation
   c. Applying a cervical collar
   d. Controlling bleeding from the scalp

Match the appropriate spinal nerve level in column A with the anatomic sensory area (dermatome) in column B.

Column A	Column B
59. _____ Thoracic 4 (T-4)	a. Groin
60. _____ Cervical 4 (C-4)	b. Nipple
61. _____ Lumbar 1 (L-1)	c. Above clavicle
62. _____ Thoracic 10 (T-10)	d. Umbilicus

63. When the spinal cord is injured at a low cervical level (C-7) or a high thoracic level (T-1), the respiratory function is most likely to be:

   a. Respiratory arrest
   b. Intercostal breathing only
   c. Diaphragmatic breathing only
   d. Normal respiration

64. When the spinal cord is injured at a high cervical level (C-2), the respiratory function is most likely to be:

   a. Respiratory arrest
   b. Intercostal breathing only
   c. Diaphragmatic breathing only
   d. Normal respiration

65. When a patient develops neurogenic shock from spinal injuries, the pulse rate is most likely to be:

   a. Slow (below 60)
   b. Normal range (60-80)
   c. Fast (above 100)
   d. Very fast (above 150)

66. The vessels of a patient in neurogenic shock are most likely to be:

    a. Constricted
    b. Dilated
    c. Normal
    d. Collapsed

67. The loss of sympathetic tone of a patient in neurogenic shock may result in a penile erection. This event is commonly called:

    a. Neuroerection
    b. Priapism
    c. Sympathetic erection
    d. Penile dilation

68. The most common cause of spinal cord injury is:

    a. Motor vehicle crashes
    b. Falls
    c. Sports-related incidents
    d. Diving incidents

69. The most common sites of vertebral injury occur where vertebrae that allow motion meet:

    a. The rib cage
    b. Vertebrae that are fixed
    c. Other mobile vertebrae
    d. Intervertebral disks

Match the type of spinal injury force in column A with the mechanisms of injury in column B.

Column A	Column B
70. _____ Compression	a. Face striking the windshield in a front-end collision
71. _____ Flexion	b. Occipital region striking the bottom of a pool during a dive
72. _____ Extension	c. The top portion of the skull striking the bottom of a pool during a dive

73. The term used to describe a hyperextension injury resulting from a rear-end collision is:

    a. Contrecoup
    b. Whiplash
    c. Posterior extension
    d. Subluxation

74. When immobilizing a spinal injury patient you should not return the neck to the neutral position if:

    a. The neck is flexed
    b. Resistance is encountered
    c. The neck is extended
    d. Contusions are noted on the neck

Match the approach to immobilization in column A to the situation in column B.

Column A	Column B
75. _____ Short board	a. Unstable driver of a car
76. _____ Long board	b. Pedestrian struck by car
77. _____ Rapid extrication	c. Stable driver of a car

Questions 78 and 79 refer to the following scenario.

A 25-year-old unconscious man was involved in a motor vehicle crash. Bystanders state that he was initially unconscious, became conscious 3 minutes after the crash, and lapsed into unconsciousness again about 5 minutes ago. He is unresponsive to pain. Physical assessment reveals left pupil dilated and nonreactive; blood pressure 200/110 mm Hg, pulse 42 beats/min and bounding, and respirations irregular at an approximate rate of 8 breaths/min. He has a contusion and crepitus in the temporal region of the skull.

78. What do you suspect is the major underlying problem?

    a. Brain contusion
    b. Epidural hematoma
    c. Concussion
    d. Subarachnoid hemorrhage

79. What is the likely cause of the change in vital signs?

    a. Increased intracranial pressure
    b. Direct injury to the brain
    c. The age of the patient
    d. A history of hypertension

Questions 80 to 85 refer to the following scenario.

A 14-year-old falls approximately 7 feet from a swing and strikes his left forehead on a soft rubber mat, causing him to become unconscious. After 30 seconds, he awakes and says he feels "all right." You find the youngster alert and breathing 24 times per minute with his abdominal muscles only. Vital signs are pulse 68 beats/min and regular and blood pressure 76/60 mm Hg. He cannot move his arms and legs and has sensation above the clavicle but none at nipple line. You also note priapism.

80. Based on the presenting signs you suspect spinal injury at the level of the:

    a. High thoracic or low cervical spine
    b. Low thoracic or high lumbar spine
    c. High cervical spine
    d. Low lumbar or high sacral spine

81. Based on the vital signs, what complication do you suspect?

    a. Increased intracranial pressure
    b. Neurogenic (spinal) shock
    c. Obstructive shock
    d. Epidural hematoma

82. The vital signs, priapism, and loss of the sweat mechanism below the clavicles are a result of:

    a. Increased parasympathetic activity
    b. Increased sympathetic activity
    c. Decreased parasympathetic activity
    d. Decreased sympathetic activity

83. His respiratory status is caused by a loss of:

    a. Diaphragm function
    b. Intercostal muscle function
    c. Abdominal muscle function
    d. Neck muscle function

84. The initial loss of consciousness is probably caused by a (an):

    a. Contusion
    b. Laceration
    c. Concussion
    d. Epidural bleeding

85. Treatment of this patient should include spinal immobilization and:

    a. Oxygen by nonrebreather mask
    b. Oxygen by nasal cannula
    c. Oxygen by Venturi mask
    d. No oxygen

Questions 86 to 89 refer to the following scenario.

A 40-year-old man was in a front-end auto collision and lost consciousness. When the ambulance arrived, the patient refused medical evaluation and treatment. A week later, the man became unconscious while watching television at home. On your arrival on the scene, the patient is unresponsive to painful stimuli. His vital signs are blood pressure 150/100 mm Hg, respirations 28 breaths/min and very deep, and pulse 80 beats/min. His left pupil is fixed and dilated and his right is mid-positional and normally reactive.

86. Based on the history and presenting signs, what do you think is the primary problem?

    a. Cerebral contusion
    b. Stroke
    c. Subdural hematoma
    d. Subarachnoid hemorrhage

87. The bleeding within the skull is most likely:

    a. Arterial
    b. Capillary
    c. Venous
    d. Arteriole

88. The initial loss of consciousness after the crash was probably caused by a (an):

    a. Concussion
    b. Contusion
    c. Laceration
    d. Abrasion

89. Based on the ventilatory status, what approach would you use to deliver oxygen?

    a. Nasal cannula
    b. Nonrebreather mask
    c. Bag-valve-mask
    d. Simple face mask

Indicate the circumstances when a helmet should be removed or left in place.

90. _____ Good fit with little or no movement
91. _____ Inability to access airway
92. _____ Proper spinal immobilization cannot be performed in place

a. Remove
b. Do not remove

93. Which of the following characteristics are typical of a sports helmet but not a motorcycle helmet?

    a. Easier access to the airway
    b. Should always be removed
    c. Has a Plexiglas face shield
    d. Should never be removed

94. During the initial step of spinal immobilization when removing a helmet, the head is stabilized by holding:

    a. Only the helmet
    b. Only the mandible
    c. Both the helmet and the mandible
    d. Only the maxilla

95. _________ is the fluid that surrounds the brain and offers some protection to it.

96. _________ is the color of the fluid that surrounds the brain.

97. _________ is the name of the soft spots that are present in the top of the skull during infancy.

98. The _________ artery supplies blood to the brainstem.

99. The term _________, used for ecchymosis around the eyes, is a sign of a fracture at the base of the skull.

100. _________ is the artery located on the inside surface of the temporal bone and may be a cause of significant bleeding if this area of the skull is fractured.

101. A period of memory loss is called _________.

TRUE OR FALSE

102. _____ During hypoventilation the carbon dioxide level in the blood decreases.

103. _____ If you reduce the carbon dioxide content of the blood the blood flow to the head will also be reduced.

104. _____ Patients who are being mobilized on a long spine board should have their heads secured to the board before their torso.

105. _____ If you need to remove a football helmet to properly manage the patient's airway, then the shoulder pads should also be removed.

106. _____ Classically, a subdural hematoma presents with a short period of unconsciousness, followed by a lucid interval and then a subsequent decrease or alteration in the patient's level of consciousness.

Across

2. Nerve cells are dependent on an adequate supply of oxygen and _____
7. Lack of sugar in the bloodstream
8. Sustained penile erection
9. The first seven vertebrae
10. Abnormal flexion
17. With hypoventilation, the _____ _____ level increases
18. Lack of oxygen after a cardiac arrest is an example of a _____ injury
20. 20% of the brain's blood flow comes from two _____ _____
24. 80% of the blood to the brain is supplied by the _____ _____
26. The _____ lobe is the center for sensory perception
27. Vomit ejected with great force; a sign of increased intracranial pressure
28. Oxygen deficiency
29. _____ skull fractures are marked by CSF leakage from the nose or ear
30. Tailbone

Down

1. Patients exhibiting neurologic dysfunction should be given high-concentration _____
3. There are five _____ vertebrae
4. If the force of an injury is applied from one direction, it is called a _____ injury
5. Airway maneuver of choice for the patient with a head injury
6. A common term used to describe an injury that results from hyperextension of the neck
8. The _____ nervous system carries messages between the brain and muscles
11. Left lateral recumbent
12. The portion of the brain posterior to the brainstem, concerned with coordination and balance
13. There are 12 _____ vertebrae
14. Semirigid short spine board
15. Most victims who sustain spinal injury do so in _____ _____ accidents
16. Abnormal extension
19. High blood pressure and slow pulse
20. The _____ nervous system controls activities that require conscious action
21. CSIDs are used to _____ the spine
22. Segments of skin innervated by nerves exiting from nearby segments of the vertebral column
23. A mnemonic for assessing a patient
25. The outer layer of membranes covering the brain, closest to the skull

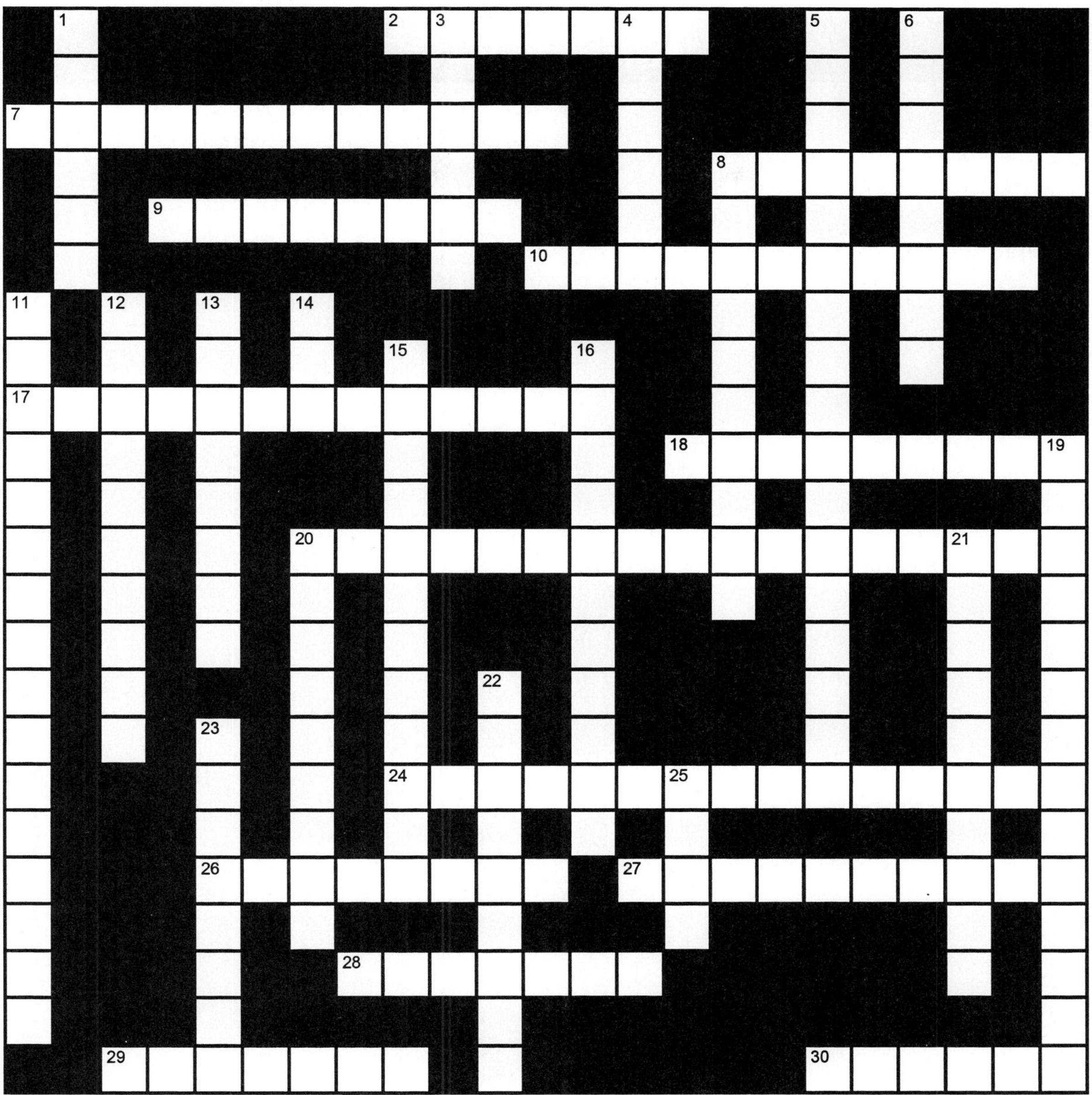

ANSWER KEY

1. a
2. d
3. b
4. d
5. a
6. c
7. b
8. a
9. d
10. a
11. b
12. a
13. b
14. a
15. a
16. b
17. b
18. b
19. e
20. a
21. b
22. d
23. c
24. a
25. d
26. c
27. b
28. a
29. a
30. b
31. c
32. b
33. a
34. c
35. d
36. b
37. d
38. a
39. c
40. e
41. c
42. a
43. a
44. c
45. a
46. b
47. b
48. c
49. b
50. c
51. a
52. a
53. c
54. b
55. c
56. b
57. b
58. b
59. b
60. c
61. a
62. d
63. c
64. a
65. b
66. b
67. b
68. a
69. b
70. c
71. b
72. a
73. b
74. b
75. c
76. b
77. a
78. b
79. a
80. a
81. b
82. d
83. b
84. c
85. a
86. c
87. c
88. a
89. b
90. b
91. a
92. a
93. a
94. c
95. Cerebrospinal fluid
96. Clear
97. Fontanelles
98. Basilar
99. Raccoon eyes
100. Middle meningeal artery
101. Amnesia
102. False
103. True
104. False
105. True
106. False

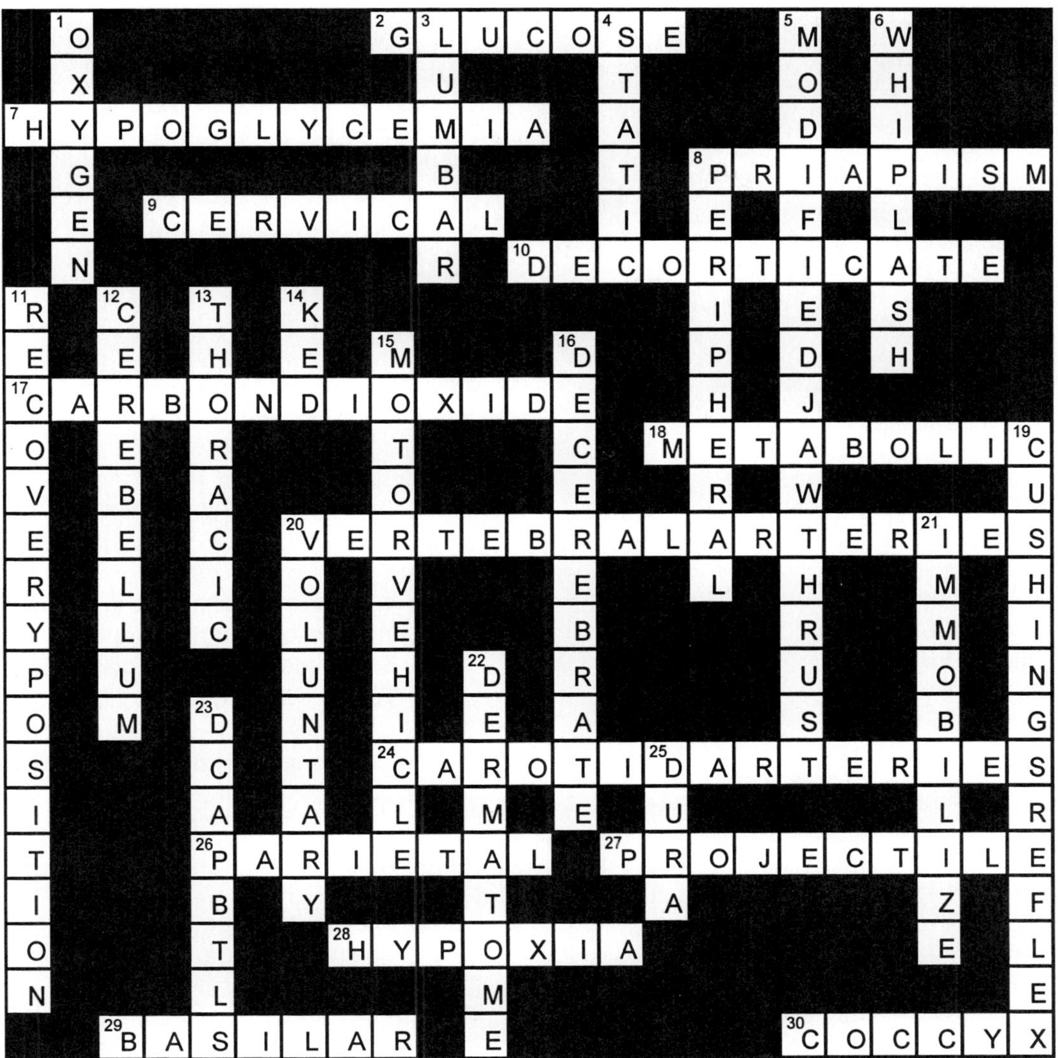

Chapter 30 Infants and Children

1. The most common cause of death in children outside the newborn period is:

   a. Sudden infant death syndrome (SIDS)
   b. Trauma and respiratory conditions
   c. Congenital heart disease
   d. Cancer

2. Most cardiopulmonary arrests in children result from failure of the:

   a. Urinary system
   b. Cardiovascular system
   c. Respiratory system
   d. Endocrine system

3. Magical thinking is primarily associated with which of the following periods of development?

   a. Infants (less than 1 year)
   b. Toddlers (15 months to 3 years)
   c. Small children (4 to 7 years)
   d. Adolescents

4. When examining adolescents it is most important to:

   a. Respect their privacy and shyness
   b. Relax them with casual conversation
   c. Be assertive to avoid resistance to questions
   d. Be upbeat and familiar with them

5. When examining small children it is a good idea to:

   a. Ask the parents to leave the room
   b. Hold them on your lap
   c. Leave them on their parents' laps
   d. Do it quickly to avoid problems

6. In small children the secondary survey should proceed:

   a. In the same manner as in an adult
   b. In a toe-to-head structure
   c. Briskly to avoid prolonged exposure
   d. Very slowly to avoid agitation

7. The narrowest part of the upper airway in infants is the:

   a. Epiglottis
   b. Trachea
   c. Thyroid cartilage
   d. Cricoid cartilage

8. To open the airway of the infant, place the head in the:

   a. Hyperflexed position
   b. Extended position
   c. Flexed position
   d. Sniffing or neutral position

9. Hyperextension of an infant's airway may result in:

   a. Kinking and obstruction
   b. Rupture of the larynx
   c. Dislocation of the cervical spine
   d. Increased intracranial pressure

10. Infants (up to 1 year) have an average respiratory rate of approximately:

   a. 12 to 20 breaths/min
   b. 20 to 25 breaths/min
   c. 25 to 30 breaths/min
   d. 30 to 40 breaths/min

11. Infants breath dominantly through the:

    a. Nose
    b. Mouth
    c. Pursed lips
    d. Cheeks

12. During ventilation you must be careful to closely observe:

    a. Pupil response
    b. Skin color
    c. Capillary refilling time
    d. Chest rise

13. When ventilating an infant, care should be taken not to overventilate because infants are more subject to:

    a. Pneumothorax
    b. Gastric distention
    c. Hemothorax
    d. Pulmonary contusions

14. Nasal flaring and retractions are signs of:

    a. Increased work of breathing
    b. Difficulty with exhalation
    c. Chest wall injury
    d. Hyperventilation

15. High-concentration oxygen therapy for children older than 1 year:

    a. Is contraindicated
    b. May cause blindness
    c. Is appropriate if needed
    d. Is never needed

16. As a general rule, the width of a blood pressure cuff applied to an infant or child should cover approximately what fraction of the length of the upper arm?

    a. 1/4
    b. 1/3
    c. 2/3
    d. 1/2

17. The American College of Surgeons considers a

    systolic blood pressure of less than _____ mm Hg with tachycardia and cool skin an indicator of shock in children.

    a. 50
    b. 70
    c. 80
    d. 90

18. Infants and children have a baseline metabolic rate

    ___________ than adults.

    a. Higher
    b. Lower

19. Early signs of dehydration in children include all the following *except*:

    a. Tachycardia
    b. Decreased urination
    c. Dry mucosal membranes
    d. Hypotension

20. Because of their healthier compensatory mechanisms, children maintain their blood pressure until they lose nearly:

    a. 20% of blood volume
    b. 30% of blood volume
    c. 40% of blood volume
    d. 50% of blood volume

21. A crowing, high-pitched sound made on inspiration that is suggestive of upper airway obstruction is called:

    a. Grunting
    b. Snoring
    c. Wheezing
    d. Stridor

22. A rhythmic sound heard at the end of exhalation that may be mistaken for whining is called:

    a. Grunting
    b. Snoring
    c. Wheezing
    d. Stridor

23. The inward depression of muscular areas and their attached ribs, which are drawn inward and reflect an increased work at breathing, is called:

    a. Thoracic paradox
    b. Myotonia
    c. Retractions
    d. Myopia

24. High pitched "musical" sounds caused by narrowing of the lower airways obstructing airflow is called:

    a. Rales
    b. Stridor
    c. Wheezing
    d. Grunting

25. All the following are common causes of upper airway obstruction in infants and small children *except*:

    a. Bronchitis
    b. Croup
    c. Foreign bodies
    d. Epiglottitis

26. A viral infection affecting the larynx, trachea, and bronchi that can cause airway narrowing, especially at the level of the cricoid ring, is called:

    a. Bronchiolitis
    b. Pharyngitis
    c. Croup
    d. Epiglottitis

27. All the following are signs of the condition described above *except*:

    a. A hoarse voice
    b. Wheezing
    c. A barking cough
    d. A low-grade fever

28. Croup is most common from ages:

    a. 6 months to 3 years
    b. Newborn to 4 years
    c. 1 year to 8 years
    d. Newborn to 11 years

29. The effective management of croup includes all the following *except*:

    a. Positioning the child supine
    b. Oxygenation
    c. Humidification
    d. Hydration in the hospital

30. Epiglottitis is an acute bacterial infection of the epiglottis that has a rapid onset of approximately:

    a. 2 to 4 hours
    b. 1 to 2 hours
    c. 10 to 12 hours
    d. 24 to 72 hours

31. Which of the following is not a common sign of acute epiglottitis?

    a. High fever
    b. Sore throat
    c. Difficulty in swallowing
    d. Absent breath sounds on one side

32. The child with epiglottitis will frequently be sitting upright and leaning forward, resting the chin on the arms. This is called the:

    a. Fowler position
    b. Recumbent position
    c. Semi-Fowler position
    d. Tripod position

33. A major contraindication in the management of acute epiglottitis is:

    a. Administering high-concentration oxygen
    b. Examining the pharynx with a tongue blade
    c. Humidifying oxygen during administration
    d. None of the above

34. When faced with a child who has a complete airway obstruction from acute epiglottitis or croup, you should:

    a. Administer back blows and chest thrusts
    b. Attempt ventilation with the bag-valve-mask
    c. Initiate rapid transport
    d. Both b and c

35. A child with a foreign body airway obstruction who is alert and demonstrating effective air exchange should be managed by:

    a. A deep finger sweep to the upper airway
    b. Back blows and chest thrusts
    c. Transport only
    d. Positive-pressure ventilation

36. The correct management of a conscious, complete foreign body airway obstruction in an infant is:

    a. Back blows
    b. Chest thrusts
    c. Finger sweep
    d. Both a and b

37. The correct position for an infant while administering back blows is:

    a. Supporting the head in your hand
    b. Resting on your arm and thigh
    c. The head in the dependent position
    d. All the above

38. Which of the following signs are associated with a partial airway obstruction with poor air exchange?

    a. A weak, ineffective cough
    b. Stridor
    c. Cyanosis
    d. All the above

39. The correct position for a chest thrust while treating an infant with a complete foreign body airway obstruction is:

    a. One fingerbreadth above the xiphoid
    b. One fingerbreadth below the nipple line
    c. The nipple line
    d. The upper half of the breast bone

40. When a conscious infant with a complete airway obstruction becomes unconscious, you should first:

    a. Attempt to ventilate and observe for chest excursion
    b. Perform a jaw lift, examine the airway, and perform a finger sweep if you visualize a foreign body
    c. Administer four back blows and four chest thrusts
    d. Check for a brachial pulse to establish the need for cardiac compressions

41. The primary disease(s) affecting the lower airways in pediatric patients is (are):

    a. Asthma
    b. Bronchiolitis
    c. Pneumonia
    d. All the above

42. Asthmatic attacks in children can be triggered by:

    a. Upper respiratory infections
    b. Allergies
    c. Medication withdrawal
    d. All the above

43. Asthmatic children with difficult breathing who become sleepy and lie down should receive:

    a. Positive-pressure ventilation
    b. Humidified oxygen
    c. Nebulized oxygen
    d. Oxygen by nasal catheter

44. Anatomically, foreign bodies that enter the lower airway are more likely to enter the:

    a. Right main stem bronchus
    b. Left main stem bronchus

45. As in the adult, the preferred method for opening the airway of an infant and child is the:

    a. Jaw thrust
    b. Head tilt/chin lift
    c. Head tilt/neck lift
    d. Chin pull

46. While performing the maneuver described above, the head should be placed in the:

    a. Hyperextended position
    b. Extended position
    c. Sniffing or neutral position
    d. Slightly flexed position

47. When providing positive-pressure ventilation in an infant, you should breathe at a rate of 1 breath every:

    a. 5 seconds
    b. 4 seconds
    c. 3 seconds
    d. 2 seconds

48. While ventilating a patient with a bag-valve-mask resuscitator, if you note air leakage through the pop-off valve, you should:

    a. Use your mouth
    b. Tape the valve closed
    c. Use a nonrebreather mask
    d. Do nothing and continue ventilating

49. When caring for a young drowning patient found in shallow water, you should automatically treat the child as if he had:

    a. Kidney damage
    b. A cervical spine injury
    c. Diabetes
    d. A bacterial infection

50. All the following are considered risk factors of SIDS except:

    a. Low socioeconomic group
    b. Adolescent mother
    c. Drug use during pregnancy
    d. Postmature baby

51. SIDS is commonly confused with:

    a. Choking
    b. Child abuse
    c. Drowning
    d. Overdose

52. A common cause of seizures in small children is:

    a. Overdose
    b. Fever
    c. Aspiration
    d. Vomiting

53. The most common internal organ injured in children is the:

    a. Heart
    b. Lungs
    c. Spleen
    d. Liver

54. The leading cause of death in children aged 1 to 14 years is:

    a. SIDS
    b. Drowning
    c. Trauma
    d. Airway obstruction

Questions 55 to 57 are based on the following scenario.

> You respond to a call and find an alert 2-year-old boy who appears to be in severe respiratory distress. On physical examination you note a barking cough, nasal flaring, intercostal retractions, and stridor. The mother tells you that he had a recent upper respiratory infection and woke up during the night with difficulty breathing.

55. Based on the history and signs and symptoms, you strongly suspect:

    a. Asthma
    b. Epiglottitis
    c. Croup
    d. Airway obstruction

56. The most important prehospital treatment of this patient is:

    a. Administering humidified oxygen
    b. Administering positive-pressure ventilation
    c. Suctioning the airway
    d. Placing in the head-down position

57. The most appropriate way to transport this patient is:

    a. Supine with the mother present
    b. Supine; no parent should accompany the patient in the ambulance
    c. Sitting on the mother's lap
    d. Sitting on the stretcher, in a position of comfort, with the mother present

Questions 58 to 60 are based on the following scenario.

> A 6-year-old boy was struck by an automobile and thrown 10 feet. He is lying supine and is responsive to painful but not verbal stimuli. There is delayed capillary refill and his skin is pale, cool, and sweaty. The vital signs are pulse 150 beats/min and thready, blood pressure 60/40 mm Hg, and respirations 34 breaths/min and shallow. There is no accessory muscle use or distended neck veins. Breath sounds are equal bilaterally.

58. Based on your assessment you suspect all the following *except*:

    a. Hypovolemic shock
    b. Tension pneumothorax
    c. Cervical spine injury
    d. Internal bleeding

59. Management of this child should include:

    a. Oxygen by nonrebreather mask
    b. Bag-valve-mask ventilation
    c. Ventilation with a manually triggered resuscitator
    d. Humidified oxygen by facemask

60. Based on the vital signs you would suspect blood loss around:

    a. 10%
    b. 15%
    c. 20%
    d. 40%

Questions 61 and 62 are based on the following scenario.

> You discover a 5-month-old child in cardiopulmonary arrest with mottling of the skin in the dependent areas of the body. The parents said they put her to bed an hour ago and found her like this when they checked on her 10 minutes before your arrival. They say she had a recent upper respiratory infection.

61. This child's condition has most likely been caused by:

    a. Abuse
    b. Choking
    c. SIDS
    d. Heart failure

62. Your action should be to:

    a. Wait for the police to arrive because the child is irreversibly dead
    b. Perform cardiopulmonary resuscitation and transport the baby to the hospital
    c. Not touch or move the baby to preserve evidence
    d. Record the parents' statements very carefully and give them to the police on arrival

Questions 63 to 65 are based on the following scenario.

> You respond to a 3-year-old girl with high fever, a sore throat, difficulty swallowing, and inspiratory stridor. She is sitting upright and leaning forward with her weight distributed on her hands, her mouth open, her tongue protruding, and her chin thrust forward. She is very restlessness and drooling and has a flushed face. Her breath sounds are diminished, but no wheezes or rhonchi are present.

63. Based on the history and signs and symptoms, you strongly suspect:

    a. Bronchiolitis
    b. Epiglottitis
    c. Croup
    d. Asthma

64. The most important immediate action is:

    a. Administering humidified oxygen
    b. Examining the lower airway
    c. Suctioning the lower airway
    d. Placing her in the supine position

65. If this patient were to become completely obstructed, you should:

    a. Perform abdominal thrusts
    b. Attempt forced ventilations
    c. Perform a finger sweep
    d. Perform back blows

Questions 66 to 69 are based on the following scenario.

> You respond to a 11-month-old girl who developed acute respiratory distress while playing with her toys in her crib. She appears to be crying, but no sounds are emitted from her airway. The parents tell you she has had no illness up to this event. Your physical exam reveals chest movements without air exchange at the mouth and nose. Her lips are cyanotic, but there are no other obvious physical signs.

66. Based on the history and signs and symptoms, you strongly suspect:

    a. Foreign body obstruction
    b. Anaphylaxis
    c. Bronchiolitis
    d. Sleep apnea

67. The most important immediate action is:

    a. Administering humidified oxygen
    b. Examining the lower airway
    c. Suctioning the lower airway
    d. Administering up to 5 back blows and 5 chest thrusts

68. You continue your efforts without success, and the baby becomes unconscious. You should first:

    a. Examine the airway
    b. Administer positive-pressure ventilation
    c. Perform chest thrusts
    d. Perform back blows

69. Two minutes later you are able to effectively ventilate the patient but you note that there is no pulse. When beginning compressions you should position your fingers:

    a. One fingerbreadth above the nipple line
    b. One fingerbreadth below the nipple line
    c. Directly at the nipple line
    d. Just above the xiphoid process

70. A best method for evaluating end organ perfusion of the brain is:

    a. Level of consciousness
    b. Capillary refill
    c. Reflexes
    d. Pupils

71. Appropriate management of seizures includes all the following *except*:

    a. Restrain the patient movements to prevent injury
    b. Place the patient on his or her side to prevent aspiration
    c. Have suction ready in case of vomiting
    d. Administer positive-pressure ventilation if needed

72. All the following are indicators of abuse *except:*

    a. Frequent calls to the same address for injuries
    b. Changes in the history depending on who gives it
    c. New bruises on the arm or leg after a fall
    d. Delay in obtaining medical care

73. Which of the following statements best describes the emergency medical technician (EMT) role in reporting child abuse:

    a. The EMT is legally responsible for reporting child abuse in every state
    b. The EMT is not legally responsible for reporting child abuse in every state but has an ethical responsibility
    c. The EMT has neither an ethical nor legal responsibility for reporting child abuse
    d. The EMT should limit his or her activities to the care of injuries and not tend to social problems

74. Caring for seriously injured children can result in psychological trauma to the health care provider. A useful method of prevention is:

    a. Treating the clinical condition without focusing on the nature of the event
    b. Involve yourself in activities that will help you forget the events that you are exposed to
    c. Seek participation in an organized debriefing process after exposure to serious childhood injuries
    d. Focus on the positive aspects of your interventions rather than the nature of the injury or illness

List the eight possible signs of early respiratory distress.

75. ______________________________

76. ______________________________

77. ______________________________

78. ______________________________

79. ______________________________

80. ______________________________

81. ______________________________

82. ______________________________

List the four key signs of respiratory failure.

83. ______________________________

84. ______________________________

85. ______________________________

86. ______________________________

Match the appearance of a bruise in column A with the age of the bruise in Column B.

Column A	**Column B**
87. _____ Yellow/brown	a. 1 to 3 days
	b. 3 to 7 days
88. _____ Red/blue	c. 7 days
	d. 3 weeks
89. _____ Brown to clearing	
90. _____ Purple	

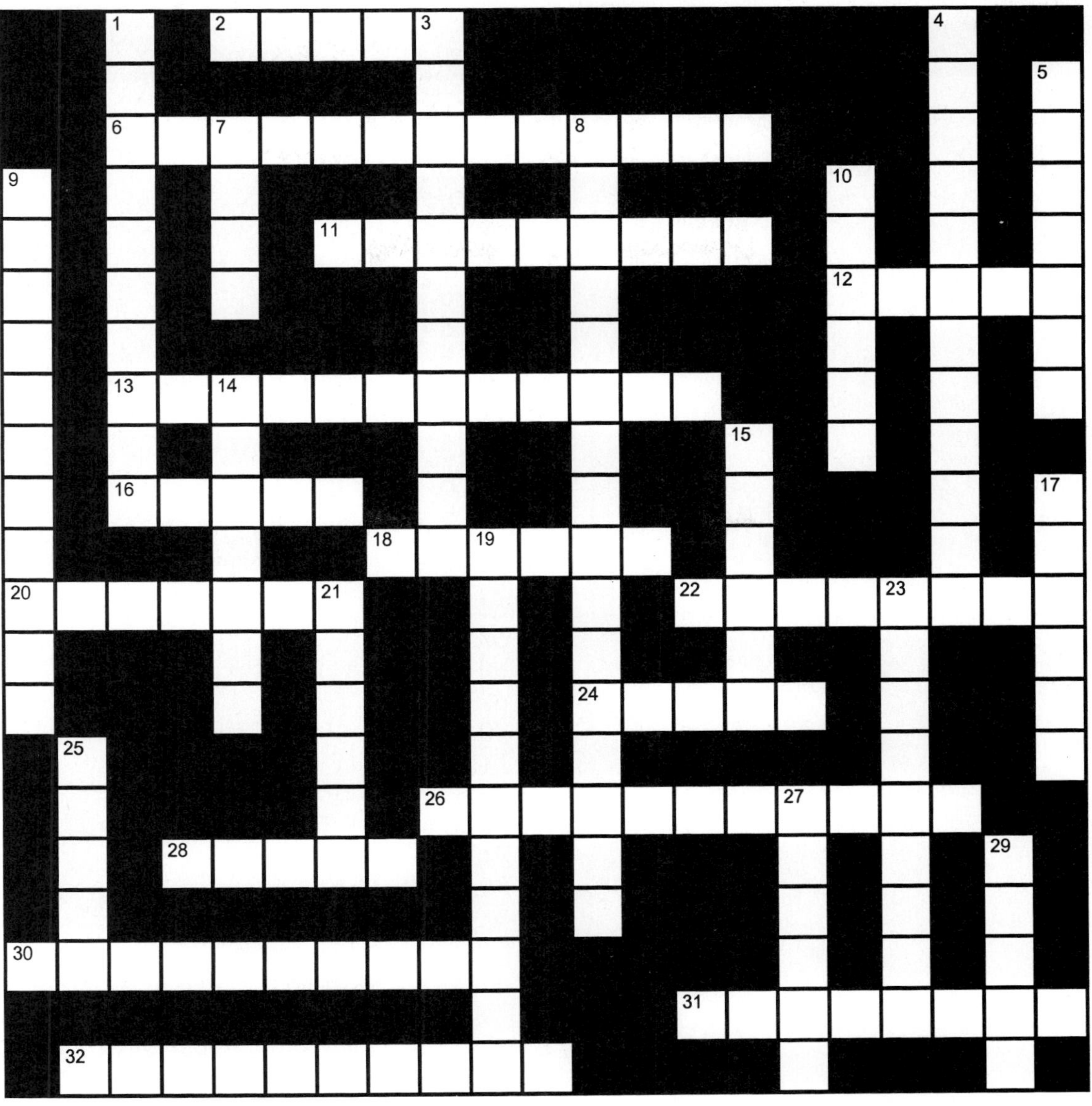

ANSWER KEY

1. b
2. c
3. c
4. a
5. c
6. b
7. d
8. d
9. a
10. c
11. a
12. d
13. b
14. a
15. c
16. c
17. b
18. a
19. d
20. c
21. d
22. a
23. c
24. c
25. a
26. c
27. b
28. a
29. a
30. c
31. d
32. d
33. b
34. d
35. c
36. d
37. d
38. d
39. b
40. b
41. d
42. d
43. a
44. a
45. b
46. c
47. c
48. b
49. b
50. d
51. b
52. b
53. c
54. c
55. c
56. a
57. d
58. b
59. b
60. d
61. c
62. b
63. b
64. a
65. b
66. a
67. d
68. a
69. b
70. a
71. a
72. c
73. b
74. c

75. to 82. Grunting
Mottling of skin
Nasal flaring
Retractions
Stridor
Tachycardia (rapid pulse)
Tachypnea (rapid breathing)
Wheezing

83. to 86. Cyanosis or mottling
Fast or slow respiratory rate relative to the age of the patient
Little or no air movement
Labored breathing and retractions

87. c
88. a
89. d
90. b
91. True
92. False
93. True
94. False
95. True
96. False
97. False
98. True

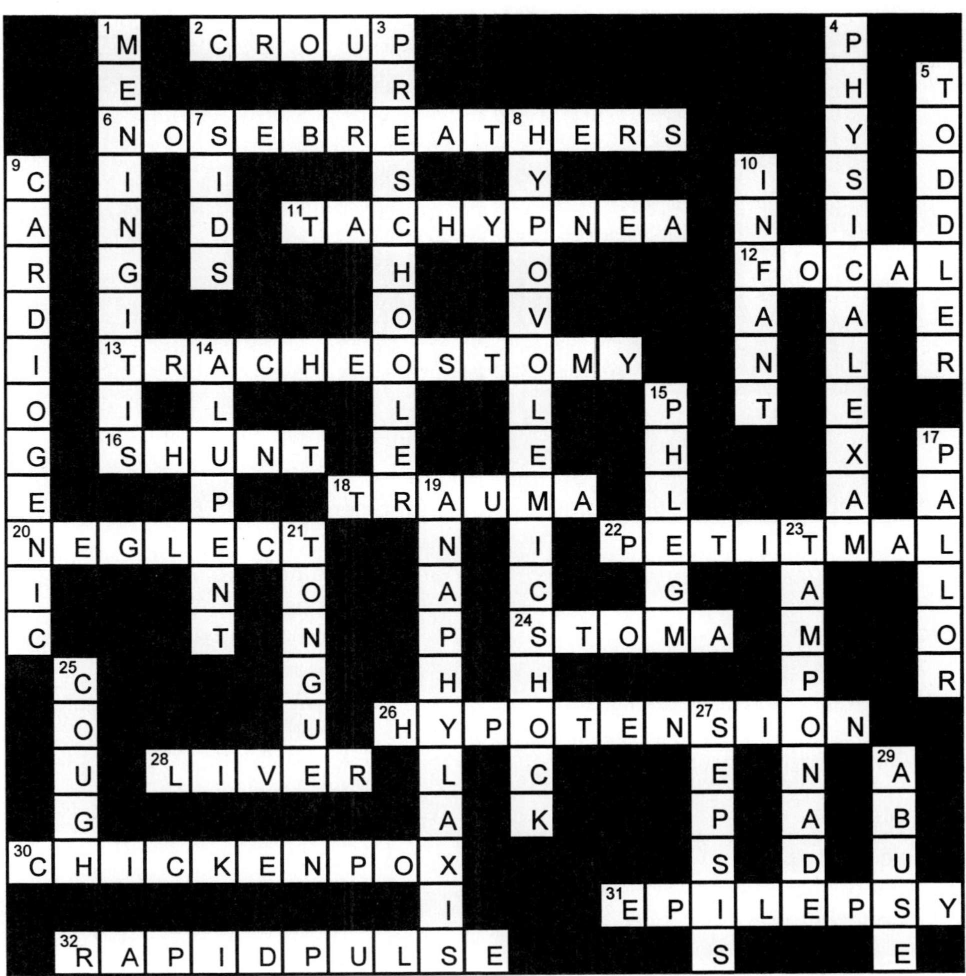

2 CROUP
6 NOSEBREATHERS
11 TACHYPNEA
12 FOCAL
13 TRACHEOSTOMY
16 SHUNT
18 TRAUMA
20 NEGLECT
22 PETITMAL
24 STOMA
26 HYPOTENSION
28 LIVER
30 CHICKENPOX
31 EPILEPSY
32 RAPIDPULSE
1 MENINGITIS
3 PRESCHOOLER
4 PHYSICALEXAM
5 TODDLER
7 SIDS
8 HYPOVOLEMICSHOCK
9 CARDIOGENIC
10 INFANT
14 ALUPENT
15 PHLEGM
17 PALLOR
19 ANAPHYLAXIS
21 TONGUE
23 TAMPONADE
25 COUGH
27 SEPSIS
29 ABUSE

Chapter 31 Ambulance Operations

1. The superior braking technique when driving an ambulance is:

   a. Left foot braking
   b. Right foot braking
   c. Dominant foot braking
   d. Alternate foot braking

2. Palming the wheel in a turn represents a:

   a. Poor driving habit
   b. Method of stable turning
   c. Method for "feeling" the turn
   d. Crash avoidance technique

3. Exemptions of traffic regulations provided by law for persons driving emergency vehicles are best described as:

   a. Necessary evils
   b. Privileges
   c. Protections from crashes
   d. Legal protections

4. The correct position of a lap belt is across the:

   a. Umbilicus
   b. Thigh
   c. Pelvic girdle
   d. Upper thigh

5. The chances of being seriously injured by a seatbelt are approximately 1 in ________ crashes.

   a. 5
   b. 10
   c. 50
   d. 200

6. Emergency lights and sirens:

   a. Are necessary to relieve the operator of liability in case of an incident
   b. Are most effective in low-light situations, such as at dawn or dusk
   c. Do not relieve the operator of liability in the event of an incident
   d. Are most effective at high speeds

7. The most effective colors for rear-facing warning lamps are:

   a. Amber and blue
   b. Red and white
   c. Red and yellow
   d. Yellow and white

8. Four-way hazard lights:

   a. Should not be used in a moving vehicle
   b. Should be turned off when the vehicle is parked
   c. Are necessary in a moving ambulance
   d. Are most effective in low-light situations

9. The most effective warning lights are mounted:

   a. Just above the rear bumper
   b. On the roof
   c. At eye level to other drivers
   d. In the outermost corners of the vehicle

10. The sound pattern of a siren in a moving ambulance is best described as:

    a. A circle with the siren at the center
    b. A square with the siren at the center
    c. A cone ahead of the vehicle
    d. A straight line in front of the vehicle

11. At 60 mph, the sound emitted from an ambulance siren:

    a. Moves more quickly through the air
    b. Barely precedes the ambulance
    c. Is louder on the sides of the vehicle
    d. Will not be heard inside the ambulance

12. The sweaty palms, rapid pulse, and tense muscles felt by the operator of an emergency vehicle when the siren is switched on can cause the operator to immediately begin speeding. This response is the result of:

    a. Endorphin release
    b. Adrenaline release
    c. Physical demands of driving
    d. Vagal stimulation

13. An escort vehicle should be used only when:

    a. The ambulance is traveling at high speeds
    b. The operator is unfamiliar with the route
    c. Police are available
    d. There is more than one ambulance

14. The two major control tasks of an emergency vehicle operator are speed control and:

    a. Vehicle balance
    b. Braking
    c. Radio communications
    d. Directional control

15. Van ambulances with raised tops:

    a. Have decreased wind resistance
    b. Have a higher center of gravity
    c. Are more stable during turns
    d. Usually have steel roof skins

16. When suddenly braking an ambulance, the rear brakes:

    a. Are considerably less effective than the front
    b. Do most of the braking
    c. Brake equally with the front brakes
    d. Allow for better directional control

17. When rolling friction is lost, you lose all the following *except:*

    a. Forward momentum
    b. Directional control
    c. Centrifugal force
    d. Stopping ability

18. When the brakes lock, the wheels stop turning and:

    a. Centrifugal force is lost
    b. The stopping distance is decreased
    c. Stopping friction is reduced
    d. Momentum is lost

19. A good way to judge the correct traveling distance between your ambulance and the vehicle in front of you in dry weather is to observe the vehicle in front of you as it passes a fixed object (such as a telephone pole) and then be able to count _______ seconds before you reach the same object.

    a. 2
    b. 4
    c. 10
    d. 12

20. On icy roads, the above rule is increased to:

    a. 6 seconds
    b. 12 seconds
    c. 20 seconds
    d. 30 seconds

21. Most emergency vehicle crashes occur:

    a. On highways
    b. At the scene of the crash
    c. En route to a crash
    d. At intersections

Match the ambulance type in column A with the descriptions in column B.

Column A	Column B
22. _____ Type I	a. Van-type ambulance
23. _____ Type II	b. Modular patient compartment with van chassis
24. _____ Type III	c. Modular patient compartment with truck chassis

25. If sterile supplies such as bandages or dressings become wet, they should be:

    a. Dried in an autoclave
    b. Air dried
    c. Discarded
    d. Dried under ultraviolet light

26. The precautions taken to prevent spread of infectious disease are called infection:

    a. Control
    b. Protection
    c. Guarding
    d. Barriers

27. The first phase of an ambulance call is:

    a. Documentation
    b. Dispatch
    c. Preparation
    d. Response

28. All the following information is needed to properly respond to a call *except*:

    a. Nature of the call
    b. Age of the patient
    c. Number of patients
    d. Severity of patients

29. The essential activities at the completion of a call before signaling your availability for the next call include all the following *except*:

    a. Ambulance disinfection
    b. Restocking
    c. Filing reports
    d. Follow-up on the status of the patient

30. All the following are important reasons for carefully preparing for the next call *except*:

    a. Lack of equipment may result in injury to a patient
    b. You may transmit an infection to yourself or the next patient
    c. The ambulance may be unsafe because of poor maintenance
    d. It will allow for a period of rest for you and your partner

31. One hour from the time of injury to arrival at definitive care is called the _________.

32. When approaching a medivac helicopter you should always approach from the _________.

Questions 33 to 35 refer to the following scenario.

> You respond to a call for a farm incident in a rural area of your county. You encounter a 32-year-old man who was operating a plow in the field when the plow rolled over, pinning the patient under the machinery by his left leg. Although you can't readily extricate the patient you observe that his arm is severely mangled and you can't feel any distal pulses. The nearest trauma center is 90 minutes away by ground ambulance and you anticipate a 30- to 60-minute extrication process.

33. Use of a helicopter for rapid transport is:

    a. Not indicated because the patient will not be extricated within the "platinum 10 minutes"
    b. Not indicated because the patient will not arrive at a trauma center within the golden hour
    c. Not indicated because the drive time to the hospital is less than 2 hours
    d. Indicated because of the patient's injury combined with the extended transport time

34. Once the patient is extricated from the machinery you learn that the helicopter has an estimated arrival time of 5 minutes. You should:

    a. Defer any further care until the helicopter personnel arrive at the scene
    b. Begin transport and cancel the helicopter
    c. Initiate any treatment indicated, package the patient, and await the arrival of the helicopter
    d. Prepare the landing zone by placing flares around the chosen landing area

35. Once the helicopter arrives you should not approach the helicopter unless:

    a. You can approach from the rear
    b. You are directed to approach by the flight team and you maintain eye contact with the pilot
    c. The helicopter is shut down and the rotors are secured by tie-down cords by the flight crew
    d. Directed by the incident commander on the scene

Questions 36 to 38 refer to the following scenario.

> You respond to a call for an injured logger. As you respond to the rural scene you round a curve in the road and see the scene blocked by a logging truck in the road. You apply the brakes immediately and as you continue pressure on the brake pedal you feel the pedal vibrating. Your vehicle is equipped with anti-lock brakes.

36. You should:

    a. Immediately take your foot off the brake to prevent an uncontrollable skid
    B. Maintain pressure on the brake pedal because this sensation is normal when the anti-lock feature is engaged
    c. Immediately pump the brake pedal to prevent an uncontrollable skid
    d. Apply the emergency brake

37. You arrive at the scene and observe that your patient is lying on his side approximately 30 yards off the road in the trees, approximately 20 feet below the level of the road. You should:

    a. Immediately summon a helicopter because this is the only way to extricate the patient
    b. Safely make your way to the patient and evaluate his injuries
    c. Wait with your ambulance until the high-angle rescue team can arrive
    d. Place the patient on a scoop stretcher and use a come-along attached to the vehicle's bumper to pull the patient up to the road

38. The optimal time from injury to arrival at the operating room is sometimes referred to as the:

    a. Prime time
    b. Critical minutes
    c. Magic minutes
    d. Golden hour

Across

2. Mechanical aid used to administer positive-pressure breathing
10. If hazardous materials are expected at the scene, park uphill and _____
11. Trained entry-level prehospital emergency care provider
14. National Institute for Occupational Safety and Health
16. One hour from the time of injury to arrival at site of definitive care
18. Material that covers a wound
20. A _____ _____ device is used primarily for immobilizing a patient with a suspected neck or back injury, who is found in a seated position
23. Force evident when operating the common high-top van ambulance
24. Device used to immobilize a suspected femur fracture
25. Material used to secure a dressing in place
26. Program sponsored by the Department of Transportation to train EMTs in the operation of emergency vehicles
27. Helicopters were first used for medical evacuation during this war

Down

1. Requirement to control both speed and direction of the vehicle
3. Used for extricating a patient in a supine position
4. Certain driving _____ are granted to emergency vehicles to expedite the delivery of care
5. A formal program that educates dispatchers in phone triage and phone-directed instructions to lay people
6. Specialized mask and regulator with portable air supply used by rescue personnel in environments that might be dangerous
7. Always approach a helicopter from the _____
8. A reasonably careful person performing similar duties under the same circumstances would act in the same manner
9. Blood pressure cuff
12. If _____ _____ is lost, directional control is lost and inertia and centrifugal force direct the movement of the vehicle
13. _____ _____ garments are air-filled pants that surround the legs and the abdomen
15. To minimize the possibility of injury, you should assume a _____ position when approaching a helicopter
17. Force that may pull a vehicle out of a curve
19. Device used for auscultation
21. 911 system with the ability to automatically identify a caller's location
22. Type II ambulance

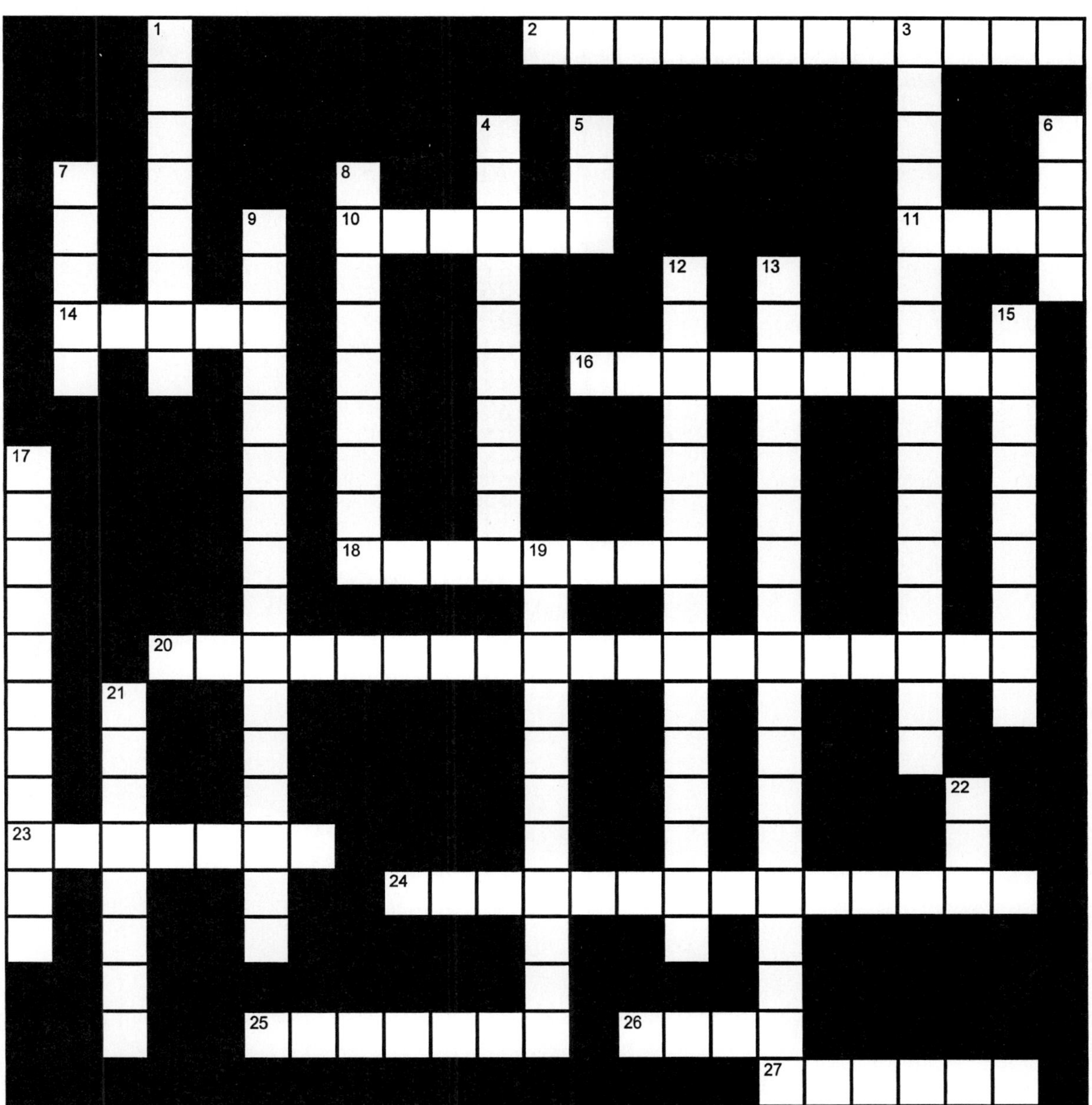
1
2
3
4
5
6
7
8
9
10
11
12
13
14
15
16
17
18
19
20
21
22
23
24
25
26
27

ANSWER KEY

1. b
2. a
3. b
4. c
5. d
6. c
7. a
8. a
9. c
10. c
11. b
12. b
13. b
14. d
15. b
16. a
17. c
18. c
19. b
20. b
21. d
22. c
23. a
24. b
25. c
26. a
27. c
28. b
29. d
30. d
31. Golden hour
32. Front
33. d
34. c
35. b
36. b
37. b
38. d

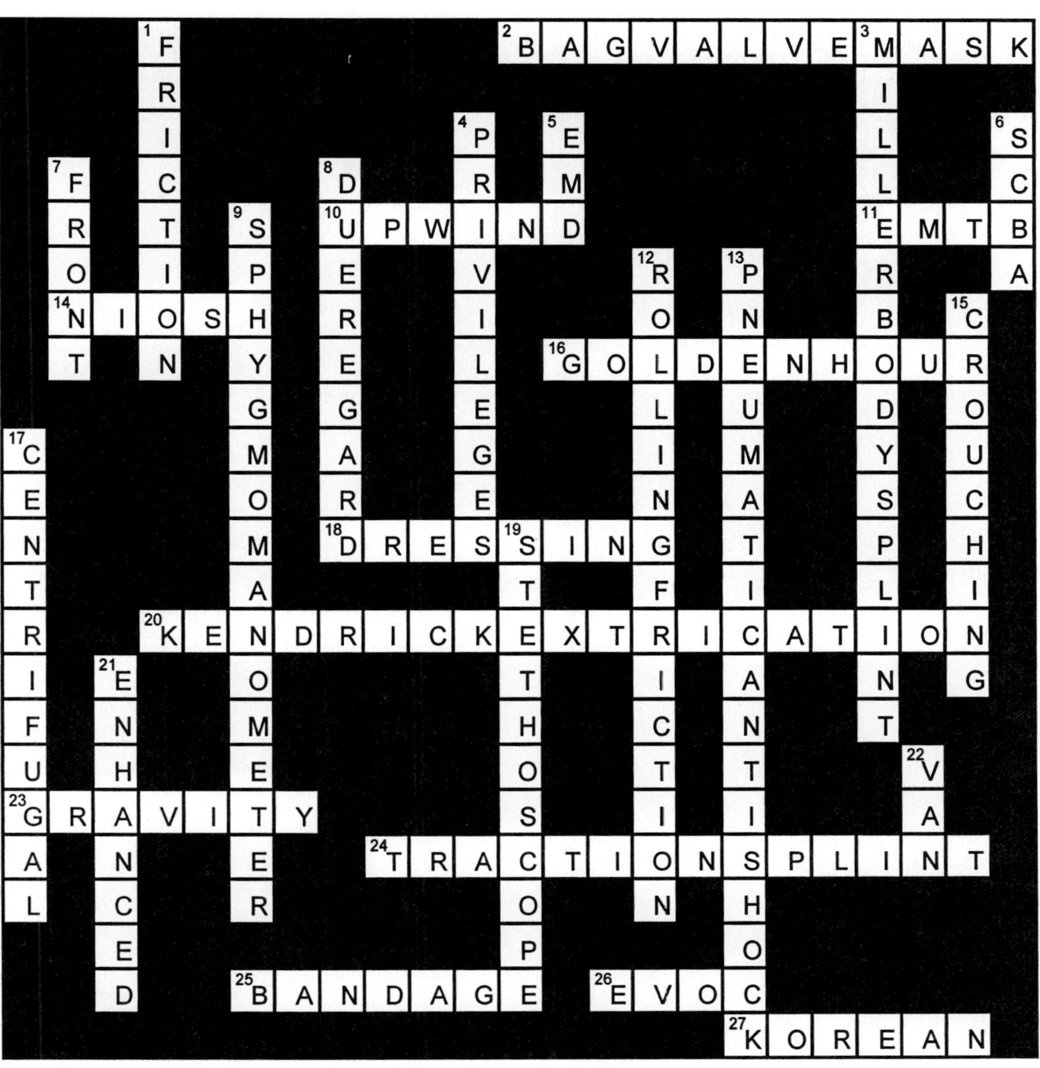
1 FRICTION
2 BAGVALVEMASK
3 MILLERBODYSPLINT
4 PRIVILEGE
5 EMD
6 SCBA
7 FRONT
8 DUEREGARD
9 SPHYGMOMANOMETER
10 UPWIND
11 EMTB
12 ROLLINGFRICTION
13 PNEUMATICANTISHOCK
14 NIOSH
15 CROUCHING
16 GOLDENHOUR
17 CENTRIFUGAL
18 DRESSING
19 STETHOSCOPE
20 KENDRICKEXTRICATION
21 ENHANCED
22 VAN
23 GRAVITY
24 TRACTIONSPLINT
25 BANDAGE
26 EVOC
27 KOREAN

Chapter 32 Gaining Access

1. The term used to describe an extrication that can be accomplished with hand tools or skills such as opening locks is called:

   a. Disentanglement
   b. Simple or light extrication
   c. Strategic access
   d. Rapid extrication

2. Because of the possibility of spilled gasoline at a motor vehicle crash site, the least appropriate method of securing the scene is through the use of:

   a. Reflectors
   b. Flares
   c. Road cones
   d. Battery operated lights

3. Blocks of wood used to stabilize vehicles are commonly called:

   a. Stacking blocks
   b. Cribbing
   c. Stabilizers
   d. Construction blocks

4. When attempting to gain further access through a window, the patient should be protected by:

   a. Moving him or her away from the window
   b. Tilting the car away from the patient
   c. Covering the patient with a rescue blanket
   d. Shattering the window from the inside out

5. On gaining access to the interior of the car, you find a patient who is short of breath, pale, cool and sweaty, hypotensive, and who has a respiratory rate of 22 breaths/min. Your immediate reaction is to:

   a. Apply oxygen and a vest-type device
   b. Rapidly extricate the patient
   c. Apply the pneumatic anti-shock garment before extrication
   d. Begin positive-pressure ventilation

6. The simplest and best method for creating room between the driver and the steering wheel is to:

   a. Cut the steering wheel away
   b. Slide the seat back
   c. Distort the steering wheel
   d. Cut the steering wheel post off

7. One method of reducing the number of glass shards when breaking a car window is to:

   a. Wet the window
   b. Tape the corners
   c. Apply contact paper
   d. Heat the window

8. If electrical wires are down at a scene, you should do all the following *except*:

   a. Retreat to a position of safety
   b. Establish a hazard zone
   c. Advise the occupants not to exit
   d. Rescue occupants with a rope

9. The first thing you should do when approaching the scene of a motor vehicle crash is to:

   a. Immediately call a tow truck for assistance
   b. Call for additional units
   c. Perform a windshield survey
   d. Park your vehicle 500 feet from the scene

Questions 10 to 12 refer to the following scenario.

> You respond to a call and find two cars in a head-on collision. You note that the passengers and driver of car #1 are ambulating and talking to bystanders. The passenger from car #2 appears in severe distress and the driver appears to be dead.

10. Your first action on leaving the ambulance is to:

    a. Evaluate the passenger of car #2
    b. Stabilize the cervical spine on the passenger from car #2
    c. Make sure the scene is safe
    d. Perform cardiopulmonary resuscitation on driver #2

11. On approaching car #2, you note that all of the doors are jammed, the windows are closed, and the passenger is too confused to cooperate in opening the door. You should gain access to the patient by:

    a. Breaking the windshield
    b. Cutting through the floor
    c. Cutting through the roof
    d. Breaking the rear driver-side window

12. After you have gained access and pried open the car door, you find the patient in severe respiratory distress, with paradoxical breathing, and pale, cool, and sweaty skin. Your immediate action should be to:

    a. Apply a pneumatic anti-shock garment
    b. Apply a short spine board
    c. Rapidly extricate the patient
    d. Perform a secondary survey

Questions 13 to 15 refer to the following scenario.

> On arriving at the scene of a motor vehicle crash, you encounter a car with flames coming from beneath the hood. You note a driver and two passengers who are trapped in the car.

13. Your immediate action should be to:

    a. Attempt to extinguish the fire
    b. Cut a flap in the door to gain access
    c. Break the front windshield to gain access
    d. Cut a roof flap to gain access

14. By the time your patients are in the ambulance, you note that they are all exhibiting signs of respiratory distress. You suspect:

    a. Cyanide poisoning
    b. First-degree burns
    c. Carbon monoxide poisoning
    d. Hyperthermia

15. The most important treatment for these patients is:

    a. Humidified oxygen by a mask
    b. Oxygen by a nonrebreather mask
    c. Nasal cannula oxygen
    d. Cool compresses to their faces

16. You respond to a call at a railroad yard and are told that two men have fallen inside a huge tanker. You climb to the top of the tanker and look down inside to see the two men approximately 15 feet below you. They do not respond when you call out to them. Your immediate action should be to:

    a. Enter the car with a nonrebreather mask on your face
    b. Allow oxygen to flow through tubing into the tanker to clear the environment, then enter
    c. Lower your partner with a rope to allow for rapid removal
    d. Maintain a safe distance from the opening into the tanker and contact a rescue unit with self-contained breathing apparatus equipment

17. The purpose of extrication is to:

    a. Free a person who is entrapped in his or her surroundings
    b. Preserve evidence at the scene
    c. Provide fracture care away from the crash site
    d. Allow for easier access to the airway

18. When specialized rescue personnel are present, the role of the EMT during extrication includes all the following *except:*

    a. Any necessary patient care before extrication
    b. Ensuring the patient is removed in a way to minimize further injury
    c. Assessment and triage of multiple patients
    d. Supervising the operations of rescue personnel

19. When the EMT is working with rescue personnel at an incident requiring patient extrication, which of the following is true?

    a. Patient care precedes extrication unless delayed movement would endanger life
    b. Extrication precedes patient care unless there are signs of uncontrolled bleeding
    c. Careful packaging of the patient for removal is the responsibility of rescue personnel
    d. EMTs should first attend to the patients who do not need extrication

20. At the scene of a motor vehicle crash, in general the greatest threat to the personal safety of the EMT is:

    a. Cuts from broken glass
    b. Oncoming traffic
    c. Fire
    d. Toxic contamination

21. All the following are examples of simple access during extrication *except*:

    a. Using a slim jim to open a door
    b. Using a punch to break a window
    c. Using power tools to pry open a door
    d. Opening an unaffected door in a crashed vehicle

22. In general, assuming side access to a vehicle (through a door or open window) is not possible, what access point represents the next best alternative?

    a. Rear or front windshield
    b. Roof
    c. Floor
    d. Trunk

23. As you approach a car that was involved in a motor vehicle crash, your quick inspection that identifies if the patients are moving or conscious is called a:

    a. Windshield survey
    b. Initial assessment
    c. Detailed assessment
    d. Focused assessment

Questions 24 and 25 refer to the following scenario.

> You respond to the scene of a vehicle rollover and find a small, late-model sport utility vehicle on its wheels after having rolled over at least once. There is only one car involved. The driver of this car is sitting behind the steering wheel and appears to be dazed. The scene appears to be safe. You are able to easily gain access to the vehicle through the driver's side door. The patient is wearing a lap/shoulder belt and the air bags have not deployed.

24. The safest way to approach the patient and provide safety from the air bag is to:

    a. Trigger the air bag before entering the vehicle
    b. Have the fire department cut the battery cables, which will ensure that the air bags can't deploy
    c. Place a protective cover over the steering wheel air bag, if one is available, and maintain a safe distance from the steering wheel
    d. There is no need for concern, the air bag can't deploy if the vehicle is stopped

25. You have provided rescuer and patient safety and begin your patient evaluation. Your patient complains of head and neck pain. His vital signs are pulse 82 beats/min and regular, blood pressure 136/78 mm Hg, respiratory rate is 16 breaths/min full and regular. The best way to remove this patient from the car is:

    a. Move the patient directly onto a long spine board
    b. Immobilize the patient in a vest-type device and then remove the patient to a long spine board
    c. Allow the patient to step out of the car and sit on your stretcher
    d. Perform a rapid extrication

Across

4. On gaining access to a motor vehicle accident victim, _____ _____ immobilization should be accomplished
5. Specialized mask and regulator with portable air supply used by rescue personnel in environments that might be dangerous
6. The process by which entrapped patients are rescued from vehicles
8. The color coding system used on a triage tag allows the EMT-B to _____ the patient
10. When approaching a scene, stop _____ and upwind
12. The EMT's primary role at the scene of an automobile accident
14. Personal protective equipment for reducing the potential for injury
15. Emergency assistance required when a patient is trapped in a collapsed building
16. When approaching a car that has been in an accident, do a _____ _____ to quickly assess the situation

Down

1. Perform a _____ _____ _____ to note potential danger to rescuers, the public, and the patient
2. A spring-loaded piece of equipment used to break glass
3. Emergency assistance required for a patient involving vertical considerations
5. Rescue from a motor vehicle using hand tools
7. Sorting patients according to priority
9. The quickest way to access an unconscious victim in a car
11. Blocks of wood used to stabilize vehicles
13. An increase in the patient's anxiety will result in an increase in the patient's oxygen consumption caused by the body's secretion of _____

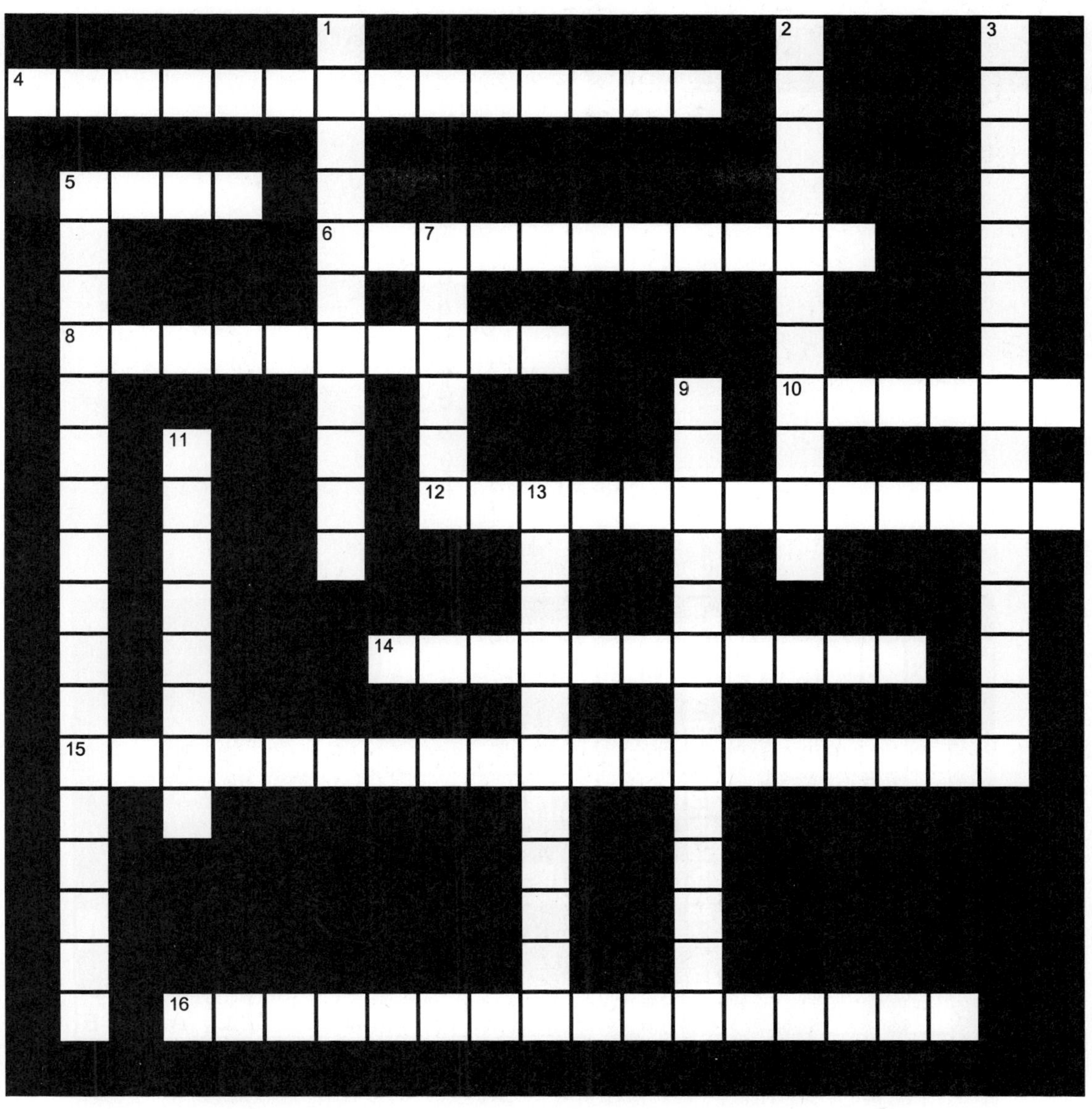
1
2
3
4
5
6
7
8
9
10
11
12
13
14
15
16

ANSWER KEY

1. b
2. b
3. b
4. c
5. b
6. b
7. c
8. d
9. c
10. c
11. d
12. c
13. a
14. c
15. b
16. d
17. a
18. d
19. a
20. b
21. c
22. a
23. a
24. c
25. b

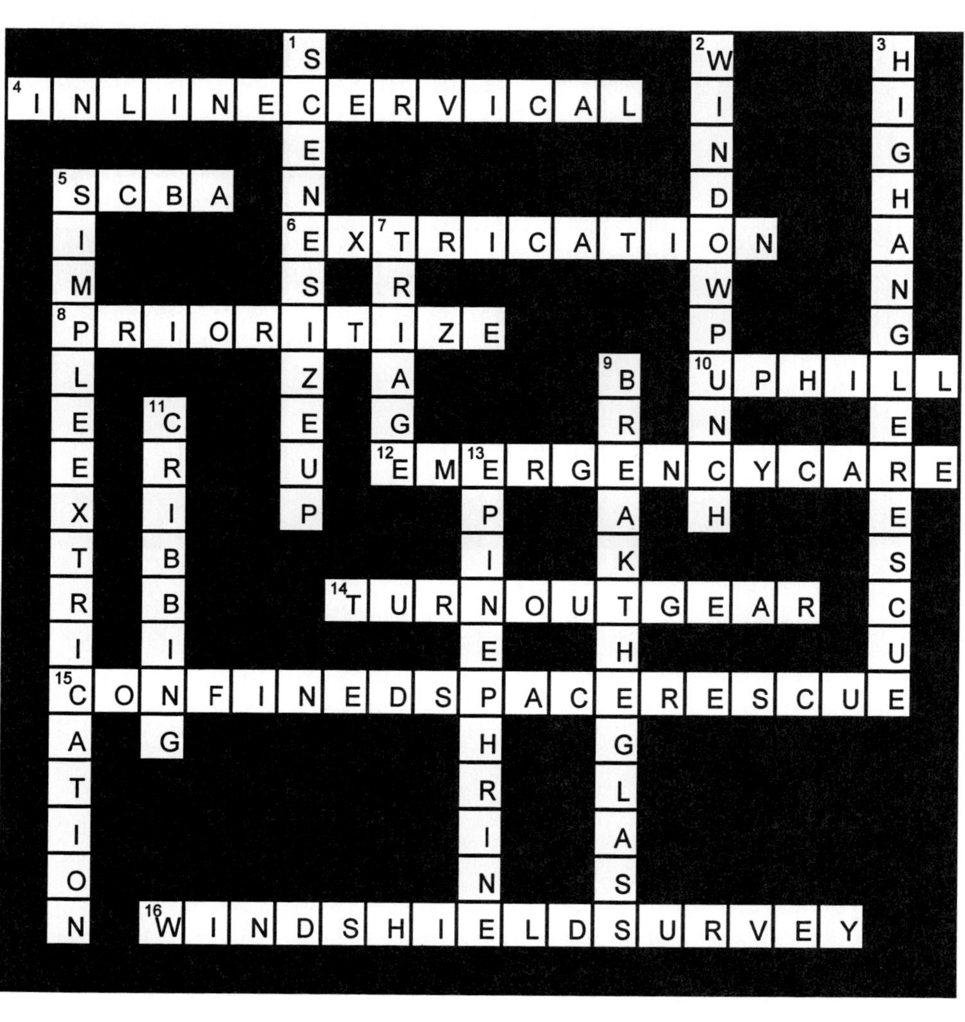

Chapter 33 Disasters and Hazardous Materials

1. The primary responsibility of an EMT at a hazardous materials incident is:

    a. Containment
    b. Decontamination
    c. Emergency medical care
    d. Removal

2. You smell a strange odor when approaching a scene involving a transportation vehicle; you should first:

    a. Relocate upwind and assess the scene from a distance
    b. Apply your self-contained breathing apparatus gear and approach the scene to perform an assessment
    c. Approach the scene and assess
    d. Contact Chemtec immediately to have an expert come to the scene

3. When reacting to a documented hazardous materials incident, it is important to establish a patient treatment and transport location called a:

    a. Command center
    b. Staging area
    c. Communications area
    d. Triage area

4. The bill of lading is most often found:

    a. In the cab of the vehicle or with the driver
    b. Posted on the back end of the vehicle
    c. Posted on the side of the vehicle
    d. Posted on the front of the vehicle

5. When approaching a potential hazardous materials scene, general clues of hazardous material from a distance might include all the following *except*:

    a. The location of the incident
    b. Noting the air temperature to detect radiation
    c. Noting the shape of the affected container
    d. Looking for placards on the container

6. To minimize damage to the environment, the EMT may assist rescue personnel to prevent runoff by use of:

    a. A dike or trench
    b. Irrigation into the sewer
    c. An ABC fire extinguisher to neutralize the runoff
    d. Vacuum devices

7. Which of the following best represents a closed disaster?

    a. A plane crash on a mountain with no access road
    b. A building collapse in a city
    c. A burning building
    d. A multiple-car collision on a highway

8. A predetermined response system with neighboring communities that ensures a large scale response of emergency vehicles during a disaster best describes a:

    a. Transfer agreement
    b. Mutual aid agreement
    c. Cross coverage plan
    d. Mass casualty incident strategy

9. The sorting of casualties of war or other disaster to determine the priority of need and proper place of treatment best defines:

   a. Categorization
   b. Stacking
   c. Triage
   d. Designation

Match the appropriate color triage tag in column A with the condition in column B.

Column A		Column B
10. _____	Red	a. An unconscious patient with a head injury
11. _____	Yellow	b. Traumatic cardiac patient
		c. Multiple pelvic fractures
12. _____	Green	d. Fractured humerus
13. _____	Black	

14. The secondary triage area is where treatment occurs and where:

    a. Patients are staged for transport
    b. Dead patients are packaged
    c. The command post is ideally located
    d. The communications center is established

15. When a patient fears death, perceives limited escape, and has no information about what happened, the likely outcome is:

    a. Suicide
    b. Depression
    c. Panic
    d. Psychosis

16. At the site of a disaster, drivers of emergency vehicles should:

    a. Participate in early triage and treatment
    b. Park as close to the scene as possible
    c. Remain with their vehicles
    d. Report to the triage officer

17. The rapid response of onlookers, rescuers, and press at the scene of a disaster that results in the blockage of traffic routes is called:

    a. Accident crowding
    b. Convergence
    c. Focal obstruction
    d. Central merge

18. The process of demobilizing response vehicles and apparatus for the purposes of returning them to normal community service is called:

    a. Recovery
    b. Remobilization
    c. Reintroduction
    d. Rehabilitation

19. The rebuilding of the community in a physical and emotional sense after a disaster, a process that includes critical incident stress debriefing, is referred to as:

    a. Reconstruction
    b. Rehabilitation
    c. Recovery
    d. Restoration

20. The three essential emergency services components of disaster management are:

    a. Command, triage, and transport
    b. Triage, patient care, and transport
    c. Triage, communications, and patient care
    d. Command, control, and triage

21. The log that records the patient distribution to ambulances and hospital destination is called the:

    a. Major event log
    b. Logistics sheet
    c. Transportation log
    d. Destination log

22. At a disaster scene, the person whose function is to control traffic flow, gather supplies, stage additional vehicles, and communicate ambulance availability to the command post is the:

    a. Supply officer
    b. Transport officer
    c. Communication officer
    d. Triage officer

23. The process by which participants are allowed to express their feelings about the incident and thereby relieve stress associated with the situation is called the:

    a. Catharsis
    b. Debriefing
    c. Critique
    d. Field exercise

Questions 24 to 29 refer to the following scenario.

> You and your partner are the first to arrive at the scene of a large airplane crash in a hilly, wooded area. At least 100 people were on the aircraft at the time of impact. The left wing of the plane is smoking. It is late fall at twilight, and it is starting to snow lightly, and the wind is blowing strong from the north. The nearest hospital is about 20 minutes away, but there is only a single small road to access the area, and several cars belonging to local residents are already beginning to block the road. Your partner is the driver.

24. This disaster can be described as:

    a. Open, active
    b. Closed, active
    c. Open, contained
    d. Closed, contained

25. As you and your partner arrive at the disaster scene:

    a. You should secure your vehicle, making sure that the road is not obstructed, and then you and your partner should begin to do a scene survey
    b. Radio for additional assistance, then both stay in the ambulance until at least one other vehicle arrives
    c. Both should drive back down the road to block further traffic and radio for assistance
    d. Radio for police, fire, and rescue assistance, then both stay with the vehicle until firemen arrive

26. As the first arriving EMT, you or your partner will temporarily become the _________ officer.

    a. Command
    b. Triage
    c. Traffic
    d. Post

27. The best place for a temporary command post at this time would be:

    a. Near the right wing of the plane
    b. 200 yards south of the plane
    c. 200 yards north of the plane
    d. In a building half a mile away

28. Your partner discovers four injured patients: a 50-year-old unconscious man with a head injury, a 16-year-old boy in cardiac arrest, a 60-year-old man with bilateral fractures of the radius and ulna, and a 35-year-old man with an open fracture of the femur. Which patient should receive priority?

    a. 50-year-old man
    b. 16-year-old boy
    c. 35-year-old man
    d. 60-year-old man

29. The 16-year-old described previously would be considered a _______________ triage category.

    a. Red
    b. Yellow
    c. Green
    d. Black

Questions 30 to 34 refer to the following scenario.

> You respond to a city street where a hot dog vendor's propane tank has exploded, causing more than 10 injuries. The truck is engulfed in flames. The scene is in absolute chaos, with people running in every direction screaming for help.

30. This disaster can be described as:

    a. Open, active
    b. Closed, active
    c. Open, contained
    d. Closed, contained

31. As you approach the disaster area, your first concern should be:

    a. Triaging and identifying the severely injured
    b. Calling for additional assistance
    c. Protecting yourself and bystanders
    d. Staying with the vehicle until firemen arrive

32. Based on the conditions described, which service is likely to assume command?

    a. Emergency medical services
    b. Fire
    c. Police
    d. Other agency

33. Your discover four injured patients: a 25-year-old man with 40% second- and third-degree burns, an unconscious 42-year-old man with a open chest wound, an 18-year-old woman in cardiac arrest, and a 58-year-old woman with a fracture of the radius. Rank these patients in order of priority treatment:

    1. 25-year-old man
    2. 42-year-old man
    3. 18-year-old woman
    4. 58-year-old woman

    a. 1, 3, 2, 4
    b. 2, 1, 4, 3
    c. 2, 3, 1, 4
    d. 1, 2, 3, 4

34. The 18-year-old described above would be considered a _______________ triage category.

    a. Red
    b. Yellow
    c. Green
    d. Black

TRUE OR FALSE

35. _____ A Level D suit provides for the highest level of respiratory protection when dealing with potential chemical contamination.

36. _____ Placards, which are affixed to the outside of the transport vehicle, identify the specific type of decontamination procedure to be followed if a patient becomes contaminated by the substance during shipping.

37. _____ Control zones are geographic areas at a hazardous materials incident that are based on safety and the degree of hazard.

38. _____ The principal patient management technique in the hot zone is patient decontamination.

39. _____ Once decontaminated, patients can be brought to the cold zone.

40. _____ The principal patient management technique in the warm zone is patient removal.

41. _____ Patients exposed to cyanide or organophosphates may require an immediate antidote.

Match the type of training in column A to the expected role that an individual would play at the scene of a hazardous materials incident in column B.

Column A	Column B
42. ____ First responder/awareness	a. Individuals who would attempt to stop the release of the hazardous substance
43. ____ Hazardous materials technician	b. Individual with the highest level of training who has specific or direct knowledge of substances being released
44. ____ Hazardous materials specialist	c. Individual who would respond to the hazardous materials incident and is trained to contain the release from a safe distance
45. ____ First responder/operations	d. Individual likely to witness or discover a hazardous incident and then initiate an emergency response

Across

1. Level of training appropriate for first responders likely to witness or discover a hazardous incident
3. Technique for quick primary triage
8. Disaster tag color for critical patients
9. Area in which contamination occurs
11. Area immediately surrounding the hot zone where decontamination occurs
14. Fully encapsulated, gas-tight body suit and SCBA are required in this classification of chemical protective clothing
18. The weight of a volume of gas compared with an equal volume of air
20. National Fire Protection Association
21. Diamond-shaped signs that identify the classification of hazardous materials
22. Rebuilding of the community, both physically and emotionally
23. Sector where ambulances receive assignments of patients and hospital destination
25. Rapid gathering of onlookers, rescuers, and members of the press at the scene of a disaster
28. Boiling liquid-expanding vapor explosion
29. Entering the body by swallowing
30. Sector where physical and psychological care is rendered to rescuers
31. Area where staging of supplies and the command center is established

Down

2. Information is gathered in the rapid trauma survey during _____ triage
4. Sector where major field medical aid is administered
5. Sector designed to deliver the equipment resources to the disaster scene
6. Drill in which participants try to solve problems in a roundtable forum
7. A 24 hour/day, 7 days/week resource for hazardous material information
10. To sort casualties in order of priority
12. Substances capable of creating harm
13. Entering the body through the skin
15. Ambulance staging and dispatch are this person's primary function
16. The EMT's primary duty at a hazardous material incident
17. Sudden, catastrophic event producing great damage, loss, and distress
19. Sector responsible for overall activities related to moving patients and resources
24. Disaster tag color generally used for ambulatory patients
26. Environmental Protection Agency
27. The person ultimately in charge of the disaster response
28. Disaster tag color for patients in cardiac arrest

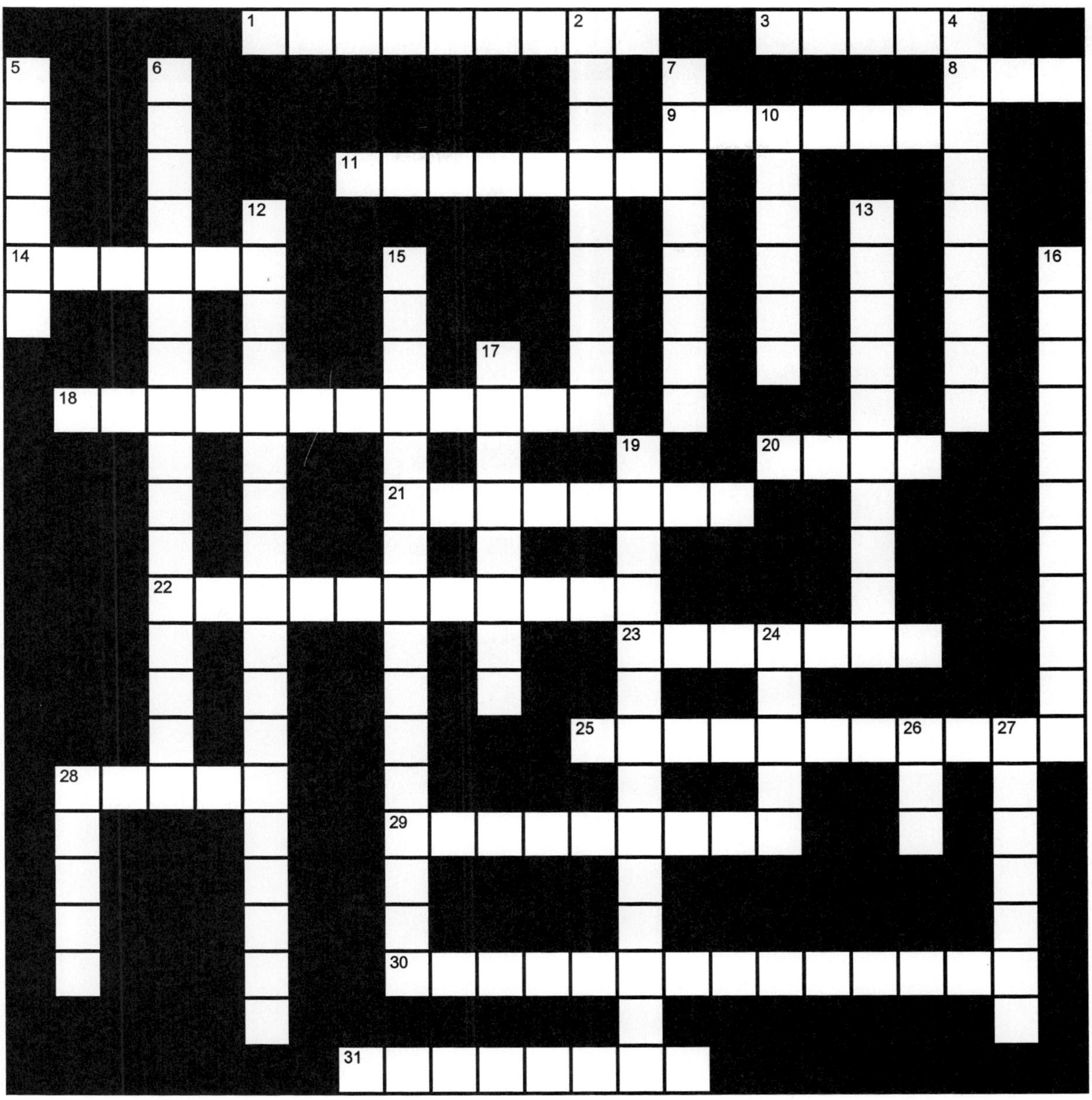
1
2
3
4
5
6
7
8
9
10
11
12
13
14
15
16
17
18
19
20
21
22
23
24
25
26
27
28
29
30
31

ANSWER KEY

1. c
2. a
3. b
4. a
5. b
6. a
7. a
8. b
9. c
10. a
11. c
12. d
13. b
14. a
15. c
16. c
17. b
18. a
19. d
20. a
21. d
22. b
23. b
24. b
25. a
26. a
27. c
28. a
29. d
30. a
31. c
32. b
33. b
34. d
35. False
36. False
37. True
38. False
39. True
40. False
41. True
42. d
43. a
44. b
45. c

1. AWARENESS
3. START
8. RED
9. HOTZONE
11. WARMZONE
14. LEVELA
18. VAPORDENSITY
20. NFPA
21. PLACARDS
22. RESTORATION
23. STAGING
25. CONVERGENCE
28. BLEVE
29. INGESTION
30. REHABILITATION
31. COLDZONE

2. SECONDARY
4. TREATMENT
5. SUPPLY
6. TABLETOPEXERCISE
7. CHEMTREC
10. TRIAGE
12. HAZARDOUSMATERIALS
13. ABSORPTION
15. TRANSPORTOFFICER
16. MEDICALCARE
17. DISASTER
19. TRANSPORTATION
24. GREEN
26. EPA
27. COMMAND
28. BLACK

Chapter 34 Advanced Airway Management

1. Which of the following does not constitute a function of the upper airway?

   a. Filtration
   b. Gas exchange
   c. Warming or cooling
   d. Humidification

2. The first bifurcation of the trachea produces the:

   a. Two bronchi, equal in length and angulation
   b. Four lobar bronchi
   c. Two bronchi, of which the left is longer and has a more acute angle than the right
   d. Two bronchi, of which the right is longer and has a more acute angle than the left

3. The primary respiratory center is located in the:

   a. Medulla
   b. Cerebral cortex
   c. Apneustic center
   d. Pneumotaxic center

4. When using a curved laryngoscope blade, it is inserted in the:

   a. Glottic opening
   b. Vallecula
   c. Carina
   d. Uvula

5. The best position to have the head in for visualization of the vocal cords is:

   a. Over the end of the bed
   b. In a neutral position
   c. Flexed forward, chin to chest
   d. In the sniffing position

6. When advancing an endotracheal tube, it should be inserted:

   a. Until 1 inch is extended from the mouth
   b. Just until the cuff is past the vocal cords
   c. Until it can't be advanced any further
   d. Until 3 inches is extended from the mouth

7. After intubation the chest is being auscultated and breath sounds are not being heard on one side. You should:

   a. Move the tube slightly ahead and reevaluate
   b. Rotate the tube and reevaluate
   c. Remove the tube completely
   d. Move the tube back slightly and reevaluate

8. In most cases, when the tube is inserted too far it will lodge in the:

   a. Left bronchus
   b. Right bronchus
   c. Terminal bronchioles
   d. Carina

9. The respiratory structure that is palpable just above the sternum is the:

   a. Bronchus
   b. Trachea
   c. Carina
   d. Bronchiole

10. The structure that covers the trachea during swallowing to prevent aspiration is called the:

    a. Pharynx
    b. Epiglottis
    c. Thyroid cartilage
    d. Cricoid cartilage

11. The narrowest part of the upper airway in infants is the:

    a. Epiglottis
    b. Trachea
    c. Thyroid cartilage
    d. Cricoid cartilage

12. To open the airway of the infant, place the head in the:

    a. Hyperflexed position
    b. Extended position
    c. Flexed position
    d. Sniffing or neutral position

13. Hyperextension of an infant's airway may result in:

    a. Kinking and obstruction
    b. Rupture of the larynx
    c. Dislocation of the cervical spine
    d. Increased intracranial pressure

14. Infants breathe dominantly through the:

    a. Nose
    b. Mouth
    c. Pursed lips
    d. Cheeks

15. On inserting an oropharyngeal airway, the patient begins to gag and choke. You next action should be to:

    a. Remove the airway
    b. Use a smaller airway
    c. Lubricate the airway
    d. Tape the airway in place

16. To ensure proper sizing, an oropharyngeal airway is measured from the center of the patient's mouth to the:

    a. Angle of the jaw
    b. Top of the ear
    c. Cheekbone
    d. Trachea

17. The endotracheal tubes for infants and small children are:

    a. More rigid
    b. More curved
    c. Different in shape
    d. Uncuffed

18. When suctioning the upper airway, you should activate the negative pressure:

    a. When the tip is in the oropharynx
    b. Before insertion
    c. At the entrance of the mouth
    d. Halfway between the teeth and the pharynx

19. Lifting at the angles of the jaw while maintaining the head in the neutral inline position best describes the:

    a. Modified jaw thrust
    b. Head tilt/chin lift
    c. Chin pull
    d. Tongue jaw lift

20. Tilting the head back with one hand while lifting the lower margin of the jaw with the index and middle fingers of the other hand best describes the:

    a. Jaw thrust without head tilt
    b. Chin pull maneuver
    c. Head tilt/neck lift
    d. Head tilt/chin lift

21. The best way to remove liquid secretions from the airway in the field is by:

    a. Finger sweeps
    b. Back blows
    c. Portable suction
    d. Abdominal thrusts

22. When using a jaw thrust in conjunction with a bag-valve-mask device, you can lift the mandible at the:

    a. Center of the chin
    b. Angle of the jaw
    c. Lower portion of the cheekbones
    d. Soft tissues of the mandible

23. To ensure proper sizing, a nasopharyngeal airway is measured from the nares to the:

    a. Angle of the jaw
    b. Top of the ear
    c. Cheekbone
    d. Larynx

24. The most common cause of airway obstruction in an unconscious patient is:

    a. A foreign body
    b. Anaphylaxis
    c. The tongue
    d. Aspiration

25. Airway obstruction caused by anaphylaxis is best managed by:

    a. Positive-pressure ventilation
    b. Back blows
    c. Chest thrusts
    d. Abdominal thrusts

26. The primary use of a nasogastric tube in the field is:

    a. When you are unable to ventilate an infant or child because of gastric distention
    b. To clear the stomach of poisons in the field
    c. To remove liquids from the stomach to avoid aspiration
    d. To prevent gastric insufflation while ventilating an infant

27. The Sellick maneuver is performed by applying pressure to the:

    a. Trachea
    b. Cricoid ring
    c. Thyroid cartilage
    d. Epiglottis

28. The primary indication for orotracheal intubation in the field is:

    a. Protecting the airway of an unconscious patient
    b. Routine prevention of aspiration of gastric contents
    c. Suctioning the lower airway of a patient
    d. Securing the airway and ventilating a patient in respiratory arrest

29. Equipment used during orotracheal intubation to maintain the shape of the tube to aid placement of the tip into the glottic opening is called the:

    a. Pilot balloon
    b. Stylet
    c. Tube cylinder
    d. Murphy's eye

30. When using a straight laryngoscope blade, it is inserted beneath the:

    a. Glottic opening
    b. Vallecula
    c. Carina
    d. Epiglottis

31. A device used to confirm placement of an endotracheal tube by monitoring gases is called a:

    a. Pulse oximeter
    b. Blood gas monitor
    c. End-tidal carbon dioxide detector
    d. Ventilator monitor

32. Which of the following endotracheal tubes is appropriate for an average adult male?

    a. 5.0 mm
    b. 6.0 mm
    c. 8.0 mm
    d. 11.0 mm

33. Which of the following methods is used to size an endotracheal tube for a child?

    a. (16 plus the age of the child) divided by 4
    b. (12 plus the age of the child) divided by 2
    c. (10 plus the age of the child) divided by 3
    d. (8 plus the age of the child) divided by 4

34. A simple alternate method for sizing an endotracheal tube for an infant or child is:

    a. Comparing the tube diameter to the little finger
    b. Comparing the tube diameter to the mouth opening
    c. Comparing the length of the tube to the child's index finger
    d. Comparing the length of the tube to the child's middle finger

35. You should continually monitor heart rate during an intubation of an infant or child with a pulse because stimulation of the airway may cause:

    a. Bleeding and shock
    b. Ventricular fibrillation
    c. Slowing of the heart rate
    d. Rapid heart rhythms

36. All the following are primary locations for confirming placement of an orotracheal tube in an infant or child *except*:

    a. Over the apex of the left and right lung
    b. At the lateral base
    c. Below the left nipple
    d. Over the epigastrium

37. Failure to note an esophageal intubation is most likely to result in:

    a. Aspiration
    b. Hypoxia and death
    c. Esophageal rupture
    d. Tear of the stomach

38. When securing the endotracheal tube, an oropharyngeal airway can be used to prevent:

    a. Occluding the tube if the patient bites down
    b. Displacement of the tongue into the airway
    c. Dislodging of the endotracheal tube
    d. Injury to the teeth and gums

39. Voice is created by movement of air past the ___________.

40. Diffusion of gases occurs between the lungs and the circulatory system in the lungs in the structure called ___________.

41. The effectiveness of ventilations is largely measured by ___________ levels in the blood.

42. The passage extending from the back of the nasal cavity down to the esophagus and larynx is called the ___________.

43. The _________ is used during positive-pressure ventilation to minimize gastric inflation and regurgitation.

Match the term in column A with the correct description in column B.

Column A	**Column B**
44. ____ Vocal cords	a. Space between the vocal cords
45. ____ Thyroid cartilage	b. Structure that creates voice
46. ____ Glottis	c. Commonly referred to as the Adam's apple
47. ____ Cricothyroid membrane	d. Disease when the alveoli are damaged or destroyed
48. ____ Trachea	e. Structure that permits movement of food to the stomach
49. ____ Esophagus	f. Lies between the cricoid and thyroid cartilage
50. ____ Emphysema	g. Structure that permits movement of air from the larynx to the bronchi

Identify which of the following are primary or secondary means of endotracheal tube placement confirmation.

51. ____ Direct visualization of the tube passing between the vocal cords
52. ____ Carbon dioxide detectors
53. ____ Pulse oximetry
54. ____ Auscultation of breath sounds
55. ____ Observation of the rise and fall of the chest with ventilations
56. ____ Esophageal detector devices

a. Primary confirmation
b. Secondary confirmation

List four complications of orotracheal intubation other than esophageal intubation.

57. ______________________________

58. ______________________________

59. ______________________________

60. ______________________________

TRUE OR FALSE

61. _____ The cuff of an endotracheal tube should generally be filled with approximately 50 mL of air.

62. _____ The small hole at the end of the endotracheal tube is called Murphy's eye.

63. _____ The small hole at the end of the endotracheal tube is used to assist in securing the tube in place.

64. _____ In general, commercial devices are more likely to secure the tube in place compared with tape.

65. ______ A towel may be used to elevate the back of the head in infants and small children to facilitate placing the patient in the sniffing position.

66. ______ The pulse oximeter may give an inaccurate reading for a patient who has carbon monoxide poisoning.

67. ______ The Esophageal Tracheal Combitube is indicated for apneic patients who are unresponsive and do not have a cough or gag reflex.

68. ______ For children younger than 8 years of age, an uncuffed endotracheal tube should be used.

69. The Esophageal Tracheal Combitube:

    a. Is designed to be used in patients older than 5 years
    b. After insertion normally is in the trachea
    c. Requires the use of the laryngoscope for proper placement
    d. Is inserted blindly

70. The most significant complication when using the Esophageal Tracheal Combitube is:

    a. Ventilation through the incorrect port after inserting the device
    b. Rupture of the trachea
    c. Trauma to the vocal cords
    d. Chipping or breaking of teeth

71. When inflating the cuffs on the Esophageal Tracheal Combitube you should use:

    a. Approximately 10 to 20 mL in each cuff
    b. Approximately 10 to 20 mL in the proximal cuff and 80 to 100 mL in the distal cuff
    c. Approximately 80 to 100 mL in the proximal cuff and 10 to 20 mL in the distal cuff
    d. Approximately 80 to 100 mL in each cuff

72. When properly inserted the laryngeal mask airway:

    a. Is inserted with the tip of the mask resting on the upper end of the esophagus and surrounding the opening of the larynx
    b. Is inserted in the trachea just below the vocal cords
    c. Is inserted in the esophagus
    d. Maintains an air-tight seal over the mouth and nose

73. The laryngeal mask airway is indicated:

    a. For patients with a respiratory rate more than 36 breaths/min
    b. For patients who do not have intravenous access and you need to rapidly administer medications through the airway
    c. For patients who are apneic and unresponsive and do not have a cough or gag reflex
    d. After the patient is successfully orally intubated with an endotracheal tube

74. Which laryngoscope blade will be more helpful when intubating a 6-month-old child?

    a. Size 1 curved blade
    b. Size 1 straight blade
    c. Size 3 curved blade
    d. Size 3 straight blade

75. You have successfully intubated a 3-year-old child. You should:

    a. Secure the tube in place with a commercial holder; the tube does not have a cuff
    b. Inflate the cuff with approximately 10 mL of air
    c. Immediately insert an oral airway because the tongue is proportionally smaller in the child than in the adult
    d. Ventilate with the appropriate sized bag-valve-mask device at least six times before auscultating breath sounds

Questions 76 to 80 refer to the following scenario.

> You arrive at the scene of a 4-year-old boy who was pulled out of a swimming pool before your arrival. The patient was found at the bottom of the pool and was removed by his babysitter. The child had been swimming and did not dive into the pool. The police on scene are performing cardiopulmonary resuscitation.

76. The best way to provide ventilation to this patient is:

    a. Open the airway with a head tilt/chin lift and ventilate with a pocket mask without supplemental oxygen
    b. Open the airway with a head tilt/chin lift and ventilate with a bag-valve-mask device connected to 15 L/min oxygen
    c. Open the airway with a jaw thrust and ventilate with a pocket mask without supplemental oxygen
    d. Open the airway with a jaw thrust and ventilate with a bag-valve-mask device connected to 15 L/min oxygen

77. The best way to determine that positive-pressure ventilation is achieving your goal of good ventilation is to:

    a. Observe for a change in skin color from blue to pink
    b. Connect this patient to a pulse oximeter
    c. Watch for adequate chest rise
    d. Perform a finger sweep

78. Despite repeated attempts at positioning your patient you continue to have difficulty adequately ventilating him. You decide to orally intubate the patient and select a:

    a. Size 4.0 endotracheal tube
    b. Size 5.0 endotracheal tube
    c. Size 6.0 endotracheal tube
    d. Size 7.0 endotracheal tube

79. This tube:

    a. Should not have a cuff and a stylet must not be used
    b. Should not have a cuff and a stylet can be used
    c. Should have a cuff and a stylet must not be used
    d. Should have a cuff and a stylet can be used

80. After passing the endotracheal tube you use an esophageal detector device to confirm tube placement. You:

    a. Connect the device to the tube, compress the bulb, and if the bulb expands, the tube is probably correctly placed in the trachea
    b. Connect the device to the tube, compress the bulb, and if the bulb expands, the tube is probably incorrectly placed in the esophagus
    c. Compress the bulb, then connect the device to the tube, and if the bulb expands, the tube is probably correctly placed in the trachea
    d. Compress the bulb, then connect the device to the tube, and if the bulb expands, the tube is probably incorrectly placed in the esophagus

Questions 81 to 84 refer to the following scenario.

> You respond to a call for a 53-year-old man who is unconscious. You find your patient on the ball field. His friends tell you that he suddenly clutched his chest and then became unconscious. You immediately evaluate the patient and determine that he is in cardiac arrest. You have your automated external defibrillator and basic/advanced airway equipment at the patient's side.

81. You should:

    a. Immediately begin positive-pressure ventilations
    b. Immediately intubate the patient
    c. Immediately connect the device to the patient
    d. Immediately begin transport

82. At the appropriate time during the call you begin to intubate the patient. You should use a:

    a. No. 2 straight blade with a 6.0 mm size endotracheal tube
    b. No. 2 curved blade with a 8.0 mm size endotracheal tube
    c. No. 4 straight blade with a 6.0 mm size endotracheal tube
    d. No. 4 curved blade with a 8.0 mm size endotracheal tube

83. Once you have intubated the patient, you auscultate breath sounds and note absent breath sounds on the left side of the chest, no sounds over the epigastrium, and good breath sounds on the right side of the chest. The endotracheal tube is:

    a. In the esophagus
    b. In the left main stem bronchus
    c. In the right main stem bronchus
    d. Properly placed

84. Based on the location of the endotracheal tube you should:

    a. Remove the tube and reintubate the patient
    b. Secure the tube where it is and ventilate the patient
    c. Push the tube a little further into the patient
    d. Pull the tube a little bit out of the patient

Across

5. Cricoid pressure used during intubation
7. Air passes through these to create voice
9. Organ that may fall back on the pharynx, causing an obstruction
10. Nostrils
11. Windpipe
14. Singular term for alveoli
16. Curved laryngoscope blade
17. Flap of cartilage that covers the larynx during swallowing
20. Structure that is inferior to the vocal cords and forms a circle just above the trachea
22. Device used to monitor oxygen saturation by measuring light transfer through capillary beds and hemoglobin
24. Combination of the vocal cords and glottis
26. Voicebox
27. Secondary means to confirm endotracheal tube placement using a _____ _____ carbon dioxide detector
28. Divider of the two compartments of the nose
29. Device used to visualize the vocal cords to insert an endotracheal tube

Down

1. Throat
2. Smallest subdivisions of bronchi, with a muscular, rather than cartilaginous, quality
3. Muscular tube from the stomach to the mouth
4. Space between vocal cords
5. Malleable metal tube inserted into the endotracheal tube to help guide the tube during intubation
6. The most effective form of airway management
8. The waste product of the body's metabolism
12. Final subdivision of the tracheobronchial tree
13. Confirmation of placement of a laryngeal mask airway is performed by observing chest rise and _____ over the epigastrium and both lungs
15. A nasogastric tube is measured from the nose around the ear to this level
16. Straight laryngoscope blade
18. First portion of the airway
19. A Miller or _____ blade is usually more helpful in intubation of an infant
21. Tubes that extend from the mouth and nose down into the lungs
23. The endotracheal tube used on children younger than 8 years of age should be _____
25. Item used to confirm placement of the endotracheal tube, using a suction mechanism, attached to the endotracheal tube

1 2 3 4 5 6 7 8 9 10 11 12 13 14 15 16 17 18 19 20 21 22 23 24 25 26 27 28 29

ANSWER KEY

1. b
2. c
3. a
4. b
5. d
6. b
7. d
8. b
9. b
10. b
11. d
12. d
13. a
14. a
15. a
16. a
17. d
18. a
19. a
20. d
21. c
22. b
23. a
24. c
25. a
26. a
27. b
28. d
29. b
30. d
31. c
32. c
33. a
34. a
35. c
36. c
37. b
38. a
39. Vocal cords
40. Alveoli
41. Carbon dioxide
42. Pharynx
43. Sellick maneuver
44. b
45. c
46. a
47. f
48. g
49. e
50. d
51. a
52. b
53. b
54. a
55. a
56. b

57. to 60. Prolonged attempts
Soft tissue trauma
Right main stem bronchus intubation
Vomiting
Slowing of the heart rate and induction of arrhythmia
Dislodgement of the tube
Self-extubation

61. False
62. True
63. False
64. True
65. False
66. True
67. True
68. True
69. d
70. a
71. c
72. a
73. c
74. b
75. a
76. b
77. c
78. b
79. b
80. c
81. c
82. d
83. c
84. d

- 5 SELLICKMANEUVER
- 7 VOCALCORDS
- 9 TONGUE
- 10 NARES
- 11 TRACHEA
- 14 ALVEOLUS
- 16 MACINTOSH
- 17 EPIGLOTTIS
- 20 CRICOIDCARTILAGE
- 22 PULSEOXIMETER
- 24 GLOTTICOPENING
- 26 LARYNX
- 27 ENDTIDAL
- 28 NASALSEPTUM
- 29 LARYNGOSCOPE

- 1 PHARYNX
- 2 BRONCHIOLES
- 3 ESOPHAGUS
- 4 GLOTTIS
- 5 STYLET
- 6 ENDOTRACHEALINTUBATION
- 8 CARBONDIOXIDE
- 12 ALVEOLI
- 13 AUSCULTATION
- 15 XYPHOIDPROCESS
- 16 MILLE
- 18 NASALPASSAGE
- 19 STRAIGHT
- 21 AIRWAY
- 23 UNCUFFED
- 25 EDD

Chapter 35 Weapons of Mass Destruction and the EMT

1. Preparation for all disasters must:

   a. Begin at the local level in each community
   b. Be established by national laws and regulations
   c. Be developed by the national disaster medical service
   d. Acknowledge that the federal response teams will comprise the first responders

List the three primary roles of the EMT relating to a potential nuclear, biologic, or chemical (NBC) event.

2. ______________________________

3. ______________________________

4. ______________________________

5. All the following are features of an NBC terrorist incident that distinguish it from a hazardous materials incident *except:*

   a. It is a deliberate attack
   b. It is an accidental incident
   c. The exact hazard is purposely hidden
   d. The incident is designed to produce mass numbers of casualties

6. Which type of incident causes the most immediate havoc and destruction?

   a. Chemical agent
   b. Biologic agent
   c. Viral agent
   d. Bacterial agent

7. The index cases in an NBC event include:

   a. The most recent victim of the attack
   b. The youngest patients
   c. The patients who are exposed but do not show any effects of the exposure
   d. Victims with severe effects or among the early fatalities

8. Identify what a "red flag" for an intentional event may be. ______________________________

TRUE OR FALSE

9. _____ Biologic agents are not infectious.

10. _____ All biologic agents are contagious.

11. _____ Use of personal protective equipment is the same for potential biologic agents as it is for general patient care.

12. _____ The use of biologic agents in warfare is a recent occurrence, dating from the 1970s.

13. _____ Antibiotics provide effective treatment and prophylaxis for many of the bacterial illnesses if they are detected early.

14. _____ Aerosolized spread of a biologic agent is the most likely means of producing large numbers of victims.

15. _____ Anthrax is a viral agent.

16. _____ The most dangerous form of anthrax is inhalational anthrax.

17. _____ Inhalational anthrax can be spread person to person.

18. You are at the scene and encounter a patient who had contact with a suspicious white powder. The powder is visible on the table. You should:

    a. Immediately transport the person who was exposed to the hospital
    b. Remain in the room until the police arrive and can determine if the powder contains anthrax
    c. Leave the area and cover your mouth and nose with a mask and keep bystanders away until the police arrive
    d. Administer an atropine injector to the exposed patient

19. Smallpox is considered to be a biologic warfare agent that:

    a. Is readily available and may be used by terrorists
    b. Is currently not considered a major threat because the population has been vaccinated against smallpox
    c. Can be spread by coughing and sneezing from an infected patient
    d. Can be prevented if the EMT wears gloves when treating all patients

20. Viral hemorrhagic fevers include:

    a. The Marburg virus and the Ebola virus
    b. Rocky mountain spotted fever and shingles
    c. Tularemia and encephalitis
    d. Meningitis and pneumococcal pneumonia

21. Tularemia is usually acquired by:

    a. Contact with poisonous plants
    b. Contact with poisonous coral in the oceans
    c. Bites by deerflies or ticks
    d. Ingestion of contaminated food

22. While not most common, tularemia used as a weapon of mass destruction would most likely be spread by terrorists through what means?

    a. Vectors such as insect bites
    b. Aerosol
    c. Distribution of contaminated powder in the mail or in public places
    d. Contaminated stockpiles of antibiotics

23. Botulism results in a:

    a. Classic feet upward, ascending paralysis
    b. Generalized paralysis that affects the entire body simultaneously
    c. Classic head downward, descending paralysis
    d. Generalized weakness in the lower extremities that slowly progresses to paralysis

24. At room temperature nerve agents are:

    a. A volatile gas
    b. A crystalline powder
    c. A liquid
    d. A solid putty material similar to clay

25. The major threat from contact with the vapors from sarin gas is:

    a. Absorption through the skin
    b. Contamination of the eyes
    c. Ingestion through contaminated food
    d. Inhalation of the gas

Match the type of chemical agent in column A with the clinical presentation of the patient in column B.

Column A	Column B
26. _____ Nerve agents	a. Pulmonary edema and shortness of breath first noticed with exertion
27. _____ Cyanide agents	b. Small pupils, muscle twitching, and secretions associated with rapid loss of consciousness, convulsions, and respiratory arrest
28. _____ Sulfur mustard	c. Loss of consciousness, convulsions, and respiratory arrest, in some cases preceded by complaints of irritation of the nasal passages and eyes
29. _____ Pulmonary agents	d. Redness or erythema of the skin that then develops into progressively larger blisters

30. The *first step* in decontaminating a victim exposed to a nerve agent, whether in vapor or liquid form, is usually:

    a. Removing the patient's clothing
    b. Quickly irrigating the patient with the patient's clothing still on
    c. Quickly irrigating the patient while neutralizing the liquid with baking soda
    d. Quickly covering the patient with a sterile burn sheet

31. The first organs in the body that will show the effects of exposure to cyanide gas are:

    a. Heart and kidneys
    b. Lungs and heart
    c. Heart and brain
    d. Brain and lungs

32. Rapid onset of hyperpnea followed by seizures, loss of respirations, and death within 6 to 8 minutes is a classic example of exposure to:

    a. Nerve agents
    b. Cyanide gas
    c. Phosgene gas
    d. Chlorine gas

33. You are a rescuer equipped with full protective equipment and encounter patients in the hot zone. In the hot zone you should provide:

    a. Full patient decontamination
    b. A complete START triage
    c. Treatment with the Mark I kit for severe nerve agent poisoning
    d. A detailed physical assessment

TRUE OR FALSE

34. _____ Mark I kits contain autoinjectors containing atropine and pralidoxime.

35. _____ Mark I kits are used to treat acute exposure to sulfur mustard.

36. _____ A patient exposed to cyanide gas has rapid respiratory and circulatory collapse. You would expect that patient to exhibit signs of cyanosis.

37. _____ A good rule of thumb regarding exposure to cyanide gas is that if the victim can walk away from the vapor to fresh air, they may escape with no need for treatment.

38. _____ The clinical effects of mustard gas tend to be incapacitating rather than lethal.

39. _____ The clinical effects of mustard gas appear within 3 to 5 minutes after exposure.

40. _____ Phosgene liquid is toxic; the vapors it forms do not pose any threat.

41. The least common type of radioactive emissions is:

    a. Alpha particles
    b. Beta particles
    c. Gamma rays
    d. Neutrons

Match the unit of measurement in column A with the description in column B.

Column A	Column B
42. _____ Roentgen	a. A measurement of the amount of radiation absorbed by the body
43. _____ Rad	b. The measurement of a charge in the air caused by ionizing radiation
44. _____ Rem	c. Unit equal to the absorbed dose in rads multiplied by modifying factors, which allows for some comparison of the effects of different types of radiation

Match the type of radiation in column A with the description in column B.

Column A	Column B
45. _____ Alpha particle	a. High-energy electromagnetic radiation rays similar to x-rays but more energetic
46. _____ Beta particle	b. Uncharged particles found in the nucleus of an atom
47. _____ Gamma rays	c. Least penetrating form of radiation that can be stopped by a sheet of paper
48. _____ Neutrons	d. Travel no more than a few feet but can be stopped by the skin where they can cause burns similar to thermal burns

List the three major factors used by rescuers to limit exposure to radiation.

49. ______________________________

50. ______________________________

51. ______________________________

52. The irreversible cardiovascular effects of acute radiation syndrome are seen if the patient has been exposed to approximately:

a. 100 rem
b. 400 rem
c. 1000 rem
d. 3000 rem

TRUE OR FALSE

53. ____ Contamination is caused by radioactive particles that are physically present.

54. ____ Irradiation is caused by radioactive energy but is not physically present on the body.

55. ____ The contaminated victim can spread radioactive materials to others; the irradiated patient cannot.

56. ____ A dosimeter is a device that is worn by individuals that identifies the type of radiation and the rate of exposure.

57. ____ The dose of radiation absorbed at a distance of 10 feet is approximately one fourth the dose that would be absorbed at a distance of 5 feet.

58. ____ Gamma rays pass through a victim and pose no threat to a rescuer once the patient is away from the radiation source.

List the three purposes of decontamination for a victim who was contaminated with a radioactive material.

59. ______________________________

60. ______________________________

61. ______________________________

62. If available, the best material to use as a shield against radiation is an apron made of __________.

63. You are the first to respond and discover a possible nuclear incident. Your first priority is to establish a __________.

64. The organized system of dealing with a mass casualty incident that identifies the role of all responders is referred to as the __________.

Questions 65 to 69 refer to the following scenario.

> You respond to a call for multiple people injured at the local shopping mall. On arrival you notice that there are two people lying on the ground in front of the entrance to the mall. You and your partner put on full protective equipment. When you approach the scene you notice at least 10 people lying on the floor inside the mall.

65. Your first priorities include:

a. Entering the mall and performing a full assessment on each patient
b. Ensuring that a safe zone is established and calling for additional resources
c. Rapidly transporting the two patients outside the mall to the hospital and allowing for units that arrive later to manage the scene
d. Immediately injecting yourself and your partner with a Mark I kit

66. You begin to evaluate the two patients outside of the mall and determine that the patients have constricted pupils, muscle twitching, and secretions. Neither is responding to verbal or painful stimuli and one begins to seize. Based on this clinical presentation you suspect an exposure to:

a. Cyanide gas
b. Mustard gas
c. Sulfur mustard
d. A nerve agent

67. The first step in decontaminating the patient is to:

    a. Irrigate with water
    b. Irrigate the patient with water and 1:100 of chlorine
    c. Remove the patient's clothes
    d. No decontamination is needed because the patients are no longer directly exposed to the contaminant that is in the mall

68. You call medical control and present the symptoms of your two patients while the hazardous materials team starts to set up to enter the mall. You would expect that medical control would instruct you to:

    a. Administer high-concentration oxygen and transport your patients
    b. Administer a Mark I kit to each patient
    c. Administer an Epi-Pen to the patient that is seizing
    d. Immediately transport the patient who is not seizing; the other patient should be triaged as a "black" triage category

69. Approximately 45 minutes after you arrive at the scene the police inform you that they have received a call from someone claiming to have released sarin gas in the mall. While this has not been confirmed, you know that if this is indeed the agent that the major threat of aerosolized sarin is:

    a. Contamination of the mucous membranes in exposed patients
    b. Inhalation of the gas
    c. That the sarin can be absorbed through the skin and strict isolation precautions are required
    d. Ingestion through contaminated food

Across

1. Viral _____ fevers cause damage to small vessels resulting in bleeding
5. If suspicion of plague exists, _____ precautions need to be implemented in addition to standard precautions
9. Mnemonic used to remember the effects of nerve agents
10. Shielding is best accomplished using _____
11. Filter that should be used while caring for patient with viral hemorrhagic fever
14. Simple Triage and Rapid Treatment
15. Agents that act by disrupting normal transmission of impulses to muscles, organs, and glands, resulting in an excess of secretions and paralysis
17. Nuclear, biological, and chemical
18. Botulism causes _____ from the head down
19. Tularemia would most likely be spread by the _____ method
21. The reduction or removal of chemical agents from a person
23. Disease caused by *Bacillus anthracis*
26. Nerve agent that evaporates at room temperature
27. WMD
31. Spread of agents through food, water, insects, and animals
32. Pulmonary agents can damage the lungs, resulting in pulmonary _____
33. In viral hemorrhagic fevers, human to human contact occurs by _____ contact with blood, secretions, organs, and semen
34. Nerve agents enter the body by inhalation, ingestion, or _____ through the skin
36. Illnesses that spread from person to person
37. Agents that have an incubation period and involve viruses, fungi, or bacteria
38. Form of nerve agents at room temperature
39. The isolation of patients exposed to or attacked by a contagious disease until they are incapable of either developing or transmitting the disease

Down

2. The absorbed dose of radiation in RADS, multiplied by modifying factors
3. Rays that do not cause contamination to the victim and the victim is of no risk to others
4. Nerve agents, as opposed to cyanide, cause pupils to be _____
6. Amount of radiation absorbed by the body
7. Phosgene and chlorine are examples of _____ _____
8. No muscle tone
12. The first principle with nuclear and chemical agents is to eliminate continued _____
13. In addition to standard precautions, droplet and _____ precautions are indicated with smallpox
14. Factors used to limit exposure to radiation are time, distance, and _____
16. With viral hemorrhagic fevers, contact and _____ precautions must be initiated in addition to standard precautions
20. Thriving in a low- or no-oxygen environment
22. The victim exposed to gamma rays is said to have been _____
24. A highly contagious virus that was thought to be eradicated in 1980
25. Agents that invade the body and then multiply and cause illness are said to be _____
28. Smallest building block of an element
29. _____ contamination occurs when the presence of radioactive materials is limited to skin and clothing
30. _____ agents cause the most immediate havoc and destruction
35. Bacterial infection exhibited in one form by a cough with bloody sputum and in another form by enlarged lymph nodes

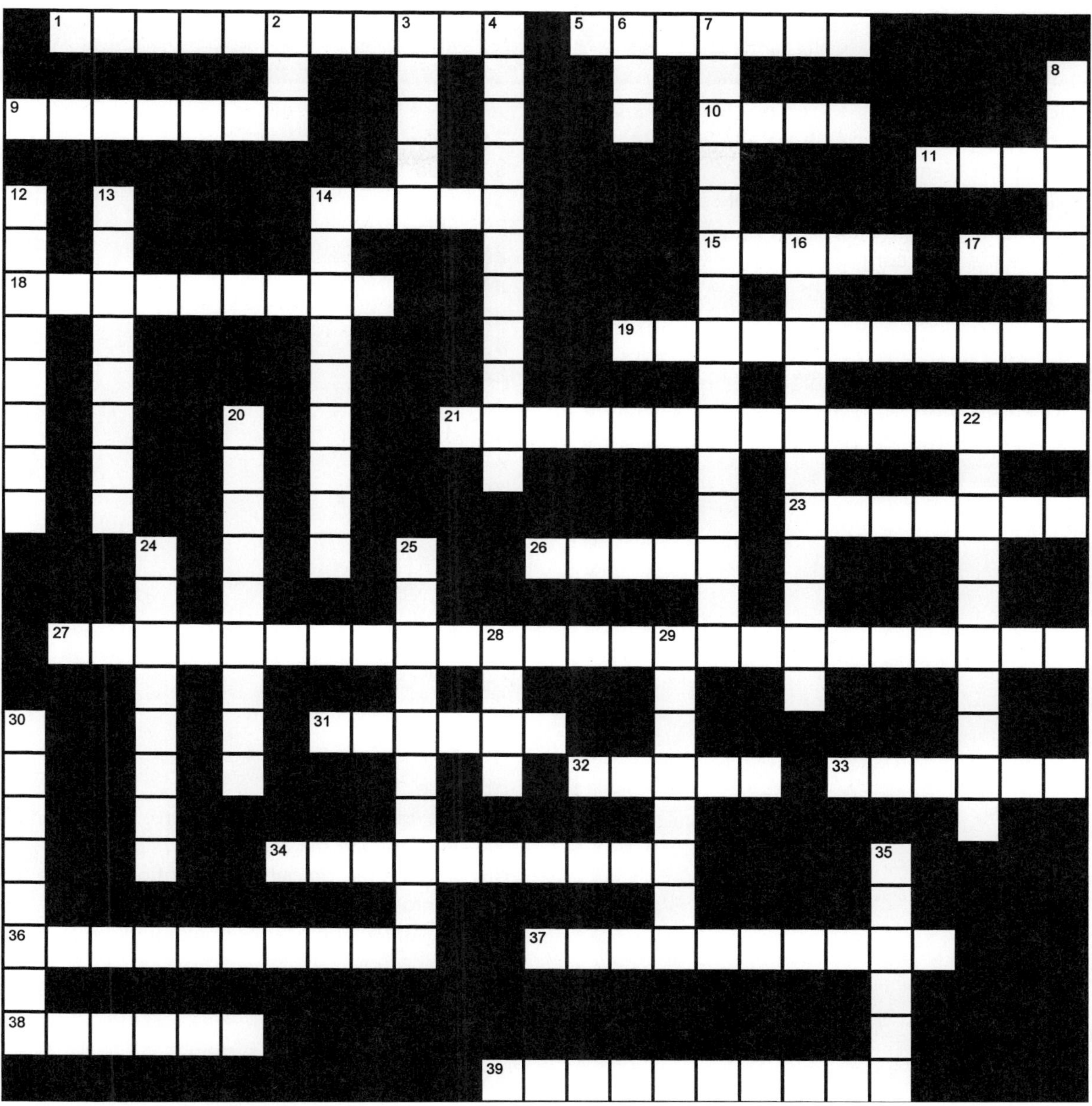

ANSWER KEY

1. a
2. Recognize a potential NBC event
3. Take actions to promote the safety of self, bystanders, and the victims
4. To provide medical care
5. b
6. a
7. d
8. Multiple casualties, all with the same complaints and who were previously well, and at a similar time of onset
9. False
10. False
11. False
12. False
13. True
14. True
15. False
16. True
17. False
18. c
19. c
20. a
21. c
22. b
23. c
24. c
25. d
26. b
27. c
28. d
29. a
30. a
31. c
32. b
33. c
34. True
35. False
36. False
37. True
38. True
39. False
40. False
41. d
42. b
43. a
44. c
45. c
46. d
47. a
48. b
49. Time
50. Distance
51. Shielding
52. d
53. True
54. True
55. True
56. False
57. True
58. True
59. Prevent or minimize transfer of contaminants to an internal site
60. Reduce the amount of radiation dosage from the contaminant
61. Prevent the spread of contamination to other persons and areas
62. Lead
63. Safety zone
64. Incident command system
65. b
66. d
67. c
68. b
69. b

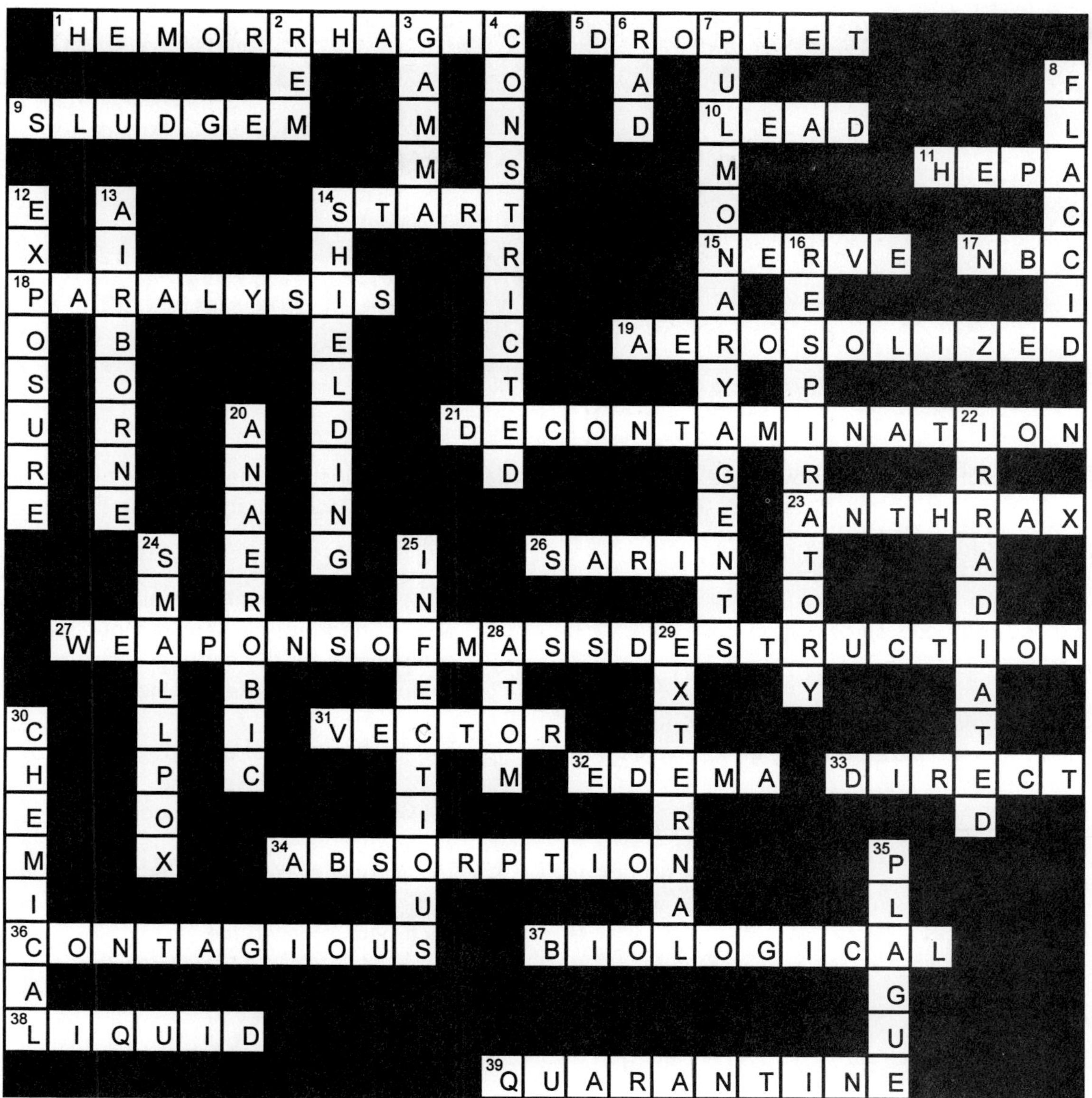
HEMORRHAGIC
DROPLET
SLUDGEM
LEAD
HEPA
START
NERVE
NBC
PARALYSIS
AEROSOLIZED
DECONTAMINATION
ANTHRAX
SARIN
WEAPONSOFMASSDESTRUCTION
VECTOR
EDEMA
DIRECT
ABSORPTION
CONTAGIOUS
BIOLOGICAL
LIQUID
QUARANTINE
REM
GAMMA
CONSTRICTED
RAD
PULMONARY AGENT
FLACCID
EXPOSURE
AIRBORNE
SHIELDING
RESPIRATORY
IRRADIATED
ANAEROBIC
SMALLPOX
INFECTIOUS
ATOM
EXTERNA
CHEMICAL
PLAGUE

Chapter 36 Geriatric Emergencies

1. The fraction of the population over age 65:

   a. Is remaining the same
   b. Is decreasing
   c. Is increasing
   d. Is decreasing because of a shorter life expectancy

Match the physiologic changes that occur with age in column A with the expected change in column B.

Column A	Column B
2. _____ Stroke volume	a. Declines with age b. Increases with age
3. _____ Vital capacity	
4. _____ Residual volume	
5. _____ Maximum pulse rate	
6. _____ Resistance of blood vessels	

TRUE OR FALSE

7. _____ The elderly have a decreased ability to regulate their thermoregulatory system and therefore are more prone to environmental changes.

8. _____ The elderly have had more diseases than the young and therefore are able to more easily compensate for severe illness.

9. _____ More than 90% of the deaths attributed to pneumonia and influenza occur in people older than 64 years.

10. _____ Drugs classified as beta-blockers or calcium channel blockers may increase the patient's heart rate.

11. _____ If you encounter an elderly patient who is hard of hearing you should shout because this will compensate for the hearing impairment and make comprehension easier for the patient.

12. The total amount of air that can be moved in and out with a given breath is called ___________.

13. The amount of blood ejected from the heart with each beat is called the ___________.

14. The amount of air that remains in the lungs at the end of an exhalation is called the ___________.

15. Hardening of the arteries is called ___________.

16. The decreased amount of bone density that occurs as a patient ages, particularly in women, is called ___________.

List three problems the elderly patient may have that make obtaining a history particularly difficult.

17. ____

18. ____

19. ____

List four conditions that the elderly patient may have that result in a diminished or confused mental state.

20. ____

21. ______________________________

22. ______________________________

23. ______________________________

24. You are treating a 75-year-old man (George Barns). The most appropriate way to refer to your patient is by calling him:

    a. Pops
    b. Grandpa
    c. George
    d. Mr. Barns

Questions 25 to 27 are based on the following scenario.

> You respond to the scene and encounter a 78-year-old woman who is sitting at her kitchen table. Her son called the ambulance because his mother "did not look right" and became very dizzy. On your examination you determine that the patient was dizzy and sweaty, but now only complains of being a little weak. There are no neurologic deficits evident. The vital signs are pulse 88 beats/min and regular, blood pressure 142/80 mm Hg, respiratory rate 14 breaths/min and normal, and the patient is alert.

25. Based on your evaluation you conclude that the patient:

    a. Has general malaise and is no apparent distress
    b. Is having an anaphylactic reaction and administer an Epi-Pen
    c. May be having a heart attack even though the patient does not complain of chest pain
    d. Is having a hypoglycemic episode and administer oral glucose

26. Based on your evaluation your treatment would include:

    a. Transport in the position of comfort; no other interventions are needed
    b. Administration of supplemental oxygen during transport
    c. Administration of oral glucose and request advanced life support intercept if available
    d. The patient is stable at this time and does not need further evaluation in the hospital

27. Your patient tells you that she does not want to go to the hospital. You should:

    a. Allow the patient to sign a refusal of medical aid form
    b. Attempt to convince the patient that hospital evaluation is needed; if she still refuses transportation, allow her to sign a refusal of medical aid form
    c. Attempt to convince the patient that hospital evaluation is needed; if she still refuses transportation, restrain and transport
    d. Attempt to convince the patient that hospital evaluation is needed; if she still refuses transportation, contact online medical direction in an attempt to have a physician convince the patient that hospital evaluation is needed

28. All the following are conditions that commonly present with a headache *except:*

    a. Stroke
    b. Subdural hematoma
    c. Acute myocardial infarction
    d. Cerebral aneurysm

29. The elderly are more prone to dehydration because:

    a. They tend to delay fluid intake and their kidney function decreases with age
    b. They tend to delay fluid intake and their kidney function increases with age
    c. They are more mobile and drink more often
    d. They are less mobile and drink more often

List three signs of dehydration that the EMT should evaluate when assessing a patient who is suspected of being dehydrated.

30. ______________________________

31. ______________________________

32. ______________________________

33. The highest rate of suicide is:

    a. For men in the 18 to 25 age range
    b. For women in the 18 to 25 age range
    c. For men older than 65 years
    d. For women older than 65 years

34. Your 82-year-old patient presents with visible bruises on her legs and back that appear to be in various stages of healing. You suspect:

    a. That this is a normal condition because of the aging process
    b. She may be the victim of elder abuse
    c. She has a bleeding disorder that requires hospital treatment
    d. Blood clots caused by arteriosclerosis

35. Factors that may lead to heat or cold emergencies in the elderly include all the following *except:*

    a. Increased basal metabolic rate
    b. Decreased ability to shiver
    c. Effects of drugs
    d. Less ability to regulate heat production and heat loss

Questions 36 and 37 refer to the following scenario.

You respond to the scene of a "man down" and encounter an 87-year-old man lying on the floor in his apartment. Your patient tells you that he fell 2 days ago and has been unable to summon help until now. Your evaluation reveals a patient with pain in the left upper leg/hip area; his left leg appears to be outwardly rotated and slightly shorter than his right leg. There are good pulses, motor, and sensation in all four extremities. The patient's vital signs are pulse 92 beats/min regular and strong, blood pressure 168/88 mm Hg, respiratory rate 16 breaths/min and regular, and the patient has full equal bilateral breath sounds. The patient's skin appears dry and "tents," and the patient has sunken eyes.

36. Based on the patient's clinical presentation you would initiate treatment that includes:

    a. A traction splint applied to the left leg for a possible fractured femur
    b. A long spine board and blankets to secure a possible hip fracture
    c. An air splint to the left leg to treat a possible femur fracture
    d. Application and inflation of the pneumatic anti-shock garment to treat a possible pelvic fracture

37. The dry skin turgor and sunken eyes are indications of:

    a. Possible dehydration
    b. A physiologic response to pain
    c. The beginning stages of hypothermia
    d. Normal status in the elderly

Across

1. Medications that promote urinary fluid loss
8. Blockage of a blood vessel by blood clots moving in the bloodstream
10. A disease similar to senile dementia that appears as early as 40 to 50 years of age
11. β-Blockers or calcium channel blockers are medications taken to treat hypertension and heart disease, which _____ the patient's heart rate
12. Elderly patients are more prone to dehydration because _____ _____ decreases with age
14. Air that remains in the lungs at the end of an exhalation
15. Cerebral aneurysms, stroke, and subdural hematomas may all present with the common complaint of _____
16. Decreased bone density occurring in the elderly, mostly women, as a result of degeneration
18. In the elderly, heart attacks frequently occur without _____ _____
19. Hardening of the arteries

Down

2. Progressive deterioration of mental status in the elderly
3. Problems encountered more by the elderly and children when exposed to environmental changes
4. A temporary blockage of blood to the brain marked by dizziness, blurry vision, and numbness on one side of the body
5. Amount of blood ejected from the heart with each beat
6. The E in SAMPLE history that stands for _____ establishing a relationship between a fall and its cause
7. The total amount of air that can be moved in and out with a given breath
9. Medication that interferes with blood clotting
13. Rapid pulse, decreased urination, and pale conjunctiva are all signs of _____
17. An abnormal respiratory sound characterized by fine crackles

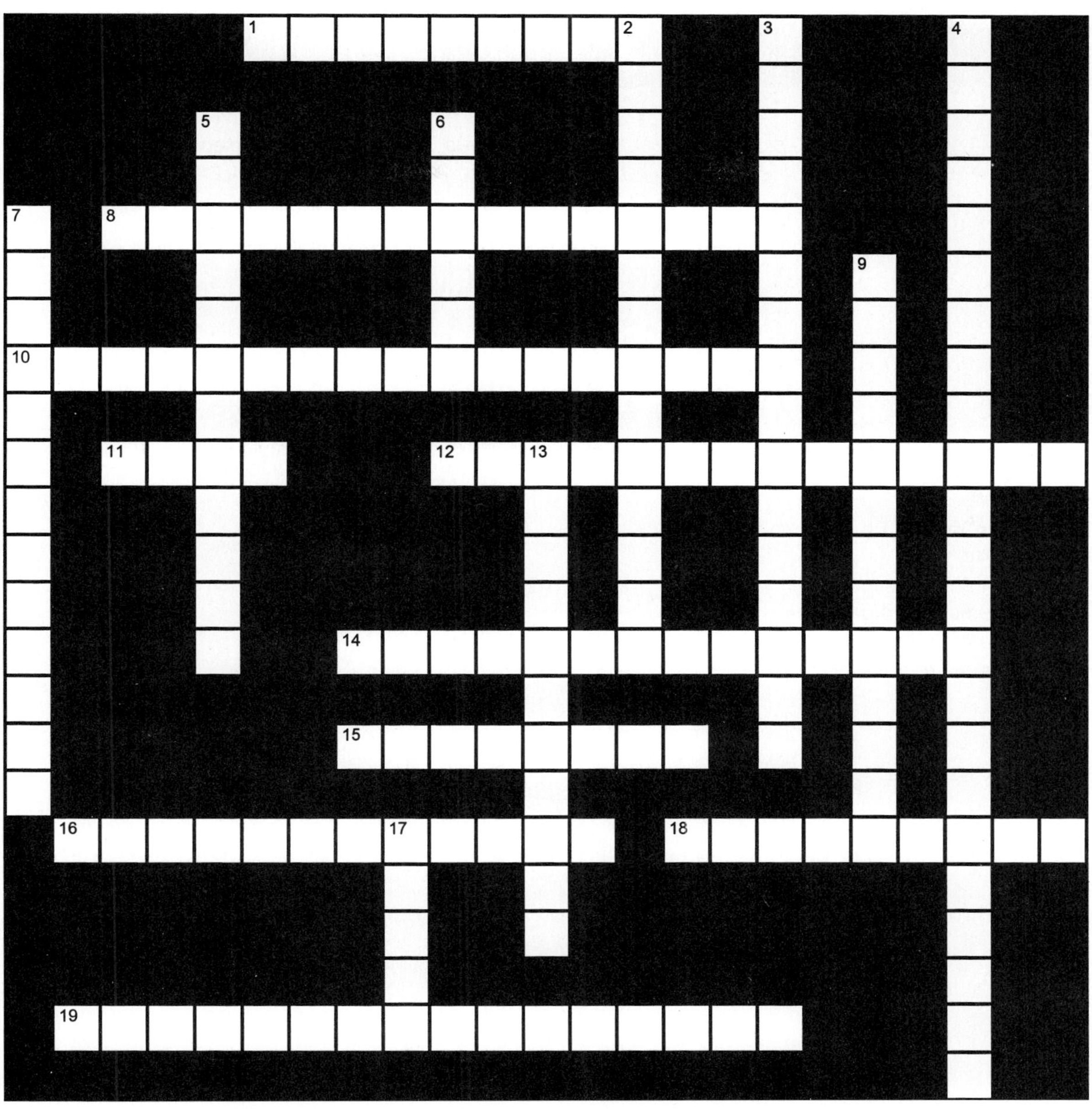
1
2
3
4
5
6
7
8
9
10
11
12
13
14
15
16
17
18
19

ANSWER KEY

1. c
2. a
3. a
4. b
5. a
6. b
7. True
8. False
9. True
10. False
11. False
12. Vital capacity
13. Stroke volume
14. Residual volume
15. Arteriosclerosis
16. Osteoporosis

17. to 19. Problems with sight
Problems with hearing
Problems in communication

20. to 23. Alzheimer's disease
Senile dementia
Organic brain syndrome
Stroke

24. d
25. c
26. b
27. d
28. c
29. a

30. to 32. Dry skin turgor
Dry oral mucosa
Sunken eyes

33. c
34. b
35. a
36. b
37. a

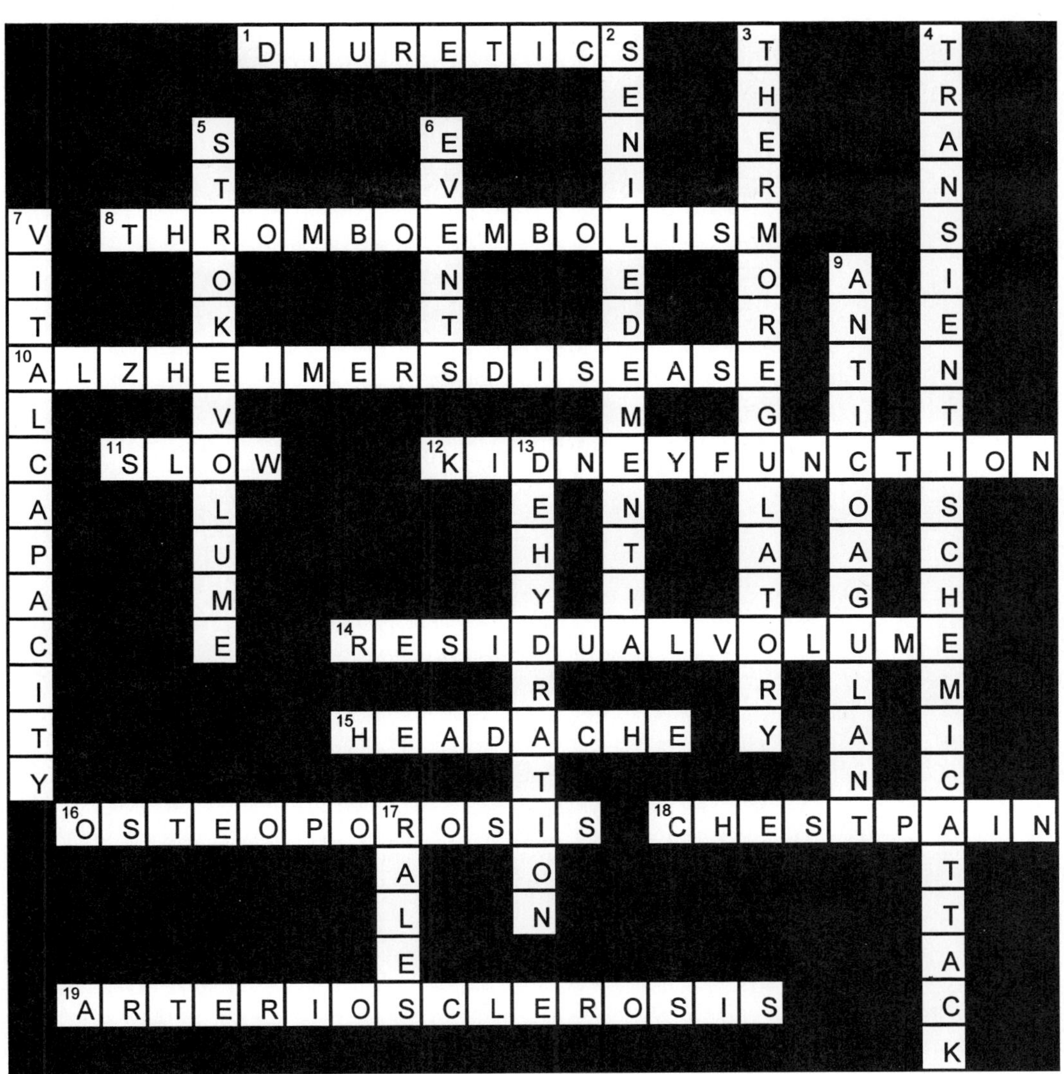
1 DIURETICS
2 SENILE DEMENTIA
3 THERMOREGULATORY
4 TRANSIENT ISCHEMIC ATTACK
5 STROKE VOLUME
6 EVENT
7 VITAL CAPACITY
8 THROMBOEMBOLISM
9 ANTICOAGULANT
10 ALZHEIMERS DISEASE
11 SLOW
12 KIDNEY FUNCTION
13 DEHYDRATION
14 RESIDUAL VOLUME
15 HEADACHE
16 OSTEOPOROSIS
17 RALE
18 CHEST PAIN
19 ARTERIOSCLEROSIS

Appendix A

Cardiopulmonary Resuscitation

All Skill Sheets from The National Registry of Emergency Medical Technicians.

1. Adult cardiopulmonary resuscitation (CPR) techniques are used on patients older than

    ___________ years of age.

2. Child CPR techniques are used on patients between

    ___________ and ___________ years of age.

3. Infant CPR techniques are used on patients younger

    than ___________ year of age.

4. The proper compression to ventilation ratio for

    adult CPR is ___________ compressions to

    ___________ ventilations.

5. The proper compression to ventilation ratio for

    child CPR is ___________ compressions to

    ___________ ventilations.

6. The proper compression to ventilation ratio for

    infant CPR is ___________ compressions to

    ___________ ventilations.

7. The proper rate for adult rescue breathing is

    1 breath every ___________ seconds.

8. The proper rate for child rescue breathing is

    1 breath every ___________ seconds.

9. The proper rate for infant rescue breathing is

    1 breath every ___________ seconds.

10. The best way to ensure adequate ventilations when treating all patients is to observe for adequate

    ___________ ___________.

TRUE OR FALSE

11. _____ When ventilating an adult patient using a bag-valve-mask connected to supplemental oxygen, a lower volume of air can be delivered compared with ventilating the adult patient with the same device without supplemental oxygen.

12. _____ Blind finger sweeps should never be used when treating a child victim of choking.

13. _____ Back blows are used to treat the adult victim who is choking.

14. _____ The automated external defibrillator (AED) should be put in the analyze mode while CPR compressions are being performed.

15. _____ The proper hand position for adult CPR is on the upper half of the victim's sternum.

16. _____ The AED can be used to determine if the adult patient has a pulse.

17. _____ AEDs designed for use in children deliver a lower energy level than that which is used in adult patients.

18. _____ The most common cause of cardiac arrest in children is cardiac arrhythmias.

19. _____ A patient in cardiac arrest has an implanted pacemaker that is visible in her upper right chest. You should not use the AED in this patient because of possible damage to the pacemaker.

20. _____ The sooner an AED is used for a victim in cardiac arrest the better the chance that the patient will be resuscitated.

Questions 21-25 refer to the following scenario.

> You respond to a church for a call of an unconscious female. On arrival, you and your partner bring the oxygen bag, airway kit, suction device, and AED into the church and find a 53-year-old woman lying on the floor. Bystanders state that the patient was sitting when she suddenly collapsed to the floor. There is no evidence of trauma and no past medical history can be obtained. You check for responsiveness and the patient does not respond.

21. Your next step should be to:

    a. connect the AED to the patient and analyze
    b. begin CPR compressions
    c. give 2 breaths
    d. open the airway and check for breathing

22. After checking for a pulse, you determine that there is no pulse and the patient is in cardiac arrest. Your next step is to:

    a. perform 1 minute of CPR and transport the patient
    b. perform 1 minute of CPR and then connect the AED to the patient
    c. immediately connect the AED to the patient
    d. deliver 5 abdominal thrusts

23. While treating your patient you determine that a pulse has returned. You determine that the pulse rate is 76 beats/min, regular and strong. The patient is breathing at a rate of 6 breaths/min. You should:

    a. attach a nasal cannula and transport the patient
    b. use a nonrebreather mask at 15 L/min and transport the patient
    c. perform positive-pressure ventilation using a bag-valve-mask without supplemental oxygen
    d. perform positive-pressure ventilation using a bag-valve-mask with supplemental oxygen

24. You are transporting this patient to the hospital and have a 15-minute estimated time of arrival to the hospital. While monitoring your patient, you can no longer feel a pulse. You should:

    a. begin CPR and continue transporting the patient to the hospital
    b. immediately press the analyze button on the AED while en route to the hospital
    c. begin CPR, instruct the driver to pull the ambulance to the side of the road, and then press the analyze button on the AED
    d. begin CPR for 1 minute and then reevaluate the patient

25. While performing CPR on this patient, a good way to determine the effectiveness of CPR compressions is:

    a. by observing for chest rise
    b. by having your partner feel for a carotid pulse while chest compressions are being delivered
    c. by having your partner feel for a radial pulse while chest compressions are being delivered
    d. by observing the patient for an improvement in skin color

Questions 26-28 refer to the following scenario.

> You and your partner are on standby at a local youth football game. A 12-year-old boy is struck in the chest by the football and immediately collapses to the field. You immediately respond to the patient's side and determine that the patient is unresponsive, not breathing, and he does not have a pulse or signs of circulation.

26. Your next step in caring for this patient is to:

    a. immediately connect the AED to the patient and analyze
    b. begin CPR and rapid transport
    c. perform 1 minute of CPR and reassess the patient
    d. place the patient in the ambulance, begin CPR, and connect the AED to the patient during transport

27. After your initial treatment the patient regains a pulse and begins to breathe adequately at 14 breaths per minute. You should:

    a. attach a nasal cannula and transport the patient
    b. use a non-rebreather mask at 15 L/min and transport the patient
    c. perform positive-pressure ventilation using a bag-valve-mask with supplemental oxygen
    d. place the patient in the recovery position; no supplemental oxygen is needed

28. If CPR compressions are required to care for this patient, they should be performed:
    a. at a rate of 80 per minute and a depth of 1 to 1½ inches
    b. at a rate of 100 per minute and a depth of 1 to 1½ inches
    c. at a rate of 80 per minute and a depth of 1½ to 2 inches
    d. at a rate of 100 per minute and a depth of 1½ to 2 inches

29. The two-hand encircling the chest technique is used when:

    a. providing one-person CPR to an infant
    b. providing two-person CPR to an infant
    c. providing one-person CPR to a child
    d. providing two-person CPR to a child

30. The location that should be used to check for the presence of a pulse in an infant is the:

    a. radial artery
    b. brachial artery
    c. femoral artery
    d. carotid artery

31. The location that should be used to check for the presence of a pulse in a child is the:

    a. radial artery
    b. brachial artery
    c. femoral artery
    d. carotid artery

32. When using the AED to analyze the patient a message is displayed to "check breathing and pulse." This means that:

    a. a pulse is present and no CPR is needed
    b. a shock needs to be delivered
    c. you must reevaluate the patient for signs of circulation and the presence of a pulse and perform CPR if needed
    d. the AED will not work for this patient and immediate transport is indicated

33. You respond to the scene of an unconscious patient that was found in a hotel room by the maid. The patient does not have any signs of circulation. You would not attempt to resuscitate this patient if:

    a. the body feels cool to the touch
    b. there is no reaction in the pupils when you examine them with a penlight
    c. rigor mortis and extreme dependent lividity are present
    d. the estimated down time is more than 8 to 10 minutes

34. You respond to a call at a private residence and find a 54-year-old woman in cardiac arrest. The patient's husband informs you that she was released from the hospital 2 days ago after undergoing coronary artery bypass surgery 8 days ago. A fresh scar is evident on the patient's sternum from the recent surgery. You would:

    a. initiate CPR as indicated in the normal fashion
    b. rapidly transport the patient without CPR because of the recent surgery
    c. pronounce the patient dead; resuscitation is futile due to the surgery
    d. perform CPR over the right anterior chest, avoiding any pressure on the sternum

35. You respond to a call in the park for an approximately 38-year-old man who was found by the police slumped on the bench. Bystanders tell you that the patient is a homeless man who frequents the park. Your evaluation of the patient identifies that his skin is very cold; the current air temperature is 34° F. You should:

    a. evaluate the patient in the same manner as you would for any other patient
    b. evaluate the patient for the presence of a pulse for an extended period of time, approximately 30 seconds
    c. immediately transport the patient; CPR is not indicated if the patient is hypothermic
    d. begin to rewarm the patient by placing heat packs on the patient's wrists

ANSWER KEY

1. 8
2. 1 and 8
3. 1
4. 15 to 2
5. 5 to 1
6. 5 to 1
7. 5
8. 3
9. 3
10. Chest rise
11. True
12. True
13. False
14. False
15. False
16. False
17. True
18. False
19. False
20. True
21. d
22. c
23. d
24. c
25. b
26. a
27. b
28. d
29. b
30. b
31. d
32. c
33. c
34. a
35. b

Appendix B

National Registry Skill Sheets

Patient Assessment/Management—Trauma

Start Time: ____________________

Stop Time: ____________________ **Date:** ________________________

Candidate's Name: ____

Evaluator's Name: ____

		Points Possible	Points Awarded
Takes, or verbalizes, body substance isolation precautions		1	
SCENE SIZE-UP			
Determines the scene is safe		1	
Determines the mechanism of injury		1	
Determines the number of patients		1	
Requests additional help if necessary		1	
Considers stabilization of spine		1	
INITIAL ASSESSMENT			
Verbalizes general impression of the patient		1	
Determines responsiveness/level of consciousness		1	
Determines chief complaint/apparent life threats		1	
Assesses airway and breathing	Assessment Initiates appropriate oxygen therapy Ensures adequate ventilation Injury management	1 1 1 1	
Assesses circulation	Assesses/controls major bleeding Assesses pulse Assesses skin (color, temperature and condition)	1 1 1	
Identifies priority patients/makes transport decision		1	
FOCUSED HISTORY AND PHYSICAL EXAM/RAPID TRAUMA ASSESSMENT			
Selects appropriate assessment **(focused or rapid assessment)**		1	
Obtains, or directs assistant to obtain, baseline vital signs		1	
Obtains SAMPLE history		1	
DETAILED PHYSICAL EXAMINATION			
Assesses the head	Inspects and palpates the scalp and ears Assesses the eyes Assesses the facial areas including oral and nasal areas	1 1 1	
Assesses the neck	Inspects and palpates the neck Assesses for JVD Assesses for tracheal deviation	1 1 1	
Assesses the chest	Inspects Palpates Auscultates	1 1	
Assesses the abdomen/pelvis	Assesses the abdomen Assesses the pelvis Verbalizes assessment of genitalia/perineum as needed	1 1 1	
Assesses the extremities	1 point for each extremity includes inspection, palpation, and assessment of motor, sensory and circulatory function	4	
Assesses the posterior	Assesses thorax Assesses lumbar	1 1	
Manages secondary injuries and wounds appropriately **1 point for appropriate management of secondary injury/wound**		1	
Verbalizes reassessment of the vital signs		1	
	TOTAL	**40**	

Critical Criteria

___ Did not take, or verbalize, body substance isolation precautions
___ Did not determine scene safety
___ Did not assess for spinal protection
___ Did not provide for spinal protection when indicated
___ Did not provide high concentration of oxygen
___ Did not find, or manage, problems associated with airway, breathing, hemorrhage or shock (hypoperfusion)
___ Did not differentiate patient's need for transportation versus continued assessment at the scene
___ Did other detailed physical examination before assessing airway, breathing and circulation
___ Did not transport patient within 10 minute time limit

Patient Assessment/Management—Medical

Start Time: ____________________

Stop Time: ____________________ **Date:** ____________________

Candidate's Name: ____

Evaluator's Name: ____

		Points Possible	Points Awarded
Takes, or verbalizes, body substance isolation precautions		1	
SCENE SIZE-UP			
Determines the scene is safe		1	
Determines the mechanism of injury/nature of illness		1	
Determines the number of patients		1	
Requests additional help if necessary		1	
Considers stabilization of spine		1	
INITIAL ASSESSMENT			
Verbalizes general impression of patient		1	
Determines responsiveness/level of consciousness		1	
Determines chief complaint/apparent life threats		1	
Assesses airway and breathing	Assessment Initiates appropriate oxygen therapy Ensures adequate ventilation	1 1 1	
Assesses circulation	Assesses/controls major bleeding Assesses pulse Assesses skin (color, temperature and condition)	1 1 1	
Identifies priority patients/makes transport decision		1	
FOCUSED HISTORY AND PHYSICAL EXAM/RAPID ASSESSMENT			
Signs and Symptoms *(Assess history of present illness)*		1	

Respiratory	Cardiac	Altered Mental Status	Allergic Reaction	Poisoning/ Overdose	Environmental Emergency	Obstetrics	Behavioral
• Onset? • Provokes? • Quality? • Radiates? • Severity? • Time? • Interventions?	• Onset? • Provokes? • Quality? • Radiates? • Severity? • Time? • Interventions?	• Description of the episode • Onset? • Duration? • Associated symptoms? • Evidence of trauma? • Interventions? • Seizures? • Fever?	• History of allergies? • What were you exposed to? • How were you exposed? • Effects? • Progression? • Interventions?	• Substance? • When did you ingest/become exposed? • How much did you ingest? • Over what time period? • Interventions? • Estimated weight?	• Source? • Environment? • Duration? • Loss of consciousness? • Effects—general or local?	• Are you pregnant? • How long have you been pregnant? • Pain or contractions? • Bleeding or discharge? • Do you feel the need to push? • Last menstrual period?	• How do you feel? • Determine suicidal tendencies • Is the patient a threat to self or others? • Is there a medical problem? • Interventions?

	Points Possible	Points Awarded
Allergies	1	
Medications	1	
Past medical history	1	
Last oral intake	1	
Events leading to present illness (rule out trauma)	1	
Performs focused physical examination	1	
Vitals (obtains baseline vital signs)	1	
Interventions *(obtains medical direction or verbalizes standing order for medication interventions and verbalizes proper additional intervention/treatment)*	1	
Transport (re-evaluates transport decision) Verbalizes the consideration for completing a detailed physical examination	1	
ONGOING ASSESSMENT (verbalized)		
Repeats initial assessment	1	
Repeats vital signs	1	
Repeats focused assessment regarding patient complaint or injuries	1	
TOTAL	**30**	

Critical Criteria

___ Did not take, or verbalize, body substance isolation precautions when necessary
___ Did not determine scene safety
___ Did not obtain medical direction or verbalize standing orders for interventions
___ Did not provide high concentration of oxygen
___ Did not find or manage problems associated with airway, breathing, hemorrhage or shock (hypoperfusion)
___ Did not differentiate patient's need for transportation versus continued assessment at the scene
___ Did detailed or focused history/physical examination before assessing the airway, breathing and circulation
___ Did not ask questions about the present illness
___ Administered a dangerous or inappropriate intervention

Cardiac Arrest Management/AED

Start Time: ____________________

Stop Time: ____________________ **Date:** ____________________

Candidate's Name: ______________________________

Evaluator's Name: ______________________________

	Points Possible	Points Awarded
ASSESSMENT		
Takes, or verbalizes, body substance isolation precautions	1	
Briefly questions rescuer about events	1	
Directs rescuer to stop CPR	1	
Verifies absence of spontaneous pulse (**skill station examiner states "no pulse"**)	1	
Directs resumption of CPR	1	
Turns on defibrillator power	1	
Attaches automated defibrillator to patient	1	
Directs rescuer to stop CPR and ensures all individuals are clear of the patient	1	
Initiates analysis of rhythm	1	
Delivers shock (up to three successive shocks)	1	
Verifies absence of spontaneous pulse (**skill station examiner states "no pulse"**)	1	
TRANSITION		
Directs resumption of CPR	1	
Gathers additional information about arrest event	1	
Confirms effectiveness of CPR (ventilation and compressions)	1	
INTEGRATION		
Verbalizes or directs insertion of a simple airway adjunct (oral/nasal airway)	1	
Ventilates, or directs ventilation of, the patient	1	
Ensures high concentration of oxygen is delivered to the patient	1	
Ensures CPR continues without unnecessary/prolonged interruption	1	
Reevaluates patient/CPR in approximately one minute	1	
Repeats defibrillator sequence	1	
TRANSPORTATION		
Verbalizes transportation of patient	1	
TOTAL	**21**	

Critical Criteria

___ Did not take, or verbalize, body substance isolation precautions
___ Did not evaluate the need for immediate use of the AED
___ Did not direct initiation/resumption of ventilation/compressions at appropriate times
___ Did not ensure all individuals were clear of patient before delivering each shock
___ Did not operate the AED properly (inability to deliver shock)
___ Prevented the defibrillator from delivering indicated stacked shocks

Bag-Valve-Mask
Apneic Patient

Start Time: ________________

Stop Time: ________________ **Date:** ________________

Candidate's Name: ______________________________

Evaluator's Name: ______________________________

	Points Possible	Points Awarded
Takes, or verbalizes, body substance isolation precautions	1	
Voices opening the airway	1	
Voices inserting an airway adjunct	1	
Selects appropriate sized mask	1	
Creates a proper mask-to-face seal	1	
Ventilates patient at no less than 800 ml volume ***(The examiner must witness for at least 30 seconds)***	1	
Connects reservoir and oxygen	1	
Adjusts liter flow to 15 liters/minute or greater	1	
The examiner indicates the arrival of a second EMT. The second EMT is instructed to ventilate the patient while the candidate controls the mask and the airway.		
Voices re-opening the airway	1	
Creates a proper mask-to-face seal	1	
Instructs assistant to resume ventilation at proper volume per breath ***(The examiner must witness for at least 30 seconds)***	1	
Total	**11**	

Critical Criteria

___ Did not take, or verbalize, body substance isolation precautions
___ Did not immediately ventilate the patient
___ Interrupted ventilations for more than 20 seconds
___ Did not provide high concentration of oxygen
___ Did not provide or direct assistant to provide proper volume/breath *(more than [2] ventilations per minute are below 800 ml)*
___ Did not allow adequate exhalation

Spinal Immobilization
Seated Patient

Start Time: ________________

Stop Time: ________________ **Date:** ________________

Candidate's Name: ________________________________

Evaluator's Name: ________________________________

	Points Possible	Points Awarded
Takes, or verbalizes, body substance isolation precautions	**1**	
Directs assistant to place/maintain head in neutral in-line position	**1**	
Directs assistant to maintain manual immobilization of the head	**1**	
Reassesses motor, sensory and circulatory function in each extremity	**1**	
Applies appropriately sized extrication collar	**1**	
Positions the immobilization device behind the patient	**1**	
Secures the device to the patient's torso	**1**	
Evaluates torso fixation and adjusts as necessary	**1**	
Evaluates and pads behind the patient's head as necessary	**1**	
Secures the patient's head to the device	**1**	
Verbalizes moving the patient to a long board	**1**	
Reassesses motor, sensory and distal circulation in extremities	**1**	
TOTAL	**12**	

Critical Criteria

___ Did not immediately direct, or take, manual immobilization of the head
___ Released, or ordered release of, manual immobilization before it was maintained mechanically
___ Patient manipulated, or moved excessively, causing potential spinal compromise
___ Device moved excessively up, down, left, or right on patient's torso
___ Head immobilization allows for excessive movement
___ Torso fixation inhibits chest rise, resulting in respiratory compromise
___ Upon completion of immobilization, head is not in the neutral position
___ Did not assess motor, sensory, and circulatory function in each extremity after voicing immobilization to the long board
___ Immobilized head to the board before securing the torso

Spinal Immobilization
Supine Patient

Start Time: ________________

Stop Time: ________________ **Date:** ________________

Candidate's Name: ______________________________

Evaluator's Name: ______________________________

	Points Possible	Points Awarded
Takes, or verbalizes, body substance isolation precautions	**1**	
Directs assistant to place/maintain head in neutral in-line position	**1**	
Directs assistant to maintain manual immobilization of the head	**1**	
Assesses motor, sensory and circulatory function in each extremity	**1**	
Applies appropriately sized extrication collar	**1**	
Positions the immobilization device appropriately	**1**	
Directs movement of the patient onto the device without compromising the integrity of the spine	**1**	
Applies padding to voids between the torso and the boards as necessary	**1**	
Immobilizes the patient's torso to the device	**1**	
Evaluates the pads behind the patient's head as necessary	**1**	
Immobilizes the patient's head to the device	**1**	
Secures the patient's legs to the device	**1**	
Secures the patient's arms to the device	**1**	
Reassesses motor, sensory and circulatory function in each extremity	**1**	
TOTAL	**14**	

Critical Criteria

___ Did not immediately direct, or take, manual immobilization of the head
___ Released, or ordered release of, manual immobilization before it was maintained mechanically
___ Patient manipulated, or moved excessively, causing potential spinal compromise
___ Device moves excessively up, down, left, or right on the patient's torso
___ Head immobilization allows for excessive movement
___ Upon completion of immobilization, head is not in the neutral position
___ Did not reassess motor, sensory and circulatory function in each extremity after immobilization to the device
___ Immobilized head to the board before securing torso

Immobilization Skills
Long Bone Injury

Start Time: ________________

Stop Time: ________________ **Date:** ________________

Candidate's Name: ________________________________

Evaluator's Name: ________________________________

	Points Possible	Points Awarded
Takes, or verbalizes, body substance isolation precautions	1	
Directs application of manual stabilization of the injury	1	
Assesses motor, sensory and circulatory function in the injured extremity	1	
Note: The examiner acknowledges "motor, sensory and circulatory function are present and normal"		
Measures the splint	1	
Applies the splint	1	
Immobilizes the joint above the injury site	1	
Immobilizes the joint below the injury site	1	
Secures the entire injured extremity	1	
Immobilizes hand/foot in the position of function	1	
Reassesses motor, sensory and circulatory function in the injured extremity	1	
Note: The examiner acknowledges "motor, sensory and circulatory function are present and normal"		
Total	**10**	

Critical Criteria

___ Grossly moves the injured extremity

___ Did not immobilize the joint above and the joint below the injury site

___ Did not reassess motor, sensory and circulatory function in the injured extremity before and after splinting

Immobilization Skills
Joint Injury

Start Time: ________________

Stop Time: ________________ **Date:** ________________

Candidate's Name: ________________________________

Evaluator's Name: ________________________________

	Points Possible	Points Awarded
Takes, or verbalizes, body substance isolation precautions	**1**	
Directs application of manual stabilization of the shoulder injury	**1**	
Assesses motor, sensory and circulatory function in the injured extremity	**1**	
NOTE: The examiner acknowledges "motor, sensory and circulatory function are present and normal"		
Selects the proper splinting material	**1**	
Immobilizes the site of the injury	**1**	
Immobilizes the bone above the injured joint	**1**	
Immobilizes the bone below the injured joint	**1**	
Reassesses motor, sensory and circulatory function in the injured extremity	**1**	
NOTE: The examiner acknowledges "motor, sensory and circulatory function are present and normal"		
TOTAL	**8**	

Critical Criteria

___ Did not support the joint so that the joint did not bear distal weight
___ Did not immobilize the bone above and below the injured site
___ Did not reassess motor, sensory and circulatory function in the injured extremity before and after splinting

Immobilization Skills
Traction Splinting

Start Time: ____________

Stop Time: ____________ **Date:** ____________

Candidate's Name: ____________________________

Evaluator's Name: ____________________________

	Points Possible	Points Awarded
Takes, or verbalizes, body substance isolation precautions	1	
Directs application of manual stabilization of the injured leg	1	
Directs the application of manual traction	1	
Assesses motor, sensory and circulatory function in the injured extremity	1	
NOTE: The examiner acknowledges "motor, sensory and circulatory function are present and normal"		
Prepares/adjusts splint to the proper length	1	
Positions the splint next to the injured leg	1	
Applies the proximal securing device (e.g., ischial strap)	1	
Applies the distal securing device (e.g., ankle hitch)	1	
Applies mechanical traction	1	
Positions/secures the support straps	1	
Reevaluates the proximal/distal securing devices	1	
Reassesses motor, sensory and circulatory function in the injured extremity	1	
NOTE: The examiner acknowledges "motor, sensory and circulatory function are present and normal"		
NOTE: The examiner must ask candidate how he/she would prepare the patient for transportation.		
Verbalizes securing the torso to the long board to immobilize the hip	1	
Verbalizes securing the splint to the long board to prevent movement of the splint	1	
TOTAL	**14**	

Critical Criteria

___ Loss of traction at any point after it was applied
___ Did not reassess motor, sensory and circulatory function in the injured extremity before and after splinting
___ The foot was excessively rotated or extended after splint was applied
___ Did not secure the ischial strap before taking traction
___ Final immobilization failed to support the femur or prevent rotation of the injured leg
___ Secured the leg to the splint before applying mechanical traction

NOTE: If the Sager splint or Kendrick Traction Device is used without elevating the patient's leg, application of manual traction is not necessary. The candidate should be awarded 1 point as if manual traction were applied.

NOTE: If the leg is elevated at all, manual traction must be applied before elevating the leg. The ankle hitch may be applied before elevating the leg and used to provide manual traction.

Bleeding Control/Shock Management

Start Time: ______________

Stop Time: ______________ **Date:** ______________

Candidate's Name: ______________________________

Evaluator's Name: ______________________________

	Points Possible	Points Awarded
Takes, or verbalizes, body substance isolation precautions	**1**	
Applies direct pressure to the wound	**1**	
Elevates the extremity	**1**	
NOTE: The examiner must now inform the candidate that the wound continues to bleed.		
Applies an additional dressing to the wound	**1**	
NOTE: The examiner must now inform the candidate that the wound still continues to bleed. The second dressing does not control the bleeding.		
Locates and applies pressure to appropriate arterial pressure point	**1**	
NOTE: The examiner must now inform the candidate that the bleeding is controlled.		
Bandages the wound	**1**	
NOTE: The examiner must now inform the candidate that the patient is showing signs and symptoms indicative of hypoperfusion.		
Properly positions the patient	**1**	
Applies high concentration oxygen	**1**	
Initiates steps to prevent heat loss from the patient	**1**	
Indicates the need for immediate transportation	**1**	
TOTAL	**10**	

Critical Criteria

___ Did not take, or verbalize, body substance isolation precautions
___ Did not apply high concentration of oxygen
___ Applied a tourniquet before attempting other methods of bleeding control
___ Did not control hemorrhage in a timely manner
___ Did not indicate a need for immediate transportation

Airway, Oxygen, and Ventilation Skills
Upper Airway Adjuncts and Suction

Start Time: ________________

Stop Time: ________________ **Date:** ________________

Candidate's Name: ________________________________

Evaluator's Name: ________________________________

Oropharyngeal Airway	Points Possible	Points Awarded
Takes, or verbalizes, body substance isolation precautions	**1**	
Selects appropriately sized airway	**1**	
Measures airway	**1**	
Inserts airway without pushing the tongue posteriorly	**1**	
NOTE: The examiner must advise the candidate that the patient is gagging and becoming conscious.		
Removes the oropharyngeal airway	**1**	
Suction		
NOTE: The examiner must advise the candidate to suction the patient's airway.		
Turns on/prepares suction device	**1**	
Ensures presence of mechanical suction	**1**	
Inserts the suction tip without suction	**1**	
Applies suction to the oropharynx/nasopharynx	**1**	
Nasopharyngeal Airway		
NOTE: The examiner must advise the candidate to insert a nasopharyngeal airway.		
Selects appropriately sized airway	**1**	
Measures airway	**1**	
Verbalizes lubrication of the nasal airway	**1**	
Fully inserts the airway with the bevel facing toward the septum	**1**	
TOTAL	**13**	

Critical Criteria

___ Did not take, or verbalize, body substance isolation precautions
___ Did not obtain a patent airway with the oropharyngeal airway
___ Did not obtain a patent airway with the nasopharyngeal airway
___ Did not demonstrate an acceptable suction technique
___ Inserted any adjunct in a manner dangerous to the patient

Mouth to Mask with Supplemental Oxygen

Start Time: ________________

Stop Time: ________________ **Date:** ________________

Candidate's Name: ____________________________________

Evaluator's Name: ____________________________________

	Points Possible	Points Awarded
Takes, or verbalizes, body substance isolation precautions	**1**	
Connects one-way valve to mask	**1**	
Opens patient's airway or confirms patient's airway is open (manually or with adjunct)	**1**	
Establishes and maintains a proper mask-to-face seal	**1**	
Ventilates the patient at the proper volume and rate *(800–1200 ml per breath/10–20 breaths per minute)*	**1**	
Connects the mask to high concentration of oxygen	**1**	
Adjusts flow rate to 15 liters/minute	**1**	
Continues ventilation at proper volume and rate *(800–1200 ml per breath/10–20 breaths per minute)*	**1**	
NOTE: The examiner must witness ventilations for at least 30 seconds.		
TOTAL	**8**	

Critical Criteria

___ Did not take, or verbalize, body substance isolation precautions
___ Did not adjust liter flow to 15 liters per minute
___ Did not provide proper volume per breath
(***more than 2 ventilations per minute are below 800 ml***)
___ Did not ventilate the patient at a rate of 10-20 breaths per minute
___ Did not allow for complete exhalation

Oxygen Administration

Start Time: ________________

Stop Time: ________________ **Date:** ________________________

Candidate's Name: ______________________________________

Evaluator's Name: ______________________________________

	Points Possible	Points Awarded
Takes, or verbalizes, body substance isolation precautions	**1**	
Assembles the regulator to the tank	**1**	
Opens the tank	**1**	
Checks for leaks	**1**	
Checks tank pressure	**1**	
Attaches non-rebreather mask to oxygen	**1**	
Prefills reservoir	**1**	
Adjusts liter flow to 12 liters per minute or greater	**1**	
Applies and adjusts mask to the patient's face	**1**	
Note: **The examiner must advise the candidate that the patient is not tolerating the non-rebreather mask. The medical director has ordered you to apply a nasal cannula to the patient.**		
Attaches nasal cannula to oxygen	**1**	
Adjusts liter flow to six (6) liters per minute or less	**1**	
Applies nasal cannula to the patient	**1**	
Note: **The examiner must advise the candidate to discontinue oxygen therapy.**		
Removes the nasal cannula from the patient	**1**	
Shuts off the regulator	**1**	
Relieves the pressure within the regulator	**1**	
Total	**15**	

Critical Criteria

___ Did not take, or verbalize, body substance isolation precautions
___ Did not assemble the tank and regulator without leaks
___ Did not prefill the reservoir bag
___ Did not adjust the device to the correct liter flow for the non-rebreather mask *(12 liters per minute or greater)*
___ Did not adjust the device to the correct liter flow for the nasal cannula *(6 liters per minute or less)*

Ventilatory Management Endotracheal Intubation

Start Time: ______________________

Stop Time: ______________________

Candidate's Name: ______________________ **Date:** ______________________

Evaluator's Name: ______________________

*NOTE: If a candidate elects to initially ventilate the patient with a BVM attached to a reservoir and oxygen, full credit must be awarded for steps denoted by "**" if the first ventilation is delivered within the initial 30 seconds*		Points Possible	Points Awarded
Takes or verbalizes, body substance isolation precautions		1	
Opens the airway manually		1	
Elevates the patient's tongue and inserts a simple airway adjunct (oropharyngeal/nasopharyngeal airway)		1	
NOTE: The examiner must now inform the candidate "no gag reflect is present and the patient accepts the adjunct."			
**Ventilates the patient immediately using a BVM device unattached to oxygen		1	
**Hyperventilates the patient with room air		1	
NOTE: The examiner now informs the candidate that ventilation is being performed without difficulty.			
Attaches the oxygen reservoir to the BVM		1	
Attaches the BVM to high-flow oxygen (15 liters per minute)		1	
Ventilates the patient at the proper volume and rate (800-1200 ml/breath and 10-20 breaths/minute)		1	
NOTE: After 30 seconds, the examiner must auscultate the patient's chest and inform the candidate that breath sounds are present and equal bilaterally and medical control has ordered endotracheal intubation. The examiner must now take over ventilation of the patient.			
Directs assistant to hyper-oxygenate the patient		1	
Identifies/selects the proper equipment for endotracheal intubation		1	
Checks equipment	Checks for cuff leaks	1	
	Checks laryngoscope operation and bulb tightness	1	
NOTE: The examiner must remove the OPA and move out of the way when the candidate is prepared to intubate.			
Positions the patient's head properly		1	
Inserts the laryngoscope blade into the patient's mouth while displacing the patient's tongue laterally		1	
Elevates the patient's mandible with the laryngoscope		1	
Introduces the endotracheal tube and advances the tube to the proper depth		1	
Inflates the cuff to the proper pressure		1	
Disconnects the syringe from the cuff inlet port		1	
Directs assistant to ventilate the patient		1	
Confirms proper placement of the endotracheal tube by auscultation bilaterally and over the epigastrium		1	
NOTE: The examiner must ask, "If you had proper placement, what would you expect to hear?"			
Secures the endotracheal tube (may be verbalized)		1	
	TOTAL	21	

Critical Criteria

___ Did not take or verbalize body substance isolation precautions when necessary
___ Did not initiate ventilations within 30 seconds after applying gloves or interrupts ventilations for greater than 30 seconds at any time
___ Did not voice or provide high oxygen concentrations (15 liters/min or greater)
___ Did not ventilate the patient at a rate of at least 10 breaths per minute
___ Did not provide adequate volume per breath (maximum of 2 errors per minute permissible)
___ Did not hyper-oxygenate the patient prior to intubation
___ Did not successfully intubate the patient within 3 attempts
___ Used the patient's teeth as a fulcrum
___ Did not ensure proper tube placement by auscultation bilaterally over each lung **and** over the epigastrium
___ The stylette (if used) extended beyond the end of the endotracheal tube
___ Inserted any adjunct in a manner that was dangerous to the patient
___ Did not disconnect the syringe from the inlet port after inflating the cuff

Ventilatory Management
Dual-Lumen Airway Device Insertion Following an Unsuccessful Endotracheal Intubation Attempt

Start Time: ____________________

Stop Time: ____________________ **Date:** ____________________

Candidate's Name: ____

Evaluator's Name: ____

		Points Possible	Points Awarded
Continues body substance isolation precautions		1	
Confirms the patient is being properly ventilated with high percentage oxygen		1	
Directs the assistant to hyper-oxygenate the patient		1	
Checks/prepares the airway device		1	
Lubricates the distal tip of the device (may be verbalized)		1	
Note: The examiner should remove the OPA and move out of the way when the candidate is prepared to insert the device.			
Positions the head properly		1	
Performs a tongue-jaw lift		1	
☐ **USES COMBITUBE**	☐ **USES THE PTL**		
Inserts device in the mid-line and to the depth so that the printed ring is at the level of the teeth	Inserts the device in the mid-line until the bite block flange is at the level of the teeth	1	
Inflates the pharyngeal cuff with the proper volume and removes the syringe	Secures the strap	1	
Inflates the distal cuff with the proper volume and removes the syringe	Blows into tube No.1 to adequately inflate both cuffs	1	
Attaches/directs attachment of BVM to the first (esophageal placement) lumen and ventilates		1	
Confirms placement and ventilation through the correct lumen by observing chest rise, auscultation over the epigastrium and bilaterally over each lung		1	
Note: The examiner states: "You do not see rise and fall of the chest and hear sounds only over the epigastrium."			
Attaches/directs attachment of BVM to the second (esophageal placement) lumen and ventilates		1	
Confirms placement and ventilation through the correct lumen by observing chest rise, auscultation over the epigastrium and bilaterally over each lung		1	
Note: The examiner states, "You see rise and fall of the chest; there are no sounds over the epigastrium and breath sounds are equal over each lung."			
Secures device or confirms that the device remains properly secured		1	
	Total	15	

Critical Criteria

___ Did not take or verbalize body substance isolation precautions
___ Did not initiate ventilations within 30 seconds
___ Interrupted ventilations for more than 30 seconds at any time
___ Did not hyper-oxygenate the patient prior to placement of the dual-lumen airway device
___ Did not provide adequate volume per breath (maximum 2 errors/minute permissible)
___ Did not ventilate the patient at a rate of at least 10 breaths per minute
___ Did not insert the dual-lumen airway device at a proper depth or at the proper place within 3 attempts
___ **Combitube**—Did not remove the syringe immediately following the inflation of each cuff
___ **PTL**—Did not secure the strap prior to cuff inflation
___ Did not confirm, by observing chest rise and auscultation over the epigastrium and bilaterally over each lung, that the proper lumen of the device was being used to ventilate the patient
___ Inserted any adjunct in a manner that was dangerous to the patient

Ventilatory Management
Esophageal Obturator Airway Insertion Following an Unsuccessful Endotracheal Intubation Attempt

Start Time: ________________

Stop Time: ________________ **Date:** ________________

Candidate's Name: ________________________________

Evaluator's Name: ________________________________

	Points Possible	Points Awarded
Continues body substance isolation precautions	1	
Confirms the patient is being ventilated with high percentage oxygen	1	
Directs the assistant to hyper-oxygenate the patient	1	
Identifies/selects the proper equipment for insertion of EOA	1	
Assembles the EOA	1	
Tests the cuff for leaks	1	
Inflates the mask	1	
Lubricates the tube (may be verbalized)	1	
NOTE: The examiner should remove the OPA and move out of the way when the candidate is prepared to insert the device.		
Positions head properly with the neck in the neutral or slightly flexed position	1	
Grasps and elevates the tongue and mandible	1	
Inserts the tube in the same direction as the curvature of the pharynx	1	
Advances the tube until the mask is sealed against the patient's face	1	
Ventilates the patient while maintaining a tight mask-to-face seal	1	
Directs confirmation of placement of EOA by observing for chest rise and auscultation over the epigastrium and bilaterally over each lung	1	
NOTE: The examiner must acknowledge adequate chest rise, bilateral breath sounds and absent sounds over the epigastrium.		
Inflates the cuff to the proper pressure	1	
Disconnects the syringe from the inlet port	1	
Continues ventilation of the patient	1	
TOTAL	**17**	

Critical Criteria

___ Did not take or verbalize body substance isolation precautions
___ Did not initiate ventilations within 30 seconds
___ Interrupted ventilations for more than 30 seconds at any time
___ Did not direct hyper-oxygenation of the patient prior to placement of the EOA
___ Did not successfully place the EOA within 3 attempts
___ Did not ventilate at a rate of at least 10 breaths per minute
___ Did not provide adequate volume per breath (maximum 2 errors/minute permissible)
___ Did not ensure proper tube placement by auscultation bilaterally and over the epigastrium
___ Did not remove the syringe after inflating the cuff
___ Did not successfully ventilate the patient
___ Did not provide high flow oxygen (15 liters per minute or greater)
___ Inserted any adjunct in a manner that was dangerous to the patient

Colophon

This catalogue is published
in conjunction with the exhibition
Melgaard+Munch

Munch Museum, Oslo
January 31 – April 12, 2015
www.munchmuseet.no

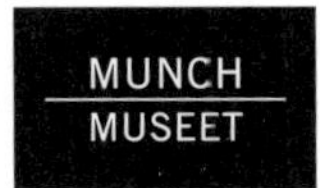

Editor: Lars Toft-Eriksen

Copyediting: Karen E. Lerheim and Tale Tveterås

Translations from Norwegian: Francesca M. Nichols

Graphic design and typesetting: Henrik Haugan
and Kim Andre Fosslien Ottesen, Snøhetta

Production: Anja Wolsfeld, Hatje Cantz

Typeface: Stanley by Optimo Type Foundry

Photography: Svein Andersen, Halvor Bjørngård,
Tone Margrethe Gauden, Jaro Hollan, Sidsel de Jong,
Jason Mandella, Adam Reich, Øystein Thorvaldsen,
Anders Valde, Stephen White, Thomas Widerberg
and Mark Woods

Paper: MultiArt Silk, 150 g/m²; Munken Pure, 100 g/m²

Printing: Offsetdruckerei Karl Grammlich GmbH,
Pliezhausen
Binding: Josef Spinner Grossbuchbinderei GmbH,
Ottersweier

Published by
Hatje Cantz Verlag
Zeppelinstrasse 32
73760 Ostfildern
Germany
Tel. +49 711 4405-200
Fax +49 711 4405-220
www.hatjecantz.com
A Ganske Publishing Group company

You can find information on this exhibition and many
others at www.kq-daily.de.

Hatje Cantz books are available internationally at selected
bookstores. For more information about our distribution
partners, please visit our website at www.hatjecantz.com.

ISBN 978-3-7757-3951-1

Printed in Germany

Acknowledgments:

—

Bjarne Melgaard acknowledges with deep appreciation
Director Stein Olav Henrichsen and the staff of the
Munch Museum, and, most especially, Lars Toft-Eriksen,
Knut Listerud, David Oramas, Svein Roar Grande,
Gabe Bartalos, Amber Halford, Jessica Scott,
Susan Cianciolo, Linda Mason, Bob Recine,
Babak Radboy, David Mandel, Nicholas Cueva,
Lauren Gregory, and Timothy Hartley Smith.

Published with generous support from:
Fritt Ord, The Freedom of Expression Foundation, Oslo

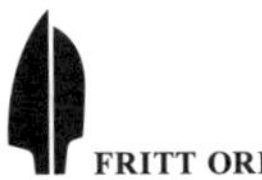

STEIN OLAV HENRICHSEN
Director of the Munch Museum

PS

With the exhibition *Melgaard+Munch* the Munch Museum introduces an ambitious two-year exhibition series called *+Munch*. Here Edvard Munch's art will be shown side by side with six other artists consecutively: Bjarne Melgaard, Vincent van Gogh, Gustav Vigeland, Robert Mapplethorpe, Jasper Johns and Asger Jorn. In other words, artists from Munch's own lifetime as well as later generations, all the way up to our own time. To present artists such as Van Gogh, Jasper Johns and Robert Mapplethorpe in a large scope for the first time here in Norway is a sensation in itself. On that level the series points to a practice that will characterise the exhibitions in the new Munch Museum, which will open in the Oslo harbor area in about five years' time. Aside from Munch's art, the new museum's exhibition program will include modernist and contemporary art. And not least, we will actively exploit the opportunities that the Munch collection affords us to present international exhibitions which we would otherwise not have been able to bring to Norway. Instead of presenting Munch as an isolated figure, we will consistently place his work in relation to other art. This will open up to new understanding and lead to a richer historical perspective on Munch's art than we have previously had the opportunity to demonstrate, as well as make it more relevant to our own time.

Edvard Munch's art is, through his art historical importance and popularity, subject to a high degree of exposure to a wide audience. However, his contemporary significance is to a lesser degree addressed. With *Melgaard+Munch*, the Munch Museum wishes to draw attention to Munch's critical relevance of today. Social, political and ethical issues are at the core of Bjarne Melgaard's oeuvre. With reference to political and social issues, often in the form of marginal and subcultural phenomena, Melgaard's art often raises provocative and critical questions. This was also the case with Munch in his time. With this exhibition the museum will put Munch's art to the test of time by placing it up against Melgaard's, through an examination of the two artists' critical and provocative power.

With great appreciation the Munch Museum acknowledges Bjarne Melgaard Studio for collaborating on making this project possible. The museum would like to sincerely thank Bjarne Melgaard, Timothy Hartley Smith, Svein Roar Grande, Rolf Hoff, David Lomas, Patricia Berman, Øystein Sjåstad, Halvor Bodin, Ina Blom, the Royal Norwegian Consulate General in New York, Hatje Cantz Verlag, Lars Bohman Gallery, Galleri Riis and Kaare Berntsen AS for their collaboration on the project. The museum also thanks Kjetil Trædal Thorsen and the staff at Snøhetta for their partnership, including Martin Gran, Filippo Gazzola, Henrik Haugan, Kim Andre Fosslien Ottesen and Aleksandra Danielak. We are very grateful to the Astrup Fearnley Museum of Modern Art and all other lenders of Melgaard's artworks, without which this exhibition would never have been realized. The museum would also like to express gratitude to the Fritt Ord Foundation and Jan Petter Collier for their generous support. Last but not least, I thank curator Lars Toft-Eriksen and the staff of the Munch Museum for their hard work and qualified contribution to this project.